BEAUTY THERAPY
Level 3

Judith Ifould
Emma Harrington

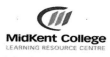
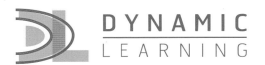

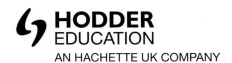

bc0015207L9

Although every effort has been made to ensure that website addresses are correct at time of going to press, Hodder Education cannot be held responsible for the content of any website mentioned in this book. It is sometimes possible to find a relocated web page by typing in the address of the homepage for a website in the URL window of your browser.

Hachette UK's policy is to use papers that are natural, renewable and recyclable products and made from wood grown in sustainable forests. The logging and manufacturing processes are expected to conform to the environmental regulations of the country of origin.

Orders: please contact Bookpoint Ltd, 130 Milton Park, Abingdon, Oxon OX14 4SB. Telephone: +44 (0)1235 827720. Fax: +44 (0)1235 400454. Lines are open 09.00–17.00, Monday to Saturday, with a 24-hour message answering service. Visit our website at www.hoddereducation.co.uk

© Judith Ifould and Emma Harrington 2012
First published in 2012 by
Hodder Education
An Hachette UK Company,
338 Euston Road
London NW1 3BH

Impression number   5 4 3 2 1
Year   2017 2016 2015 2014 2013 2012

Whilst the advice and information in this book are believed to be true and accurate at the date of going to press, neither the authors nor the publisher can accept any legal responsibility or liability for any errors or omissions that may be made, or any injury that may result from performing the treatments described. In particular (but without limiting the generality of the preceding disclaimer) every effort has been made to check the technical accuracy of instructions for use of electrical equipment; however, it is still possible that errors have been missed. For these reasons the reader is strongly urged to consult manufacturers' printed instructions before using any electrical equipment or carrying out any of the treatments recommended in this book.

Cover photo Larysa Dodz/Getty Images
Illustrations by Barking Dog Art
Typeset in Palatino Light 11/13 by Pantek Media, Maidstone, Kent
Printed in Italy

A catalogue record for this title is available from the British Library

ISBN 978 1444 168 358

CONTENTS

The following additional chapters can be accessed online at **www.hodderplus.co.uk/beautytherapy** using the following: username: btl3; password: therapies.

Chapter	NVQ units covered	VRQ units covered
Checking the likely success of a business idea	G11	Check the likely success of a business idea
Eyelash extensions	B15	Apply individual permanent lashes
UV tanning	B21	Provide UV tanning
Self-tanning	B25	Provide self-tanning
Intimate waxing	B26; B27	Intimate waxing for male clients; Intimate waxing for female clients
Nail technologies	N6; N7; N8	Enhance and maintain nails using UV gel; Enhance and maintain nails using wraps; Nail enhancements and advanced hand and nail art techniques; Apply and maintain nail enhancements
Nail art	N9; N10	Nail enhancements and advanced hand and nail art techniques
Glossary		
Answers to Test yourself questions		

Introduction

Welcome to this new book – **Level 3 Beauty Therapy**.

A new book needed a new collaboration – this time between one of our established authors, Judith Ifould, and a new face, Emma Harrington.

We are so excited about this new book as we have covered all the units on the Beauty Therapy general and massage routes, as well as those for the Nail Services. There are also further chapters online at www.hodderplus.co.uk/beautytherapy.

We have taken many of the features of the already successful Level 2 book and included them here:

The NVQ and VRQ units covered are listed at the beginning of each chapter.

The NVQ evidence requirements, including the range you must cover, are clearly stated.

The VRQ evidence requirements, including the range you must cover, are clearly stated for the relevant VRQ units.

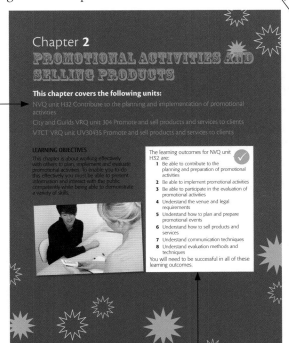

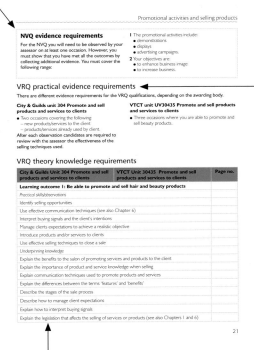

All of the learning outcomes for the NVQ unit are listed.

A table at the beginning of each chapter shows you where you can find all of the necessary knowledge to cover the knowledge requirements of the listed VRQ qualifications.

Green circles next to headings show the NVQ learning outcome number covered by that particular section (a full list of the learning outcomes is given at the beginning of the chapter), allowing you to easily find the information you need to fulfil each learning outcome.

Key terms boxes explain unfamiliar words and terminology.

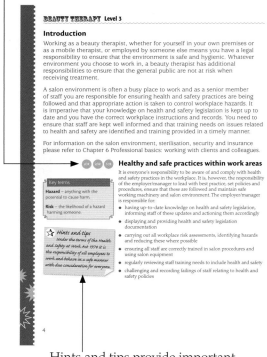

Hints and tips provide important and relevant information.

Short activities are included to check your learning.

Remember boxes remind you of the key points within the treatment procedure, for example link selling.

Beauty therapy is a fascinating and ever changing industry that can engage your interest with new treatments and product developments, and can bring you close to celebrity through employment opportunities in beauty salons, nail bars, health clinics, spas, cosmetic houses, cruise ships and working overseas.

The beauty therapy industry is just one of six industries within the 'Hair and Beauty sector' that are controlled by the skills sector professional body, HABIA. You will see that we refer to and advise you throughout the book of their recommendations of what is considered to be the industry's standards of work and good practice. The six industries are:

- Beauty therapy
- Hairdressing
- Nail services
- Barbering
- Spa
- African-type hairdressing.

At the end of each chapter you will find a 'Want to know more' section, to expand the topic, introduce new technologies and feed your thirst for more.

An NVQ assessment checklist is provided at the end of each chapter, so you can check you have all the necessary knowledge and practical skills for the unit.

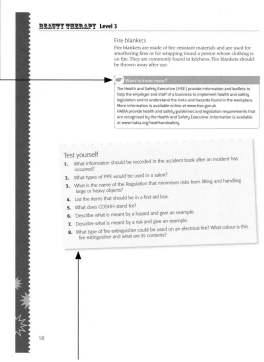

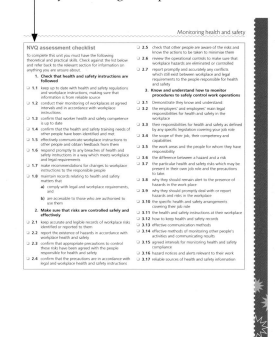

Short tests at the end of each chapter are provided to help you practise for your theory assessment.

Meet the professional

These case studies will give you a real insight into what it's really like to work within the industry.

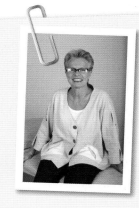

Meet the professional

Angela Barbagelata-Fabes, Chairman of The Carlton Group Beauty & Spa Ltd.

Angela attended Northbrook College in Worthing as a mature student and qualified with an International Beauty Therapists' Diploma in 1992.

Working alongside her late husband, Rod Fabes, Angela aided the development of the Carlton Professional range of machines and supplied training and demonstrations on the equipment to colleges and salons both in the UK and overseas.

Since 2000, Angela has been Chairman of The Carlton Group. During this time, she has developed a variety of Electrotherapy and Microdermabrasion machines under the Carlton Professional banner, as well as seeking out new international innovations, which Carlton has distributed to the UK market.

In 2007, Angela created SEBTA, the Student Electrotherapy Beauty Therapist Award, the first award to celebrate excellence in Electrotherapy. Now in its sixth year, SEBTA continues to grow, with more applications from colleges all over the UK every year.

Meet the professional

Sam Biddle, Independent International Educator, International Educator Ez Flow Nail Systems, Elite Master Educator IBD

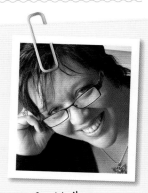

Sam Biddle is a renowned nail technician, living in Dorset, England; she has found success within her speciality design and colour. Internationally published, Sam regularly contributes to trade and national press worldwide. She has also achieved eight front covers in the UK, Europe and USA.

Sam is an international judge and competition winner, and in 2008 and 2009 was finalist for Nail Professional of the Year. She is now on the judging panel for Nail Professional of the Year awards. Having featured on the BBC, ITV and in the national press, Sam hopes to bring colour and help technicians find inspiration to express their creativity, which helps develop their careers by utilising new skills.

As an independent global educator, Sam brings a new way of learning to nail technicians all over the world. Sam loves to teach and sees it as an exchange of knowledge: 'For every lesson I give, I learn as much as the students'. Sam also works with various distributors and product houses internationally, developing brands and providing training.

With a career that has taken her across the globe, Sam started within this industry in 2000 as a mobile nail technician, before going on to owning her own salon and successful nail academy. Fully aware of the highs and lows of running a successful business on the high street, Sam can empathise with her students, and help them find creative ways to build their business. In 2004, after a bout of cancer, Sam's priorities changed – now working with a different agenda, her desire to give something back to the industry, helping it grow and showing nail technicians that there can be alternative ways to realising their own potential.

Now with her own company 'Be Inspired' Sam brings a series of tools to develop technicians move forward within their craft. Sam has designed specialised and advanced workshops and DVDs, plus publications to support nail technicians. The aim of 'Be Inspired' is to show that anything is possible, giving you the tools you could need to realise your dreams and ambitions. Sam also has an international distribution company Jealous Cow Ltd. Run with her business partner Rebecca Orme, Jealous Cow has various in-house brands for both the consumer market and the professional. Brands such as Be Creative, which has a range of unique items such as the pigments, nail art pen, Jealous Cow was also the first company to launch gel paints into the UK. Original Sugar is a consumer brand which has featured in Cosmopolitan, More and Closer magazines because of its fantastic nail art products for use at home.

Outside the industry Sam continues to wow people with her creations, giving them an example of just how far you can take the art of nails. She has worked on photo shoots for couture magazine spreads and with supermodels such as Erin O'Conner. Although most of these fantastical pieces of art are not for the average customer, it goes a long way to inspire them.

Guide to beauty therapy qualifications

Qualifications types

This book provides you with the knowledge and skills you need when completing two types of beauty therapy qualifications:

- NVQs/SVQs – work-related, competence-based qualifications that allow you to work and train in a salon. Your progress is measured by ongoing assessments.

- VRQs – preparation for work qualifications that assess the skills and abilities required in the workplace, particularly the underpinning knowledge and understanding. They are assessed through a series of practical and written assignments.

Training to a high standard to enable you to access the wide and varied employment opportunities within the Hair and Beauty sector anywhere in the United Kingdom or overseas is essential.

National Vocational Qualifications (NVQs) and Scottish Vocational Qualifications (SVQs)

National Vocational Qualifications (NVQs) and **Scottish Vocational Qualifications (SVQs)** are designed to assess your ability to do a particular job according to a set of standards for beauty therapy called the National Occupational Standards (NOS). The NOS are set by the beauty therapy industry's professional body HABIA. This organisation is made up of employers, industry experts, educators and trainers, so it is our industry that decides the standards by which we must be trained and perform beauty therapy treatments. When you have successfully completed an NVQ/SVQ and apply for a job, the employer will immediately know what you are capable of doing.

NVQs/SVQs are based on assessment of **practical skills**, **knowledge** and **understanding** at Levels 1, 2, 3 or 4.

Level	Description
1	An introduction to beauty therapy involving the application of knowledge and skills that is routine and predictable. You might be an assistant helping therapists in a salon.
2	The application of knowledge and skills to varied work activities in a variety of contexts that are non-routine and with some individual responsibility, but also working as part of a team. Basically, performing treatments on clients in the salon.
3	More complex treatments requiring advanced skills and knowledge, as well as considerable responsibility and the control or guidance of others such as an assistant manager or supervisor.
4	Knowledge and skills in a broad and complex nature with a high degree of responsibility for self and others as well as resources, such as the management of stock, money and people, including training.

An NVQ/SVQ qualification is made up of **units**, which describe a particular treatment or job within the salon, for example B20 'Provide body massage treatments'. Each unit is made up of several **outcomes** that break up that treatment into stages and these are broken down further into **performance criteria (PCs)** that reflect our industry's standards. These PCs are what you **must do** to perform the treatment; what you **must know** is a list of **essential knowledge** that supports the practical performance. An NVQ/SVQ requires you to show 'competence' over a period of time so this requires you to perform a treatment more than once to cover a **range** of different circumstances and clients.

To gain an NVQ/SVQ you will be taught to the national standards by your teacher, either in the workplace or at a recognised training centre, such as a college of further education through demonstrations, followed by practice on clients in the salon, as well as through theory lessons to provide you with the necessary knowledge needed to support the practical activities.

It is necessary to make an action plan at the beginning of your course to enable you to watch your progress in both your learning and assessment and to review what you have achieved. Assessment takes place when you and your assessor agree that you have sufficient learning and understanding through practice on clients, written work and collection of supplementary evidence (such as client record cards) to perform a treatment to the industry's standard.

Your candidate logbook will help you plan for assessment and your assessor will discuss with you what the assessment process involves.

The assessor will usually be your teacher, who will advise you on assessment opportunities such as:

- observation of practical work
- oral questioning
- written tests
- case studies
- assignments or projects.

The assessor will discuss the assessment with you before it takes place and agree how the assessment will be carried out. You will then perform the treatment on a **paying client** while your assessor watches you work. This is called an **observation** and will be judged against the performance criteria and recorded in your assessment logbook at the time of your assessment, along with the range you have covered performing that treatment.

The assessor will need to be sure that you understand what you are doing and why. This will involve asking you questions. This is called **oral questioning**. As most of your work involves a client this will usually be done after your client has left, unless the assessor wishes to confirm something with you during the treatment.

You will collate evidence of assessment into a **portfolio**. The type of evidence can be divided into **performance evidence** and **knowledge evidence**. Performance evidence includes items such as client record cards, photographs, case studies and witness testimonies, which help to confirm that you can carry out a task. Knowledge evidence will be such things as written tests and assignments or projects, which show that you have gained knowledge of a subject. You are required to provide a guide for your assessor so that the information contained in your portfolio is organised. This is called **referencing**.

To ensure the quality of your work reaches the standard for our industry and to ensure that the assessment is fair, a process called **verification** is carried out. This involves someone who is trained to observe assessments watching the assessment process and reviewing the marking of written tests, assignments and/or projects. Initially this is carried out by the **internal verifier** who will sign off units as you complete them and then your portfolio before you can claim certification from the awarding body. The training centre will retain your portfolio and assessment logbook for the **external verifier**, who does a further check on behalf of the awarding body.

Awarding bodies offering NVQ/SVQs include City & Guilds; Edexcel and Vocational Training Charitable Trust (VTCT), all of which provide NVQ/SVQs with the same PCs, range, essential knowledge and evidence requirements following the NOS.

Progression

Below is a chart indicating **NVQ/SVQs** in beauty therapy at the different levels:

Level 1	Level 2	Level 3
Diploma in Beauty Therapy	Diploma in Beauty Therapy – general route	Diploma in Beauty Therapy – general route
Diploma in Hairdressing and Beauty Therapy	Diploma in Beauty Therapy – make-up route	Diploma in Beauty Therapy – make-up route
	Diploma in Nail Services	Diploma in Nail Services
		Diploma in Beauty Therapy – massage route
		Diploma in Spa Therapy

Note that the NVQ Level 1 Hairdressing and Beauty would also allow entry into an NVQ Level 2 Hairdressing or Barbering qualification.

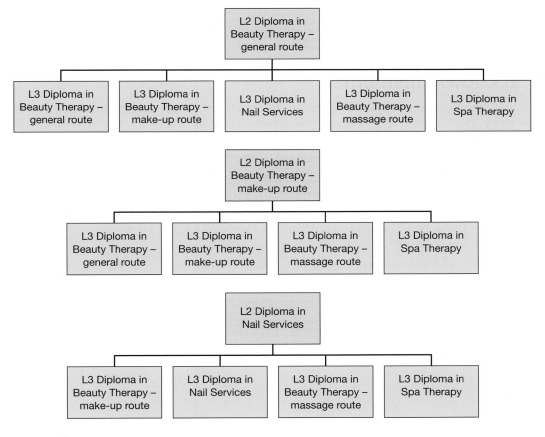

△ Progression routes

Career options

An NVQ/SVQ in Level 2 Beauty Therapy general make-up routes or in Nail Services offers employment opportunities within the hair and beauty sector.

On completion of a Level 2 in Beauty Therapy – general route or in Nail Services you can obtain insurance and therefore employment in a salon, spa, clinic or nail bar performing the treatments in which you are competent, while taking NVQ Level 3 as an apprenticeship. Your training can be delivered through a training agency or local further education establishment or given by your employer with the aid or a peripatetic assessor and/or internal verifier.

This is also true of the Beauty Therapy – make-up route; with employment opportunities being found in departmental stores for a particular 'cosmetic house' or indeed in salons, clinics or health centres.

Vocational Related Qualifications (VRQs)

There are other qualifications besides the NVQ/SVQ that are recognised for employment by the beauty therapy industry. These qualifications are written by awarding bodies in line with the NOS and approved by HABIA; these are called Vocational Related Qualifications (VRQs). Throughout this book we have included all the relevant underpinning knowledge and assessment requirements needed in order to be successful in these types of qualifications and have cross-referenced their unit requirements at the beginning of each chapter. The information contained in this book will meet the needs of all students of beauty therapy, regardless of which qualification they are working towards.

Author acknowledgements

Both of us would like to send our special thanks to our partners, family and friends for all their support and patience during the writing of this book. It has been a labour of love and an experience that we have thoroughly enjoyed. We are extremely proud of the final book and we hope it enhances your learning and inspires long and dynamic careers in beauty-related industries.

To our wonderful students, Annabelle, Eloise and Paige, who gave up two days of their holidays to model and assist with the photo shoot; thank you so much for your help and ensuring the days were great fun. A special thank you to Teresa Dickson, who is a truly talented nail technician, for allowing us to use her skills and nail art for the shoot. Thanks to Paul, the photographer, for his patience with the required level of perfection to the photos.

Thank you to Gemma and Stephen at Hodder Education for their guidance and assistance throughout the whole writing process.

Finally we would like to thank all the professionals within the industry who have contributed to the book and enabled us to make careers in this industry exciting, relevant and realistic.

Jude Ifould and Emma Harrington

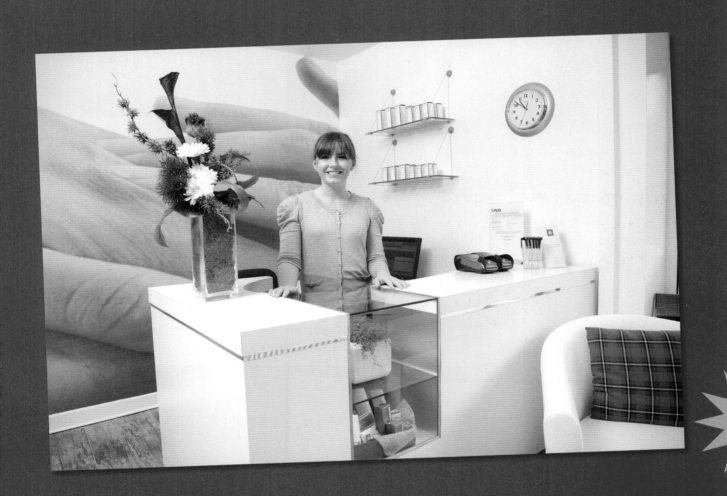

Chapter 1

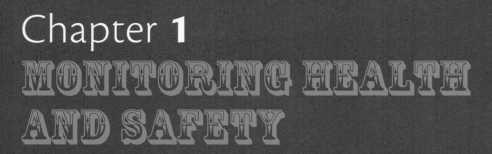

MONITORING HEALTH AND SAFETY

This chapter covers:

NVQ unit G22 Monitor procedures to safely control work operations

City and Guilds VRQ unit 302 Monitor and maintain health and safety practice in the salon

VTCT VRQ unit UV30491 Monitor and maintain health and safety practice in the salon

LEARNING OBJECTIVES

As a senior member of staff working in a salon environment, it is your legal responsibility to monitor the operational health and safety of not just yourself and staff, but of other people who enter the business. Health and safety is not the manager's or proprietor's responsibility alone. This chapter will guide you in making sure that statutory and workplace instructions are carried out to ensure the monitoring of health and safety.

The learning outcomes for NVQ unit G22 are:

1. Check that health and safety instructions are followed
2. Make sure that risks are controlled safely and effectively
3. Know and understand how to monitor procedures to safely control work operations

You must consistently show competence in these outcomes when applied to the practical skills and services within this qualification.

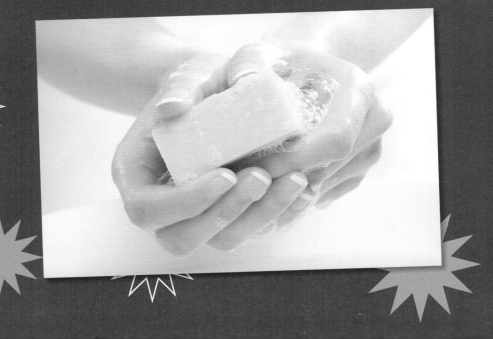

VRQ knowledge requirements

City & Guilds Unit 302 Monitor and maintain health and safety practice in the salon	VTCT Unit 30491 Monitor and maintain health and safety practice in the salon	Page no.
Learning outcome 1: Be able to carry out a risk assessment		
Practical skills		
Carry out risk assessments and take necessary actions		15–16
Underpinning knowledge		
State the reason for carrying out risk assessments		15–16
Describe the procedures for carrying out a risk assessment		15–18
Describe when risk assessments should be carried out		15–18
Outline necessary actions to take following a risk assessment		15–18
Learning outcome 2: Be able to monitor health and safety in the salon		
Practical skills		
Monitor and support the work of others to ensure compliance with health and safety requirements		5–18
Underpinning knowledge		
Outline the health and safety support that should be provided to staff		5–18
Outline procedures for dealing with different types of security breaches (Chapter 6)		187–8
Explain the need for insurance (see also Chapter 6)		185–6

Introduction

Working as a beauty therapist, whether for yourself in your own premises or as a mobile therapist, or employed by someone else means you have a legal responsibility to ensure that the environment is safe and hygienic. Whatever environment you choose to work in, a beauty therapist has additional responsibilities to ensure that the general public are not at risk when receiving treatment.

A salon environment is often a busy place to work and as a senior member of staff you are responsible for ensuring health and safety practices are being followed and that appropriate action is taken to control workplace hazards. It is imperative that your knowledge on health and safety legislation is kept up to date and you have the correct workplace instructions and records. You need to ensure that staff are kept well informed and that training needs on issues related to health and safety are identified and training provided in a timely manner.

For information on the salon environment, sterilisation, security and insurance please refer to Chapter 6 Professional basics: working with clients and colleagues.

Healthy and safe practices within work areas

It is everyone's responsibility to be aware of and comply with health and safety practices in the workplace. It is, however, the responsibility of the employer/manager to lead with best practice, set policies and procedures, ensure that these are followed and maintain safe working machinery and salon environment. The employer/manager is responsible for:

- having up-to-date knowledge on health and safety legislation, informing staff of these updates and actioning them accordingly
- displaying and providing health and safety legislation documentation
- carrying out all workplace risk assessments, identifying hazards and reducing these where possible
- ensuring all staff are correctly trained in salon procedures and using salon equipment
- regularly reviewing staff training needs to include health and safety
- challenging and recording failings of staff relating to health and safety policies

> **Key terms**
>
> **Hazard** – anything with the potential to cause harm.
>
> **Risk** – the likelihood of a hazard harming someone.

> ☆ *Hints and tips*
> Under the terms of the Health and Safety at Work Act 1974 it is the responsibility of all employees to work and behave in a safe manner with due consideration for everyone.

- providing and reviewing the accident book to reduce future hazards
- ensuring a safe and healthy workplace environment is maintained.

Keeping health and safety records

The accident book

The recording of all accidents is essential for any workplace, and it is the responsibility of the employer/manager to ensure that the accident book is regularly reviewed to improve workplace practices and identify trends. Entries into the accident book need to be completed immediately after the accident has occurred, by the staff member who witnessed the accident.

The accident book should include details of:

- the date and time of the accident
- contact details of all those involved with the accident
- where the accident occurred
- details of the accident and injury suffered
- what first aid was given (if applicable)
- a signature of the staff member or first aider making the recording
- the initial after-effect: this may be the person going home or seeking further medical treatment (i.e. going to hospital).

If the person injured requires qualified medical treatment the accident is deemed to be serious and therefore an incident report form is also required. You have a duty to report any serious accidents to the Health and Safety Executive (HSE) in accordance with the Reporting of Injuries, Diseases and Dangerous Occurrences Regulations 1985 (RIDDOR). RIDDOR states that any activity taking place in the workplace, where an incident occurs that leads to injury, serious injury where absence from work is required or death, must be reported to the HSE within 10 working days.

Specific legislation

There is a vast amount of health and safety legislation and regulations that apply to those working in the beauty industry. Everyone working within the organisation has a duty and legal responsibility to follow health and safety requirements, although it is the employer/manager's responsibility to stay abreast of developments, provide training and display relevant health and safety documentation. Below are the responsibilities outlined in important pieces of health and safety legislations and regulations that directly relate to working in the beauty therapy industry.

Key terms

Accident – An unforeseen or unfortunate event or occurrence which usually results in harm, injury or damage.

Incident – The individual occurrence of something happening.

Occupational health – the effect of work on a person's health and the effect that their health has on their work.

Remember...
If the accident is a result of negligence a prosecution may be made against both you and your employer.

Activity

Design a page in an accident book. Make sure you include all the details stated here so an incident can be recorded clearly and precisely. Include a space for reviewing the incident so that measures can be taken to reduce the likelihood of the accident happening again in the future.

Hints and tips
HABIA provide the beauty and nail industry's Code of Practice and their website is a great source of information (www.habia.org).

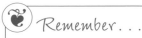

Remember...

You can be fined or imprisoned for breaking health and safety law.

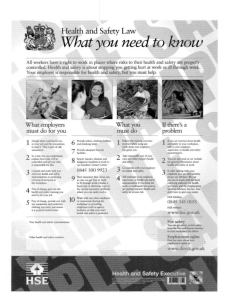

△ This health and safety law poster must be displayed in the workplace where it can be easily read. This new version of the health and safety law poster was published in 2009 and employers have until 5 April 2014 to replace their old copies with this health and safety law poster and leaflet.

(Source: Health and Safety Executive)

Hints and tips
The HSE website is a valuable source of information: visit www.hse.gov.uk.

The Health and Safety at Work Act 1974

The Health and Safety at Work Act (HASAW Act) states that all workers have the right to work in an environment where the risks to health and safety are properly controlled. It identifies the duties and responsibilities of employers and employees while at work and is reviewed regularly to ensure it remains relevant to the changing workplace. The Act states the minimum standards for health and safety for all areas of the workplace and covers a whole range of legislation relating to health and safety. All individuals have responsibility for health and safety while at work and must cooperate with employers on all health and safety related matters. The Health and Safety Executive (HSE) is responsible for enforcing the act and they will send their environmental health officers (EHOs) to investigate and enforce health and safety law.

As a senior member of staff it may be your responsibility to ensure all staff are familiar with the HASAW Act and have read and know where to find the poster and leaflets.

Management of Health and Safety at Work Regulations 1999

These Regulations are addressed to the employer/manager (including self-employed people) in the workplace and relate to how to consult and involve employees on health and safety matters at work. They explain to the employer/manager their duties under the Regulations and require them to assess the risks posed to workers and any others who may be affected by their work or business.

The Regulations focus on risk assessments and how they can be used effectively to identify potential hazards and risks and the measures that can be applied to prevent such dangers. They provide information on the management and surveillance of health and safety and outline the procedures that should be followed in the event of any health and safety issues. Examples of issues covered by the Regulations include the following:

- If a worker becomes pregnant, a risk assessment should be carried out and any necessary actions taken. Legally this risk assessment must be recorded if there are five or more people employed.

- If a worker is below the school leaving age a risk assessment must be carried out to identify any potential risks. This must be recorded and kept safe.

The Regulations also provide guidance for employees about their health and safety responsibilities if they are pregnant, a temporary worker or a young person.

Health and Safety Information for Employees Regulations 1989

These Regulations require the employer to provide health and safety information to all employees. This may include displaying a poster or giving leaflets to employees informing them of what they need to know regarding health and safety. The Regulations set out the general duties that employers have towards employees and members of the public and the duties employees have to themselves and to each other.

The employer/manager is required by law to consider what the risks are in the workplace and take sensible and reasonable measures to prevent them occurring. The main requirement on the employer/manager is to carry out a risk assessment and an organisation where five or more people are employed must retain records of the findings from such risk assessments.

The employer/manager also needs to:

● implement the health and safety measures identified in the risk assessment

● set up emergency procedures, such as fire evacuation and escape routes

● provide clear information and training to employees.

Control of Substances Hazardous to Health Regulations 2002 (COSHH)

Under the terms of COSHH an employer is required to regulate employees' exposure to substances that may cause hazards to health. A risk assessment must be carried out by the employer/manager, formally stating the risk posed. Training, safety procedures and any personal protective equipment (PPE) must then be given to employees to use when dealing with these substances. The COSHH risk assessments should be updated regularly to include any new substances and, if possible, hazardous substances should be replaced by a product which is less harmful. COSHH hazard warning symbols appear on the packaging of hazardous substances and on notices around the workplace.

Substances can take many forms and can include:

● chemicals

● products containing chemicals

● fumes

● dust

● vapours

● mists.

COSHH does not cover the use of lead, asbestos or radioactive substances as they have their own specific regulations.

Activity

Look at the labels on all the different substances that you have in the salon. How many are there? Which ones have the COSHH warning symbol on them?

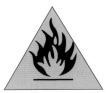
Highly Flammable

Harmful

Explosive

Toxic

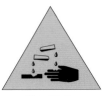
Corrosive

Oxidising

△ COSHH warning symbols

Material Safety Data Sheets

Material Safety Data Sheets (MSDSs) are documents that contain details of the composition, safety, handling, storage, disposal and transport of a material and other regulatory information. They are intended to provide guidance on handling or working with a product in a safe manner and every beauty product supplier is legally required to produce them and have them available on request. They are routinely used in performing risk assessments for chemicals or other products used in a working environment, in compliance with COSSH Regulations.

Electricity at Work Regulations 1989

The beauty therapist uses a wide range of electrical equipment, from computers and electronic couches, to wax pots and face and body machinery. Every piece of electrical equipment must be tested by a qualified electrician, based on their frequency of use. If equipment is constantly in use this can be every six months to a year, with a maximum of every five years for something less frequently used. Portable appliance testing (PAT) is an important part of any health and safety policy. A green and white sticker will usually be placed on each item, showing the date it was tested, when it is to be re-tested and the name of the person who conducted the test. A record of equipment inspection and servicing must be kept and made available on request.

Electrical equipment must be checked for:

- worn and exposed cables and flexes
- sufficient sockets to reduce overloading
- broken plugs and sockets.

Any piece of electrical equipment that is not safe should be reported and removed from use immediately.

Health and safety

'25% of all reportable electrical accidents involved portable appliances' according to the Health & Safety Executive (source: www.pat-testing.info, 2011).

Personal Protective Equipment at Work Regulations 2002

The main requirement of the PPE at Work Regulations 2002 is that personal protective equipment is supplied by the employer and used by the employees when at work wherever there are risks to health and safety that cannot be adequately controlled in other ways.

Examples of PPE include:

● uniform, aprons, disposable gloves, eye goggles and masks for use by therapists and nail technicians

● protective covers to protect the client where necessary.

An employer is not allowed to charge an employee for PPE, whether it is returnable or not.

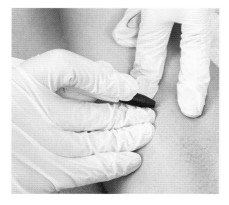

△ Example of PPE: gloves

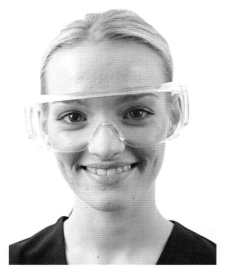

△ Example of PPE: goggles

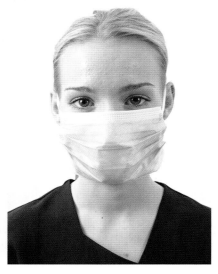

△ Example of PPE: mask

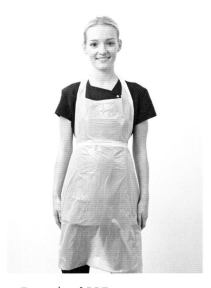

△ Example of PPE: apron

The PPE Regulations also require that the PPE is chosen carefully before use to ensure it is suitable, that it is maintained and stored properly and that instructions are given to the employee so they know how to use it safely and correctly.

The salon will have a set of professional work wear for all staff, commonly a tunic with trousers. The salon uniform should present a clean and professional image as well as protecting the therapist. The uniform should be washed and changed daily and only be worn in the salon, to avoid cross contamination and odours.

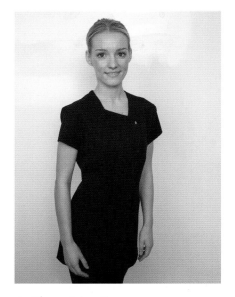

△ Therapist uniform

Manual Handling Operations Regulations 1992

These Regulations are intended to prevent musculoskeletal damage to employees and minimise risks from lifting and handling large or heavy objects. The employer should conduct a risk assessment for any activity which requires the manual handling of large or heavy objects. The risk assessment should include:

- load weight and frequency of handling
- the physical impact of the manual lift
- environmental factors, such as floor surface, condition and obstacles
- carry distance.

Therapists and nail technicians should also be advised on correct posture, since incorrect posture requires greater muscular effort and can lead to fatigue, especially when the position is held for a long period of time such as when providing a set of artificial nail enhancements. The employer/manager should ensure that equipment such as couches and stools can be raised or lowered to meet the needs of the individual therapists.

> ☆ *Hints and tips*
> *Always ask someone to help you when lifting a heavy load. Two pairs of hands are better than one and will reduce the risk of injury.*

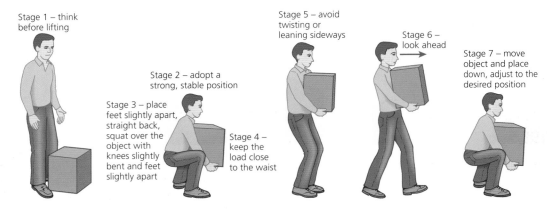

Stage 1 – think before lifting

Stage 2 – adopt a strong, stable position

Stage 3 – place feet slightly apart, straight back, squat over the object with knees slightly bent and feet slightly apart

Stage 4 – keep the load close to the waist

Stage 5 – avoid twisting or leaning sideways

Stage 6 – look ahead

Stage 7 – move object and place down, adjust to the desired position

△ Lifting heavy objects

Local Government (Miscellaneous Provisions) Act 1982 (Local Authority Licensing)

Some treatments that a therapist carries out require increased vigilance to hygiene, for example, epilation and extractions using micro-lances, because of the high risk of cross infection from blood or body fluids. The salon must be licensed by the local authority and meet the required standards of the EHO, who will inspect the premises to check hygiene procedures. Once these required standards are met the salon will be registered and receive a certificate. Activities such as ear-piercing, epilation and acupuncture also require this licensing.

Cosmetic Products (Safety) Regulations 2008

Cosmetic products that are intended to be placed in contact with the human body for protection, cleaning, perfuming, changing its appearance or correcting body odours fall under the terms of these Regulations. The Regulations are part of consumer protection legislation and state that every cosmetic product placed on the market must have undergone a safety assessment to ensure that the product complies with correct labelling, has a safe formulation and is fit for the purpose intended.

Labelling

Cosmetic product labels must include an address within the European Union from where the product information is available and a full list of ingredients shown in weight order.

Cosmetic ingredient

A cosmetic ingredient is any substance of a synthetic or natural origin used in the composition of a cosmetic product.

Fit for purpose

Cosmetics must be fit for purpose and clearly state the general use for the product. Clear instructions regarding safe use must be identified, for example, if the manufacturer has stated that the product may irritate the eyes and has warned against applying the product to the eye area the manufacturer cannot be held responsible if the consumer chooses to ignore the warnings.

Provision and Use of Work Equipment Regulations 1998

These Regulations apply to employers and the self-employed who provide equipment at work; they do not apply to equipment that is used by the general public. The Regulations require that equipment (both old and new) provided for use at work, including machinery, complies with safety guidelines. The Regulations state that the equipment must be suitable for its intended use, that it is safe, well maintained and inspected to retain its condition. They go on to identify that only those trained to use the equipment are able to do so, following adequate instruction and training. Suitable safety measures should also be in place.

Regulatory Reform (Fire Safety) Order 2005

This is the latest fire safety legislation and replaces most fire safety legislation with one Order. It applies to every type of building and structure including open spaces. It places the responsibility for fire safety on the 'responsible person', which means that any person with some level of control over the building must take reasonable steps to reduce the risk from fire and make sure people can escape should

> ⭐ **Hints and tips**
> Look out for the British Kitemark on equipment. This registered certification mark symbolises quality and safety.

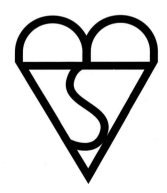

△ The British Kitemark

the need arise. The responsible person must carry out a fire-risk assessment that includes:

- reducing the risk of fire
- considering who will be at risk
- taking measures to ensure flammable or explosive materials are stored correctly
- creating a plan to follow in an emergency
- providing appropriate signs to enable safe escape
- ensuring that effective fire detection equipment is provided and maintained.

Fire authorities no longer issue fire certificates and those previously in force no longer have legal status; however, you still need to ensure a fire-risk assessment has been carried out.

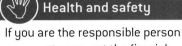

Health and safety

If you are the responsible person you must carry out the fire risk assessment. If you pass this task onto a competent person to complete on your behalf you are still legally responsible for meeting the order.

Health and Safety (First Aid) Regulations 1981

The Health and Safety (First aid) Regulations 1981 apply to all workplaces in Great Britain, including those who are self-employed and businesses with fewer than five employees. It identifies the aspects of first aid that employers need to address and aims to help employers understand and comply with the Regulations. An employer can provide a first aider for a workplace; this person must have a valid certificate in first aid to prove competence. If a first aider is not provided an appointed person should take charge of checking over first aid equipment and calling the emergency services when required to do so.

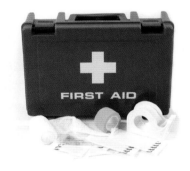

△ A first aid box

The first aid box

It is a requirement by law to have a first aid box and it is the employer's responsibility to provide the contents and maintain the first aid box. Although there is no mandatory list of items to be included in a first aid box the following are recommended:

- a leaflet containing general guidance notes
- assorted sterile plasters that are individually wrapped
- sterile triangular bandages
- sterile eye pads
- medium and large sterile dressings
- safety pins
- disposable gloves.

Scissors, adhesive tape and individually wrapped wipes can also be included if deemed necessary.

First aid procedures for minor accidents

- **Fainting**: lie the person down with their legs raised. Open a window for fresh air if possible.

- **Minor cuts**: wearing disposable gloves, apply pressure to the wound with one of the clean dressings.

- **Epilepsy**: do not restrain someone who is having a seizure. Ensure that their airway is clear and remove any objects or furniture that they may injure themselves on. Once the seizure has ended cover the person with a blanket to keep them warm and allow them time to rest.

- **Burns or scalds**: place the area under cold running water for at least 10–15 minutes. Do not burst any blisters or remove clothing stuck to the burn. Apply a sterile dressing and send casualty to hospital.

- **Electric shock**: do not touch the person. Disconnect any appliance at the mains immediately and use a wooden or plastic implement to push the person away from the electrical source. Check they are breathing and call 999 immediately.

- **Product in the eyes**: perform an eye bath immediately, allowing the water to rinse through the eyes. Do not allow the person to rub their eyes. Depending on the severity, send casualty to hospital.

Safe working environment

Employers have a duty to ensure the environment of the workplace is safe and suitable for its purpose; an employer must maintain the workplace and relevant machinery. They need to provide adequate ventilation, lighting and working temperature and the means to dispose of waste materials. Under the terms of the HSE's 'Welfare at Work' (a summary of the Workplace, (Health, Safety and Welfare) Regulations 1992), adequate and appropriate welfare facilities must be provided. These include drinking water, washing and sanitary conveniences, rest and changing facilities and somewhere clean to eat and drink.

Washing and sanitary facilities

Adequate washing and toilet facilities must be provided. There must be enough toilets and wash basins for people to use and if possible there should be separate facilities for men and women. Toilet paper must be supplied and a hygienic means of disposing of sanitary dressings should be available for women. There must be hot and cold running water and soap for hand washing. Paper towels or a hand dryer must also be supplied.

Health and safety

First aid does not include giving out medicines or tablets and it is recommended that these are not kept in the first aid box.

Hints and tips
A first aid certificate is only valid for three years. After this period of time the first aider must undergo requalification.

Remember . . .
Record any accidents in the accident book (see page 5).

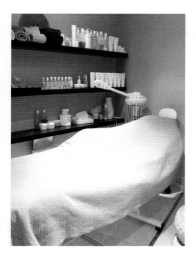

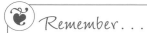
△ A clean and tidy treatment room environment is essential

Remember . . .

Under the terms of the Local Government (Miscellaneous Provisions) Act 1982 (Local Authority Licensing), an environmental health officer can inspect the hygiene and cleanliness of your salon at any time.

Health and safety

Any spillages should be wiped up immediately to reduce the risk of slipping over.

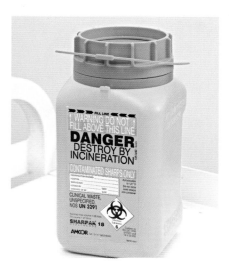
△ Sharps box

Salon hygiene

A clean and tidy salon helps to prevent the spread of infection and promotes a professional image; it is everyone's responsibility to follow hygiene procedures. Recognising skin diseases and disorders, sterilising equipment and using new laundry and disposable items are essential for each client. Disposing of waste correctly and keeping a clean and tidy environment is part of everyday routine for a therapist.

Everyone is required to participate in salon cleaning and this should be done on a daily basis. A rota system is often used to enable staff to take it in turns to perform different roles; this also places responsibility on staff members. General cleaning should include the windows, reception area, product display cabinets, treatment room cupboards, trolleys and work surfaces, staff areas, toilet facilities, stock rooms and all floors. A disinfectant should be used at all times during cleaning.

Floors should be wiped or vacuumed daily, with a clear sign displayed if the surface may still be damp. Carpets, tiles, wood flooring and vinyl should be checked on a regular basis to ensure they are in good, safe working order.

Clean laundry should be placed neatly onto shelving units and wash baskets should be provided for dirty towels. Laundry should be washed on a regular basis, at a high temperature with sufficient washing detergent.

Waste disposal

The correct methods for waste disposal must be provided by your employer. These should include general waste bins, contaminated waste bins and a sharps box.

Each treatment room and work area must have a general waste bin with a lid and ideally a foot pedal to avoid using your hands to open it. These bins should be emptied at the end of each day and disposed of in a large general waste bin which will be collected by the local council at regular intervals.

Contaminated waste is lined with a yellow bin bag and should be used to dispose of waste which contains blood or bodily fluids, such as wax strips and consumables used for waxing and epilation. This waste must be handled with care and is removed and incinerated as required by your local authority.

A sharps box is a small yellow plastic container which is used for the disposal of any 'sharps'; this will include epilation probes and micro-lances. It must be handled with care and is also removed and incinerated as required by your local authority.

Inspection and registration

Under the terms of the Local Government (Miscellaneous Provisions) Act 1982 (Local Authority Licensing), an environmental health officer can inspect the hygiene and cleanliness of your salon at any time. Should the inspector identify any hazards, an improvement notice will be issued. In such a case any hazards identified must be dealt with by the employer within a set period of time. Failure to do so will lead to prosecution, which may result in closure of the business via the issue of a prohibition notice.

Taking appropriate action to control workplace hazards LO2 LO3

Hazards and risks

As a senior member of staff you may find yourself responsible for health and safety practice in the salon. This consists of assessing the risks and hazards in the salon and controlling them by implementing policies and procedures to minimise them.

- A hazard is the potential to cause harm.
- A risk is the likelihood of harm.

Control is used to minimise or eliminate the risk. For example, spilt water on the floor presents a *hazard*; the *risk* would be someone slipping on the water and hurting themselves. Controlling the risk would be for whoever spilt the water to clear it up straight away before it poses a risk to anyone.

A senior therapist needs to be acutely aware of other hazards within their workplace and anticipate these by implementing methods of control wherever possible. Other examples of hazards in a salon environment include:

- electrical machinery
- substances hazardous to health such as chemicals
- trailing wires
- stacked stock in storage rooms
- essential oils
- lifting heavy objects.

Evaluating the risk

Risk assessments

As identified in the relevant legislation described earlier, there are many risk assessments that need to be conducted by the employer/manager in the workplace and it is their responsibility to action and implement the necessary controls.

There are certain treatments that have a higher potential for risk than others, including anything involving the use of electrical equipment, hair removal or extractions and any treatment that involves the use of chemicals, such as soaking off an artificial nail structure.

A therapist also needs to be aware of hazards that are not related to performing treatments but are linked to the workplace, such as trailing wires and spilt water. If a hazard is low risk then it will be the responsibility of the therapist to deal with it, such as cleaning up water spillages. If a hazard is high risk then the therapist will need to report it to the relevant person and place a warning sign to inform others.

Safe working practices play an important part in reducing the risks from hazards and the following rules apply:

- Do not ignore a hazard. If it falls within the realm of your responsibility deal with it; if not, report it to the relevant person.
- Always read and follow manufacturers' instructions.
- Do not perform treatments that you are not trained or qualified to do.
- Always keep accurate and thorough client records.
- Always follow strict hygiene and health and safety procedures.
- Always seek relevant help if you do not know how to do something that may put you or someone else at risk.

There are, however, times when unforeseen accidents occur. At these times it is imperative that you follow salon procedures in dealing with and recording the accident to reduce further injury.

Emergency procedures

Every member of staff must be trained and prepared for an emergency situation. All staff must be aware of their level of responsibility and respond to the situation professionally and in a calm manner.

Staff training on emergency procedure is the responsibility of the employer/manager. New staff should be given a full induction that includes information on:

- health and safety polices and systems of work in the salon
- fire prevention and evacuation procedures
- risks and hazards, including the level of risks and who to report them to
- emergency procedures in the event of an accident
- where the accident book is kept and how to make a recording
- first aid or details of who is the responsible person/first aider.

Every salon should have clear and well signposted emergency exits and fire escapes. Staff should also be aware of the fire-fighting equipment that is kept on the premises and should know where it is and how to use it.

Key term

Safety management system – a term used to describe the management of occupational safety and health in the workplace.

⭐ *Hints and tips*

It is a good idea to have practice runs of emergency procedures so that all staff know what to do and where to go. They will then be more confident in the event of a real situation.

NVQ evidence requirements

For the NVQ you will need to be observed by your assessor on at least one occasion. However, you must show that you have met all the outcomes by collecting additional evidence. You must cover the following range:

1 The promotional activities include:
- demonstrations
- displays
- advertising campaigns.

2 Your objectives are:
- to enhance business image
- to increase business.

VRQ practical evidence requirements

There are different evidence requirements for the VRQ qualifications, depending on the awarding body.

City & Guilds unit 304 Promote and sell products and services to clients

- Two occasions covering the following:
  - new products/services to the client
  - products/services already used by client.

After each observation candidates are required to review with the assessor the effectiveness of the selling techniques used.

VTCT unit UV30435 Promote and sell products and services to clients

- Three occasions where you are able to promote and sell beauty products.

VRQ knowledge requirements

City & Guilds unit 304 Promote and sell products and services to clients	VTCT unit 30435 Promote and sell products and services to clients	Page no.
Learning outcome 1: Be able to promote and sell hair and beauty products		
Practical skills/observations		
Identify selling opportunities		26–7
Use effective communication techniques		29; 183–4
Interpret buying signals and the client's intentions		28
Manage clients expectations to achieve a realistic objective		24
Introduce products and/or services to clients		29
Use effective selling techniques to close a sale		28; 207–8
Underpinning knowledge		
Explain the benefits to the salon of promoting services and products to the client		22
Explain the importance of product and service knowledge when selling		30
Explain communication techniques used to promote products and services		29
Explain the differences between the terms 'features' and 'benefits'		30
Describe the stages of the sale process		28
Describe how to manage client expectations		29
Explain how to interpret buying signals		28
Explain the legislation that affects the selling of services or products		22–23

City & Guilds unit 304 Promote and sell products and services to clients	VTCT unit 30435 Promote and sell products and services to clients	Page no.
Learning outcome 2: Understand how to evaluate the promotion of products and services		
Practical skills/observations		
Review effectiveness of selling techniques		30–1
Underpinning knowledge		
Explain the importance of reviewing selling techniques		30–1
Explain different methods of evaluating selling techniques		30–1
Describe how to implement improvements in their own selling techniques		31
Evaluate the effectiveness of advertising services and products to a target audience		30–1
Explain the importance of how to set and agree sales target/objectives		44–6

Introduction

Performing promotional activities and selling products offers many benefits to a business. From low-cost promotional techniques to big budget events, promotions come in a wide range of guises. A promotion is the business of communicating with clients. It provides the opportunity and information for clients to make a decision on whether or not to purchase a product or service. It allows for demonstrations of services and products to be seen, enabling clients to see at first hand the features, benefits and effects of a particular product or service.

In terms of business productivity, promotional activities and selling allow for increased sales and business, enhance the business' image and profile and may help to gain business in quieter times of the year. They enable you to validate your professionalism and knowledge and maximise the efficiency of staff, products and often your environment.

Contribute to the planning and preparation of promotional activities

Legal requirements

There are six specific legal requirements that directly relate to this chapter on planning and delivering promotional activities. More detail can be found on legislation and regulations by referring to Chapter 1 Monitoring health and safety and Chapter 6 Professional practices.

The six specific legal requirements are:

1 Data Protection Act 1998: regulates the use of personal data.

2 Trade Descriptions Act 1968: protects the consumer from false trade descriptions.

3 Sale and Supply of Goods Act 1994: prohibits the use of false trade descriptions.

4 Consumer Protection Act 1987: protects the client against the selling or use of defective products.

5 Consumer Safety Act 1978: makes further provision with respect to the safety of consumers and others.

6 Prices Act 1974: prices should be clearly marked to not give a false impression.

Much of your health and safety planning will be implemented when you conduct your general planning for a promotional event. However, it is essential that you know the legal requirements for your promotional activities and all relevant health and safety procedures, including:

- roles and responsibilities for public and staff safety in the event of an emergency, if using an external venue
- fire evacuation procedures and routes
- electrical safety for any items of electrical equipment needed
- risk assessments.

Remember that a risk assessment follows a procedure that:
- identifies all hazards that could cause harm
- decides what the risks are of the harm and who might be affected
- assesses the risks
- takes action to minimise the risks.

Always make sure you are fully insured for your promotional event or activity (information on insurance can be found in Chapter 6 Professional practices, page 181).

Choosing a venue

You may be holding your promotional activity in your normal salon or spa environment, to which you should already hold the correct insurance, health and safety requirements and risk assessments. You may, however, find that you are conducting your promotion at an external venue. This could range from a hotel conference room, a large exhibition hall or even a stall in a local shopping precinct. When choosing a venue consider the following:

- availability and cost of hiring the venue
- access to the venue, particularly for guests with disabilities
- amenities and facilities the venue has to offer
- capacity of the venue (i.e. the number of people it can hold)
- type of insurance already held by the venue.

It is essential to check the venue has its own public liability insurance and entertainment license. Read and familiarise yourself with any contractual obligations, as it may state requirements you must abide by and which

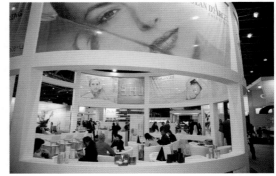

△ A promotional stand

could invalidate your insurance if not adhered to. Be aware of the contract requirements of any local bye-laws and legislation which could restrict your promotional activity in the venue.

Identify who are your points of contact at the venue and make a note of their contact numbers somewhere safe and easily accessible.

Ensure that you know the following about your chosen venue:

- access dates and times
- first aid and emergency procedures
- electrical supplies and requirements for microphones, overhead projectors and equipment
- amenities and facilities available
- hospitality arrangements for guests, to include drinks, food and seating
- floor plan and decor of venue
- background music needs.

Promotional planning

Promotional event planning and preparation can be a sizable task depending on the event you are organising. It is imperative you know and appreciate the value of detailed and accurate planning. Start your organisation several months before the event and arrange a meeting with all those involved to discuss your objectives, agree a schedule and set a time scale. You may also want to allocate:

- an organising committee for the smooth and safe operation of the event
- an event manager who will be in overall charge of the event
- a safety officer with overall responsibility for safety matters.

At your initial meeting you will either need to decide on your objectives or review them if they have been set by your organisation. An effective way of ensuring you meet all your objectives is to ensure they are SMART:

- **S**pecific: Give yourself a specific goal – one which will identify who is involved, what needs to be accomplished and explains why the event is being held.
- **M**easurable: Distinguish criteria for measuring progress towards the attainment of your objectives.
- **A**chievable: Ensure that the objectives are appropriate, agreed and achievable to complete within the time available.
- **R**ealistic: Ensure the objectives planned are realistic so they can be met.
- **T**ime bound: Give a reasonable time frame to plan, perform and evaluate the event.

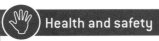

Health and safety

You must ensure you do not overcrowd your venue. It is essential to know the safe maximum number of people that the venue can hold to control hazards and enforce health and safety requirements.

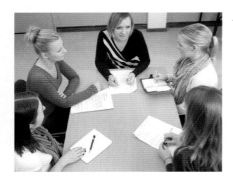

△ Team meeting

☆ Hints and tips

It is a good idea to identify one competent person and appoint them to be the event manager to oversee the whole planning process. The event manager is then responsible for coordinating the event effectively and making all final decisions.

In the planning stages you will also need to:

- decide on your venue

- choose the dates and times your event will be open

- decide whether admission will be free, by pre-sold tickets or by payment on arrival

- identify your target audience and how you will attract their interest

- estimate the approximate number of clients expected to attend

- choose suppliers for hospitality and decor (if required)

- carry out risk assessments and obtain specialist advice if necessary

- identify methods of evaluating your event at this stage (via websites, focus groups or word of mouth).

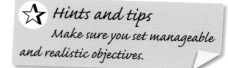
☆ *Hints and tips*
Make sure you set manageable and realistic objectives.

Resources

Material resources

There will be a vast array of resources that you will need for your activity to take place effectively. Some of these will need to be ordered in advance, like extra stock; others you may need to research how to obtain them, such as an overhead projector and microphones. Other resources will come from your salon. Types of resourcing requirements for an event include tools, equipment, materials and consumables.

Human resources

Clearly define the roles and responsibilities of those involved with the event. Ensure they are matched to their individual's level of competence and inform everyone of who is responsible for what. Gain each person's commitment and agreement to participate in the activity. Ensure that:

- specific responsibilities are allocated to each member of the team for before, during and after the event, and cascade these to all members of the team

- there is confirmation in writing and minutes of meetings of everyone's job roles

- any training needs are identified and completed before the activity commences

- models have been identified and organised as required

- on the day everyone is fully aware of their responsibilities.

☆ *Hints and tips*
Always make sure you have enough resources for the number of guests you are expecting. Running out of resources such as products and leaflets will make you look unprofessional and disorganised and may even lose you a sale. Plan how you will transport your resources to the venue. You may need to hire a van and may need help to load and carry heavy pieces of equipment.

Working to a budget

It is important to be aware of the budget you have for your activity and what resources you can afford. A large organisation will generally outline a budget for marketing activities in an annual business plan. However, smaller business will need to decide what money can be allocated to promotions and plan for this accordingly. It is essential that you stick to a budget as running out of money in the middle of planning an activity could result in the event being cancelled and all money lost.

☆ *Hints and tips*
Make sure you have planned for foreseeable problems that may occur and have back-up plans in place to resolve them.

Types of promotional activities

There is a huge range of promotional activities. Factors that influence an organisation's choice of activity include the budget available, the target audience and the product or service that is being promoted. Below are the three promotional activities that are required in the range for this chapter: demonstrations, displays and advertising campaigns. Other methods of promotional activities include using customer loyalty point accumulation systems, coupons, limited time discounts and money off products with purchases.

Demonstrations

Demonstrations are used widely throughout promotional activities to physically demonstrate to clients the product or service. They vary immensely, depending on the situation and environment the demonstration is being delivered in. A demonstration can be performed to an individual in a small surrounding or a large group of people in an extensive setting. You may be able to perform the demonstration on the client or you may require a model to perform the demonstration in front of an audience. The success of the demonstration will depend on:

- the person demonstrating being fully prepared with all resources and props required
- ensuring equipment is in full working order
- the knowledge and confidence of the person delivering the demonstration.

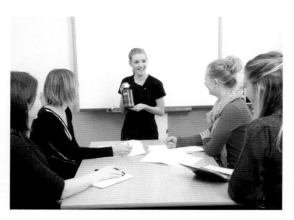

△ A demonstration

Displays

Displays help to boost product recognition, client interest and sales. Promotional displays can be effective for themed promotions throughout the year, such as Valentine's Day, Mother's Day and Christmas. Displays must look professional, be clean and tidy and undamaged. They should be placed in an area that is widely seen, such as in windows and the reception area. They should be changed on a regular basis to ensure clients are kept interested. Many professional product companies will supply promotional material for displays, such as leaflets, posters and stands.

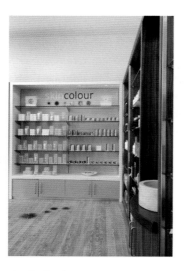

△ A display

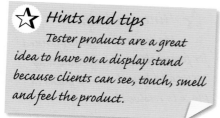

☆ *Hints and tips*
Tester products are a great idea to have on a display stand because clients can see, touch, smell and feel the product.

Advertising campaigns

Advertising campaigns create interest and a want and need for a product or service. They are used to launch a new product, increase brand awareness and boost sales. An advertising campaign is a series of messages that share and support a theme or idea. The planning and delivery methods of a campaign will lead to its success or failure. For example, you may choose to focus your campaign at a quieter time of year to stand out from your competitors, although there may be fewer clients to target. A budget should be allocated to your campaign at the initial planning stages which will dictate your methods and volume of advertising.

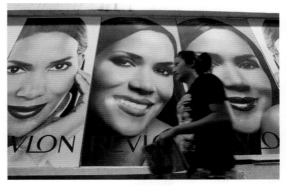

△ Advertising campaign

Advertising and marketing your event

New and existing clients will not know about your event unless you inform them. Not marketing your event properly means there is a risk it will fail. Make sure you allocate enough time to advertise your promotional activity in order to spark interest in your target audience. There are many different advertising methods and it is important that you match your activity with the relevant advertising material. Common methods of advertising events include:

- emailing and texting existing clients
- posters
- letters
- flyers
- brochures
- leaflets
- press release
- newsletter.

Word-of-mouth and telling people in person are other ways of marketing your event, but these methods cannot be relied upon alone. It is good practice to use a mixture of different methods as this also enables you to target your advertising at a particular segment of your target audience. The level, amount and method of advertising will depend on your budget and your objectives.

Activity

Research successful advertising campaigns in the beauty and nail industries. Identify what is being advertised, where and when it was advertised, and why it was such a success.

Remember . . .

Your advertising will only be successful if you reach your target audience and effectively communicate a message that makes them want to buy or find out more about your products or services.

Implement promotional activities

Before the event

In the run-up to your event you should hold further meetings with your organising committee, events manager and safety officer to ensure all is proceeding as planned. At this point you should review your budget to check you are within your allocation and are not overspending. Check that the risk assessments have been carried out and that all insurance is in place. This is your opportunity to review

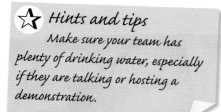

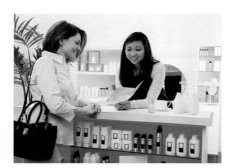

△ Positive buying signals

the current plans, raise any issues and make the relevant changes before it is too late. Ensure that any changes are cascaded to your team and notes are kept of changes to refer back to if needed.

Event day

On the day of the event collect your team together at a set time and place before the activity starts to check everyone knows their roles and responsibilities. Everyone should have a floor plan and schedule and know where their nearest facilities and amenities are. Have a rota for lunch and breaks, so your event is always fully manned.

Make sure everything is going according to plan and check the environment is appropriate for the event. Check any machinery you will be using and complete a 'walk-through' around the area to examine the displays, resources, décor and set up. Position yourself ready for the event to begin. Remember to smile, be helpful and enthusiastic.

Selling skills

There are different selling skills that can be utilised during promotional activities. It will be up to you to identify the most suitable for the activity and tailor these skills to meet individual client needs and interests.

You need to know how to identify customer's buying signals and how to close a sale. Customer's buying signals include:

- making eye contact with whoever is selling or promoting
- spending time looking at the product
- asking detailed questions
- asking about price
- using positive body language
- asking other people's opinions to seek confirmation.

You can close a sale by:

- recognising the buying signals described above
- listening to the customer and answering any concerns and questions
- staying positive
- giving the customer time to think
- identifying the features and benefits of the product/service
- offering the customer an alternative, such as 'would you like to book this treatment, or the other one?'

Communication techniques

There are two methods of communication:

1 Verbal communication, which includes use of language, tone of voice and questioning techniques.

2 Non-verbal communication, which includes listening techniques, body language, eye contact and facial expressions.

Always use positive forms of communication, such as appropriate and correct language and a varied and interested tone of voice. Make sure you smile and use eye contact. Part of effective communication is knowing how and when to participate in discussions. Wait for natural pauses in conversation and when responding to questions. Although you may be leading a demonstration or presentation, identify how and when to make openings to encourage others to ask questions. Know how to manage the answers to questions and queries in a way that maintains goodwill.

You can also communicate by creating a visual impact; this can be through your choice of décor, set-up and personal presentation. This is another form of non-verbal communication.

More information on communication techniques can be found in Chapter 6 Professional Practices.

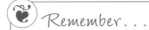

Remember...
It only takes a few seconds to make a first impression so make it a positive one!

Presentation techniques

At some point in your promotional activity it is likely that you will take part in a presentation. This may be a formal presentation as a speaker discussing a specific topic or while demonstrating a service or use of a product. Tailor your presentation to meet individual needs and interests. Consider the following points:

- Introduce yourself to your audience at the beginning of your presentation and clearly identify your objectives.

- Timing: the average attention span of an adult is 20 minutes. Keep to your schedule and do not go over time.

- Pace: do not speak too quickly or move on too fast but equally do not take too much time to explain your points.

- Use of voice: think about the tone and language used.

- Use of graphics: these can help elaborate and explain the points you make and retain the audience's interest.

- Closing statement: briefly summarise your presentation at the end, pulling together all the points you have made.

- Environment: have enough chairs for people to sit on and make sure the room temperature is comfortable.

Hints and tips
Make eye contact with your audience and speak slowly and clearly.

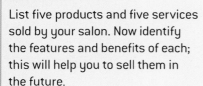
Features and benefits

When selling a product or service you need to be able to explain its features and benefits to your client. Features and benefits are an essential part of the sales process and when both are clearly identified they offer maximum impact and will hopefully lead to a sale.

Look at the following example:

'This moisturiser contains a sun protection factor which means it will protect the skin from sun damage such as pigmentation.'

In this statement the sun protection factor is the *feature*; the protection from sun damage such as pigmentation is the *benefit*.

Participate in the evaluation of promotional activities

An evaluation needs to be conducted as soon as possible after the promotional event has taken place. This will be completed by the employer/manager or whoever has been responsible for the promotional activity. The evaluation process enables you to measure the success of the activity and the importance of this process should never be underestimated.

You will need to identify the areas of the promotional activity that should be evaluated. This could include whether the desired target audience were captured, a review of the selling techniques used and the effectiveness of the venue used. You must also consider whether everyone involved fulfilled their individual roles and responsibilities competently, and the overall cost of the activity. Finally, evaluate the overall success of the activity, for example what amount of retail sales or bookings were sold because of the activity.

Feedback

Customer feedback is one of the most important and useful ways of evaluating how successful the activity has been. Feedback can be obtained from:

- clients who attended
- the targeted market
- people involved with the planning process
- sponsors
- external companies involved with the event.

The most productive and successful methods of gaining feedback are:

- forms or questionnaires
- face-to-face discussions
- focus groups
- telephone conversations

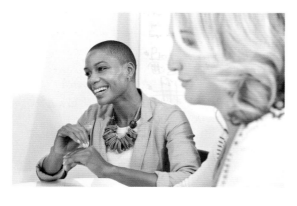

△ Focus group

- website or paper feedback comments
- tracking the increase in sales/services.

You will need to decide which method is the most suitable way of gathering your feedback, based on the type of promotional activity. You may choose to adopt two or three methods to offer choice to clients and to provide a wide breath of evidence.

Analysis

Analysing your feedback means collating, reviewing and summarising your activity in a clear and concise way. Analysing your promotional activity will give you information on the overall costs involved, levels of increased public awareness, improved sales and levels of repeat business.

Analysing customer feedback may provide pointers or suggestions that you did not envisage or suggestions that do not relate directly to the activity.

In your analysis you should consider the businesses strengths and weaknesses, where the areas for improvement are, and any outstanding staff training needs. A good place to start is to conduct a SWOT analysis.

Taking a few minutes to conduct a SWOT analysis on the event can help to create a broad and justified analysis and may lead to a future strategy that helps you distinguish yourself from your competitors, enabling your organisation to compete successfully in the beauty and nail-related industries.

Evaluation report

Creating a written report is a more formal way of evaluating your event. This may be a requirement of the organisation you work for; it may also be used to present evidence of the measured success of the promotion to senior managers of a large corporation.

You may find you are given a deadline to submit the report. Make sure you gather as much evidence as possible at the event. The more data you can refer to, the stronger your report will be. Remember to make your report honest, informative, clear and concise.

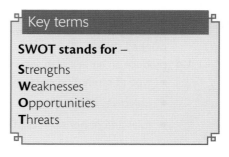

Key terms

SWOT stands for –
Strengths
Weaknesses
Opportunities
Threats

Activity

Next time you are involved in a promotional activity or event, complete a SWOT analysis as part of your evaluation process.

☆ *Hints and tips*
An important part of the evaluation report is the requirement to be critical and analyse where things did not go so well. What recommendations can you make and what would you do differently next time?

Want to know more?

Why not attend one of the large trade show exhibitions to see for yourself how the professionals sell and promote? You will not be able to see the months of planning and preparation but you will be able to see for yourself the implementation of the promotional activity. Exhibitions are also a great way of keeping abreast with developments in the industry and seeing companies showcase and demonstrate new products and services. Professional Beauty hold exhibitions throughout the year in London, Manchester and Dublin. Information on these can be found at www. professionalbeauty.co.uk
Olympia Beauty also holds exhibitions – visit their website at www. olympiabeauty.co.uk

NVQ assessment checklist

To complete this unit you must have the following theoretical and practical skills. Check against the list below and refer back to the relevant section for information on anything you are unsure about.

1. Be able to contribute to the planning and preparation of promotional activities

❑ **1.1** make recommendations to the relevant person (s) for suitable promotional activities, identifying the potential benefits for the business

❑ **1.2** identify and agree specific, measurable, achievable, realistic and time bound objectives and target groups for the activity with the relevant person(s)

❑ **1.3** agree requirements for the activity with all relevant person(s) in sufficient detail to allow the work to be planned

❑ **1.4** produce an agreed plan showing the
- type of promotional activity
- objectives of the activity
- roles and responsibilities of others involved
- resource requirements
- preparation and implementation activities
- timescales
- the budget
- methods of evaluation

❑ **1.5** agree a plan that takes into account any legal requirements, when necessary

❑ **1.6** make sure resources are available to meet the planned timescale

2. Be able to implement promotional activities

❑ **2.1** implement promotional activities to meet the agreed plan

❑ **2.2** adapt promotional activities, when necessary, in response to changed circumstances and/or problems

❑ **2.3** use resources effectively throughout the promotional activities

❑ **2.4** communicate the essential features and benefits of products and services to the target group

❑ **2.5** use methods of communication that are suitable for the type of promotional activity being undertaken

❑ **2.6** present information in logical steps

❑ **2.7** encourage the target group to ask questions about the services and products being promoted

❑ **2.8** respond to questions and queries in a way which promotes goodwill and enhances the salon's image

❑ **2.9** actively encourage the target group to take advantage of the services and products being promoted

❑ **2.10** clear away products and equipment at the end of the promotional activity, when necessary, to meet the requirements of the venue

3. Be able to participate in the evaluation of promotional activities

❑ **3.1** use the methods agreed in the promotional activity plan to gain feedback from the relevant sources

❑ **3.2** collate and record the information gained from the feedback using a clear and concise format and method of presentation

❑ **3.3** draw accurate and clear conclusions on the effectiveness of the promotional activity in meeting the agreed objectives

❑ **3.4** participate in discussions giving a clear and well-structured summary of the results of the evaluation

❑ **3.5** make recommendations for improvements to any future promotional activities based upon the outcomes of the evaluation

4. Understand the venue and legal requirements

❑ **4.1** explain the practical requirements and restrictions of any venue

❑ **4.2** describe the contract requirements, local bye-laws and legislation which could restrict the promotional activity in any venue used

❑ **4.3** explain the importance of considering health and safety and other legal requirements

❑ **4.4** explain the health and safety procedures applicable to any venue used

❑ **4.5** explain the potential hazards that must be considered when working at any venue

❑ **4.6** describe the steps that should be taken to minimise risks when working at an external venue

5. Understand how to plan and prepare promotional events

❑ **5.1** explain the purpose and value of detailed and accurate planning

❑ **5.2** explain the type of resourcing requirements necessary for promotional activities

❑ **5.3** explain how the nature of the target group can influence the choice of promotional activity

❑ **5.4** explain how to match types of promotional activities to objectives

❑ **5.5** describe how to present a plan for promotional activities

❑ **5.6** explain why it is important to consider methods of evaluation at the planning stage

❑ **5.7** explain how to write objectives that are Specific, Measurable, Achievable, Realistic and Time Bound (i.e. SMART objectives)

❑ **5.8** explain the importance of working to a budget

❑ **5.9** explain where and how to obtain resources

❑ **5.10** explain the importance of clearly defining the roles and responsibilities of those involved in promotional activities

❑ **5.11** describe the importance of allocating roles and responsibilities to match an individual's competence levels

❑ **5.12** explain the importance of gaining an individual's commitment and agreement to undertake a role in the promotional activity

❑ **5.13** explain the types of foreseeable problems that occur and ways of resolving them

6. Understand how to sell products and services

❑ **6.1** explain how to recognise buying signals and to close sales

❑ **6.2** identify the difference between the features of a product or service and the benefits of a product or service

❑ **6.3** describe the features and benefits of products and/or services being promoted

❑ **6.4** describe how to tailor the presentation of the benefits of products and/or services to meet individual needs and interests

7. Understand communication techniques

❑ **7.1** explain how and when to participate in discussions

❑ **7.2** describe how to give a short presentation

❑ **7.3** compare different methods of presenting information

❑ **7.4** explain how and when to make openings to encourage others to ask questions

❑ **7.5** describe how to answer questions and manage queries in a way likely to maintain goodwill

8. Understand evaluation methods and techniques

❑ **8.1** explain the purpose of evaluation activities

❑ **8.2** explain the areas of the promotional activity which should be evaluated

❑ **8.3** describe the most suitable methods of gaining feedback for the promotional activities in the range

❑ **8.4** explain how to collate, analyse and summarise evaluation feedback in a clear and concise way

❑ **8.5** explain suitable ways of formatting and producing an evaluation report

Test yourself

1. State three pieces of legislation that directly relate to promotional activities and selling.

2. Name the three job roles you may want to identify when planning an event.

3. State three points to consider when choosing a venue.

4. What is meant by SMART objectives?

5. Identify four ways that you can advertise and market your event.

6. What are the two methods of communication?

7. Identify four methods of positive communication.

8. What are features and benefits of products or services?

9. What methods can be used to gain feedback after an event has taken place?

10. What is a SWOT analysis?

Chapter **3**

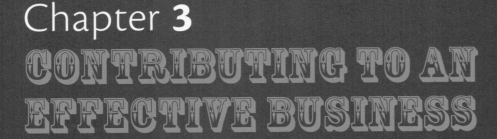

CONTRIBUTING TO AN EFFECTIVE BUSINESS

This chapter covers the following units:

NVQ unit G11 Contribute to the financial effectiveness of the business

VTCT VRQ unit UV30449 Contribute to the effective running of business

LEARNING OBJECTIVES

This chapter is about the monitoring and effective use of salon resources and meeting productivity and development targets to enable you to make a positive contribution to the business. You are also responsible for ensuring that individuals who assist you to deliver services to clients are working effectively too.

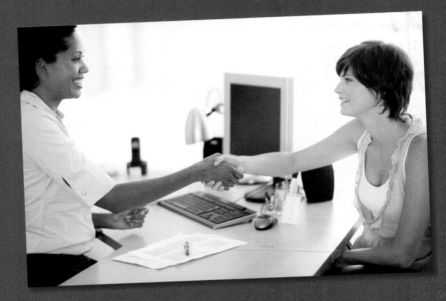

The learning outcomes for NVQ unit G11 are:

1 Contribute to the effective use and monitoring of resources
2 Be able to meet productivity and development targets
3 Understand salon procedures and legal requirements
4 Understand the use, monitoring and recording of resources
5 Understand effective methods of communication
6 Understand work and time management
7 Understand productivity and development targets

You will need to be competent in all of these outcomes.

NVQ evidence requirements

For the NVQ you will need to be observed by your assessor on at least one occasion. However, you must show that you have met all the outcomes by collecting additional evidence. You must cover the following range:

1 Resources, to include:
- human
- stock
- tools and equipment
- time.

2 Productivity and development targets for:
- retail sales
- technical services
- personal learning.

VRQ practical evidence requirements

The evidence requirements for the VRQ qualification for VTCT are shown below (note: there is no equivalent for City & Guilds for this chapter).

VTCT unit UV30449 Contribute to the effective running of business
- Three occasions

VRQ knowledge requirements

VTCT unit UV30449 Contribute to the effective running of business	Page no.
Learning outcome 1: Be able to make a positive contribution to run a business effectively	
Practical skills/observations	
Communicate effectively with colleagues and clients	37
Use effective communication skills to gather and present productivity and development targets	44–6
Assist others to resolve problems	37–8
Provide support and guidance to contribute to the effective running of the business	37–8
Use resources in a way which complies with legal and salon requirements	37, 210–13
Maintain accurate records for effective running of a business	40–1
Follow safe and hygienic working practices	181–2
Underpinning knowledge	
Describe the benefits of effective team work when running a business	193–4
Describe the requirement for productivity and development targets	44–5
Describe how the effective use of resources contribute to the effective running of a business	36–43
Describe health, safety, legal and salon requirements within the workplace	210–13
Describe the requirement for accurate records to be established for client base, stock and resources	36–43

Introduction

Contributing to the financial effectiveness of a business is part of every therapist's job role. Whether you are working for yourself, for a small salon or as part of a large organisation you must follow salon procedures for monitoring the resources in the range stated. Knowing how to communicate effectively is a large part of making a successful contribution, as is ensuring the effective working of individuals who may assist you to deliver services to clients. However, you must also recognise the limits of your responsibility and know who to report to when dealing with a situation outside your remit.

Meeting productivity and development targets will help to ensure that you continue to develop as an individual, contribute as an active team member and ensure that the financial effectiveness of the business is maintained. Not contributing effectively is likely to have serious repercussions for both the therapist and the business and the two outcomes of the occupational standards are therefore closely related.

Contribute to the financial effectiveness of the business

For current legal requirements relating to this unit please refer back to Chapter 1 Monitoring health and safety. You also need to be aware of current legislation relating to the sale of retail goods and employment legislation and this information can be found in Chapter 6 Professional practices.

Resources

All businesses require resources to implement their workplace procedures. The four main types of resources are:

1 human

2 stock

3 tools and equipment

4 time.

Successful use of resources contributes to the financial effectiveness of a business and all resources, whether human, physical (such as stock, tools and equipment) or time, need to be monitored and managed effectively. This is likely to be by the employer/manager, although other members of the team may

> **Key term**
>
> **Resources** – these are used to achieve the organisation's objectives and are usually assets or materials from which benefit is produced.

be given responsibility for resources such as stock taking. It is the responsibility of the employer/manager to provide each member of staff with the salon's procedures for monitoring the use of resources and your responsibility to ensure you follow these procedures. Always know the limits of your authority relating to resources, and who you should refer to if you have any concerns or recommendations to make.

Human resources

Human resources (HR) is a term that describes the individuals within an organisation. Skilled and qualified individuals are the most important element of any business. People are different from any other form of resources as they have thoughts, feelings and needs. Maximising and investing in an organisation's human capital will ensure effective use of human resources.

All members of staff should be given a full induction on commencing their employment. This should be performed by a senior member of staff who can clearly inform them of all the salon's policies, workplace procedures and relevant duties under health and safety legislation. Along with their contract, employees should receive a job description which details their individual role and responsibilities. They should be given regular performance development reviews (PDR) and targets to aim for. The Employment Protection Act 1978 states that each employee should have access to the business' disciplinary and grievance procedure (this is a framework that provides a clear and transparent structure for dealing with difficulties which may arise in the workplace).

Information on staff working hours, break entitlements and annual leave are covered in the section on 'Working within the law' in Chapter 6 Professional practices, page 210.

Communication

Therapists and nail technicians have direct contact with clients, so they need to be customer focused, professional and happy. Effective team working and successful communication with both clients and colleagues is vital.

More information on effective communication techniques can be found in Chapter 2 Promotional activities and selling methods, page 29 and Chapter 6 Professional Practices.

Make sure both your verbal and written forms of communication are clear and precise. Any instructions should be given accurately and in a timely way. Always check that colleagues understand what you are saying and clarify any points in a professional way. Respect should be shown to all members of staff, no matter what hierarchy is in place.

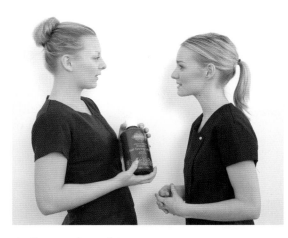
△ Beauty therapists

Key term

Human resources – a term that describes the individuals within an organisation.

★ **Hints and tips**
A large organisation usually has its own HR department that oversees the wellbeing of the staff employed within it. The HR responsibilities of a large company include recruitment and disciplinary matters, payroll, benefits and keeping up to date with tax law.
Staff wages will be one of the largest costs to a business within the beauty and nail industries. However, it is important that good staff are paid accordingly, with the opportunity to earn commission. This will help to ensure they work productively and staff retention levels will remain high.

 Remember...
When communicating with others use positive techniques, such as smiling, eye contact and suitable hand gestures and tone of voice.

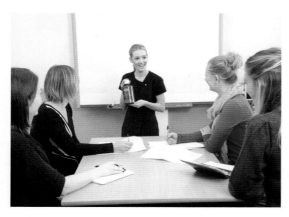

△ Staff meeting

Showing value to all employees will encourage them to work effectively on your behalf, remain loyal and improve staff retention levels.

Meetings

Staff meetings should be held on a regular basis, in a suitable area, and at a time that enables all team members to attend. The meetings should be chaired by a senior member of staff who plans the agenda. Team meetings are a chance for all staff to come together and be informed of changes and updates that may be occurring. They can also be used to discuss ideas and concerns and may even be utilised for training purposes.

Someone should be responsible for taking minutes of each meeting which are then circulated to all staff after the meeting has taken place. This is an effective way of keeping staff informed of what was discussed even if they were unable to attend.

Staff training

After induction training has taken place all staff should continue to receive ongoing training. Investing in staff through training is an essential process to ensure development and up-skilling of the workforce, and is part of continuous professional development (CPD). Enhanced knowledge and abilities help the business to achieve its objectives.

Training should be identified for each individual during their PDR and through analysis, in order to meet organisational and personal objectives. A training and development plan should be created from all employees' PDRs and this plan should be reviewed annually. This will set out how the training needs can be addressed and will assess the budget allocated for training courses. It may be that a member of staff is sent on an external course or in-house training may be provided within the salon environment.

Stock

Managing stock effectively is important for every business, as services and sales are unable to be performed without the required stock.

Cost effective use of resources and good retail sales contribute considerably to the financial profitability of a business. There are many processes involved with stock, so it is recommended that one person is responsible for stock sourcing, ordering, checking, unpacking and rotation. In addition, because of the high level of accountability required for this job role, the staff member should be in a senior or managerial role. However, it is everyone's responsibility to ensure cost-effective use of products and consumables, to sell retail products and to oversee the security of stock.

Sourcing and ordering stock

Stock can be sourced and ordered from a number of different channels. The supplier you choose must be reliable and cost effective and you may find you source different stock from different suppliers. Providers of stock include the following.

Wholesalers

Wholesalers' prices are direct from the manufacturer so costs can be kept down. Wholesalers should be seen as a service provider to distributors and businesses. They do not create demand for products; they efficiently respond to demand and they offer cash-and-carry operations.

Distributors

Distributor prices are higher than those of the wholesaler because they get their product from the wholesaler or the manufacturer and sell it on to the retailer or consumer; therefore they also need to make a profit. They usually distribute from factories and carry large amounts of stock.

Company representatives

Certain companies will have their own representatives, known as 'reps' who represent the company and showcase and sell their products and machinery. It is their job to visit businesses and sell directly to them. They offer specific product knowledge and will notify you of new products and promotional activities. They can also deliver and book training and support your business with strategies for financial effectiveness.

Before choosing your stock supplier you will need to consider what their delivery time is, what their delivery costs are and what terms of payment they require (you may be required to pay on order or you may be able to set up a credit account to pay later).

When sourcing and ordering retail stock, it is also a good idea to consider the following points:

- Where else is the range sold in your area? Do you want to be selling distinctive items if they are also available in other salons?

- Can you take goods on a sale or return basis? If not, you need to be sure you can sell every item or absorb the cost?

- Do your suppliers have any seasonal price breaks or offer price deals or incentives? (Some manufacturers have periods when they reduce the price of their products; knowing when these are to place orders makes financial sense.)

- Does the supplier offer any promotional material such as leaflets, posters, bags and display stands?

Key terms

Company representative – a person who represents a company and showcases and sells their products.

Distributor – company that gets its products from the wholesaler or manufacturer and sells them on to the retailer or consumer; known as the 'middle man'.

Wholesaler – company that orders direct from the manufacturer, enabling costs to be kept down.

Hints and tips
Buying stock in bulk (storage space permitting) is cost effective as it is often cheaper.

Hints and tips
You can order stock via the telephone, internet websites, postal order forms, through your representative or by visiting a wholesaler.

Remember . . .
When displaying stock for effective selling, remember 'eye level is buy level'!

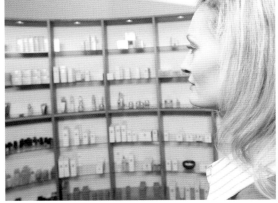
△ Retail stock

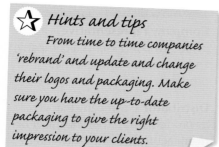

Remember . . .

Make sure you allow adequate time when placing an order to guarantee you do not run out of stock.

Stock control

The basic principles of stock control are to ensure sufficient stock is held for the smooth running of the business. This requires careful planning and regular reviewing to ensure the business has sufficient levels at the required time. The table below describes some of the problems associated with holding too much or too little stock.

Problems associated with holding too much stock	Problems associated with holding too little stock
Wastage, e.g. passing use by/sell by dates	Dissatisfied clients
Risk of theft	Limits services that can be provided
Increased storage space required	Loss of business/revenue
Ties up business capital that could be spent elsewhere	Poor reputation

Stock levels need to be maintained to a suitable level for the business but this may change according to trends, the time of year and any promotional activities that are carried out. Regular re-evaluation of stock levels should be carried out to ensure both customer and business needs are met. Stock levels are generally monitored by the following ways:

- **Maximum stock level**: The most stock that the business is willing or able to have.

- **Minimum stock level**: The level below which it is felt to be unsatisfactory for the business to operate with.

- **Re-order stock level**: The point at which the business re-orders stock.

- **Re-order quantity**: The amount of new stock that will be ordered when stocks fall to the re-order level.

Stock control should be conducted on a regular basis by the allocated person. It is essential to keep detailed, accurate and up-to-date records, including:

- name of the product, including its code and size required

- minimum and maximum stock level

- stock re-order level

- how much is currently in stock

- what has been used and what has been sold

- what has arrived in the stock order.

Stock control may be recorded either manually or via computerised stock control systems.

Manual systems

This is a paper recording system in which a new form is manually completed every time a stock take is conducted. The form must be completed accurately and clearly and kept in a safe and confidential area along with all the previous stock-take records.

The main disadvantages of this method are the problem of human error and the fact that it is a time-consuming process. For these reasons, one person should be solely responsible for stock taking as they will become familiar with the procedure and therefore more efficient and are likely to make fewer errors.

Stock control form

Company: _The Beauty Shop_

Date: _12/6/2012_

Performed by: _J. Hall_

Product size and name	Max. stock level	Min. stock level	Re-order level	No. currently in stock	No. sold	No. arrived in order
Moisturiser 50 ml	10	3	5	8	1	0
Hot wax 450 g	12	5	6	7	3	2
Disposable sponges 100	8	2	3	3	1	0
Clary sage 10 ml	10	3	5	8	2	3

△ Manual stock control paperwork

Computerised systems

These offer similar principles to manual control systems, but are more flexible and reliable (provided the information is correctly input) and information is easier to process and read. A computerised system is a good route for businesses who deal with large amounts of stock. They also offer additional benefits of:

- automatic stock monitoring and identification once re-order level is reached
- bar code reading systems which accelerate processing and recording
- storage of previous stock records and the ability to print a paper copy if required.

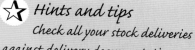

⭐ **Hints and tips**
Check all your stock deliveries against delivery documentation and report any inaccuracies or damaged products to the supplier immediately. Do not assume that your delivery will be accurate.

Stock handling

When lifting or moving stock to its storage area you must ensure you adhere to the requirements of the Manual Handling Operations Regulations 1992. By doing so, you will minimise the risks from lifting and handling large or heavy objects and prevent damage to your musculoskeletal system. If an object is heavy or a difficult shape to lift on your own you should seek help.

For more information on the correct handling of heavy objects and The Manual Handling Operations Regulations 1992, see Chapter 1 Monitoring health and safety, page 10.

Stock rotation

Stock rotation follows the basic principal of first in first out (FIFO). When new items of stock are delivered they should be placed behind existing stock on the shelves, with the older stock being brought forward to the front of the shelf to be sold first.

Stock should be stored in a safe and dry place, away from heat sources and out of direct sunlight. Any stock that has passed its sell-by date or shelf life, or has changed colour or smells unpleasant, should be disposed of accordingly and in line with COSHH regulations.

Stock security

Stock should be stored in a safe but conveniently accessible place. Regular stock takes by the allocated person will help to reduce stock theft. Security of your stock should be taken very seriously and if you suspect a theft and have evidence you should call the police immediately. Your salon should have a policy to follow in the event of theft; make sure you are familiar with this policy.

Some of the measures a business can take to reduce the risk of theft are listed below.

- Explain the consequences of theft to all staff at their induction.
- Never leave the reception area unattended.
- Use closed-circuit television (CCTV) at reception, retail and stock storage areas.
- Store stock and retail products in a safe and lockable area and only allow access by designated staff.
- 'Dummy' products should be displayed in lockable glass cabinets.
- Tester products should be clearly identified and kept to a minimum.
- Stock should be checked, moved and stored quickly after it is delivered.
- Stock levels should not exceed the stated maximum stock level.

Key term

FIFO (first in first out) – a process of stock rotation: new stock is placed behind older stock so that older stock is sold first.

⭐ *Hints and tips*

If stock is going to be displayed in cabinets ask your supplier if they make 'dummy' copies for display purposes. That way money is not wasted on products that will deteriorate while on display.

If products are used as testers in reception areas, place a neat and professional looking 'Tester' label on them so they can be clearly identified and monitored by the reception team.

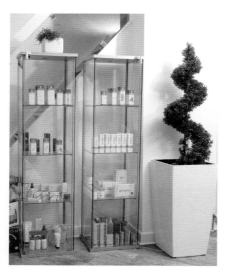

△ Retail glass cabinet containing stock

Tools and equipment

Every workplace needs sufficient and suitable tools and equipment to perform effectively. Tools and equipment are physical resources that need to be sourced, purchased, maintained and eventually replaced. They can vary in size and cost, from a small set of cuticle nippers to a large freestanding unit such as a body electrical machine.

There must be an adequate number of tools and equipment for employees to use and they must be maintained in accordance with the Provision and Use of Work Equipment Regulations (PUWER) 1998. Equipment needs be suitable for its intended use and it must be safe to use, well maintained and regularly inspected to ensure its condition is retained. Any pieces of equipment should only be used by those trained to do so and the employer should identify suitable safety measures where necessary.

Electrical equipment must also conform to the Electricity at Work Regulations 1989 which states that electrical equipment must be regularly tested by a qualified electrician, based on their frequency of use. A record of equipment inspection and servicing must be kept and made available if requested.

Equipment can also be purchased from wholesalers, distributors and company representatives. Before committing to any equipment purchases it is important to critically evaluate if there is a want and need from your client base. You should also:

- examine the equipment in use
- experience the equipment first-hand by having someone use it on you
- conduct market research to ensure there is a want and need for the equipment
- identify the cost and ascertain whether it would be more cost effective to buy or lease the equipment
- find out what support is provided by the company for repairs, warranty and insurance (if the machine is very expensive).

Any faulty tools or equipment should be removed from use immediately and either disposed of correctly or stored with a clear sign on it indicating that the equipment is faulty until it is possible to have it repaired.

Tools and equipment should also be maintained by sterilising as appropriate; large pieces of machinery need to be wiped over with a disinfectant before and after use. When not in use all tools and equipment should be stored correctly.

Hints and tips

If you know the provision of tools and equipment is inadequate, inform your manager so they can check the budget to see if it will be possible to purchase more.

Health and safety

Faulty equipment should be reported immediately to the relevant person. Do not use equipment if you have concerns about its safety.

Activity

List all the tools and equipment that you need in order to perform your treatments effectively (the list will be longer then you anticipate!) Do you know where the tools and equipment were sourced from?

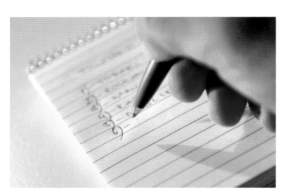

△ Writing a list

Time

Good time management is essential for productivity and effective work. You should prioritise your tasks in order of importance: identify what is urgent and ensure these are completed before other less crucial tasks are performed. Writing lists and recording what needs to be done is another good approach to time management. Keeping your lists in one place, be it a book or computer program, will enable you to refer back if you need to double check a task has been completed.

Senior members of staff should delegate tasks to other team members, provided the task falls within the remit of their job role and level of competence. For example, if a therapist has had a cancellation they could clean their treatment area or change a display stand.

Each person is responsible for their own time management, but in a salon environment it is often the reception team that are in control of a therapist's treatment schedule. Therefore the receptionist must know the allocated treatment timings to ensure enough time is assigned for each service and treatments do not overrun. When using a manual paper appointment schedule or computerised program, therapists' working hours must be identified correctly with their break times clearly blocked out. Furthermore, any salon closures for training, maintenance or staff holidays must also be arranged as soon as possible so the receptionists can work around them effectively and accommodate clients' needs.

The therapist must arrive at work on time. They should check their treatment schedule at the beginning of each working day and prepare their service area in advance. Working in a tidy and organised way will ensure time is utilised more effectively. The therapist should also make sure the salon is clean and tidy before they leave for the day, because returning the next day to a chaotic work area is unprofessional and an example of poor working practice.

Each therapist must adhere to the salon's service timings: clients should not be undercut in their treatment time or kept waiting because the therapist is overrunning. If the client has arrived late, the appointment schedule should be looked at to see if the treatment can still be provided. If not, it may be possible to modify the treatment to fit in the remaining time or the client may choose to reschedule.

Meet productivity and development targets

Meeting productivity and development targets are an important part of ensuring the effectiveness of a business. Failure to meet targets will result in the business losing money, which could result in cuts in both jobs and resources or even the closure of the business.

All targets need to be SMART:

- **S**pecific: Decide what exactly needs to be accomplished by the target.
- **M**easurable: Distinguish the criteria for measuring progress towards the attainment of the target.

- **A**chievable: The target must be agreed and possible to complete.

- **R**ealistic: Ensure your target is realistic so it can be met.

- **T**ime bound: Set a reasonable timeframe in which to meet the target; this might be within a week, a month or longer.

If you believe your targets to be unrealistic you must discuss this with your manager. Being provided with targets that are not SMART will reduce your productivity and personal confidence.

Productivity targets

These relate directly to the business and will be set by the manager during PDRs. They are derived from the annual business plan and overall business targets. Every member of staff should be set productivity targets because everyone should take an active role to increase the productivity of the organisation they work for. Productivity targets are capital-based and can include:

- selling a minimum number of retail products

- up-selling to a certain amount of advanced treatments

- selling courses of treatments instead of individual ones

- performing a minimum number of services.

Some businesses will offer commission on retail products sold or treatments performed. This will be a percentage of either the cost or a general business commission percentage and is often a great way of encouraging staff to increase productivity to ensure targets are met.

Development targets

These relate to expanding the education and ability of staff to meet productivity targets and will often be identified during the PDR. It is important to realise that learning is lifelong and does not stop the moment you gain your industry qualification; training supports your continuing professional development. Regular training keeps staff up to date in their professional field, instils confidence, makes them feel valued and stops them from becoming complacent and feeling jaded. Development targets are personal and can include:

- communication and team working skills

- customer and client care development

- improving 'housekeeping' tasks within the salon

- working on time keeping

- refining services skills

- developing sales skills.

> **Remember...**
>
> The goal of the business is ultimately to make money. If this is not the case it will not be feasible for the business to continue.

Target opportunities

A therapist needs to be aware of the opportunities that are available to achieve their productivity and development targets, including:

- add-ons to services and sales
- promotion of new products and services
- promotional activities and events
- seasonal promotions, such as Mother's Day and Christmas
- special offers
- awareness of trends for new products and services
- participating in training to develop your selling skills.

Performance development review (PDR)

Having regular reviews with a senior member of staff is not only important for identifying training needs but will also provide you with feedback on how effective your overall performance is. Gaining feedback from others is essential for personal development.

Reviews can make you feel anxious but they should largely be a positive and valuable experience. It is good practice to plan for your review by writing down what you wish to discuss with your manager. Remember to take your notes with you so you do not forget anything.

During your review you can discuss and negotiate agreed productivity and development targets. Current targets should also be reviewed and adjustments made if necessary.

Your PDR also gives you an opportunity to discuss any matters that you wish to raise, such as:

- your identified training needs
- any areas that are affecting your performance ability
- additional duties and responsibilities you would like to take on
- identifying your strengths and targets that you have achieved.

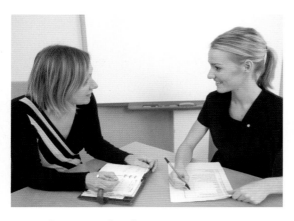

△ Performance development review

NVQ assessment checklist

To complete this unit you must have the following theoretical and practical skills. Check against the list below and refer back to the relevant section for information on anything you are unsure about.

1. Contribute to the effective use and monitoring of resources

❏ **1.1** follow salon procedures for monitoring the use of resources

❏ **1.2** ensure information relating to stock levels is obtained from colleagues in time to coincide with the salon ordering system

❏ **1.3** use resources in a way which complies with legal and salon requirements

❏ **1.4** check deliveries against order documentation, reporting any inaccuracies and/or damages

❏ **1.5** identify and resolve any problems with resources within the limits of own authority

❏ **1.6** report any resource problems they cannot resolve to the relevant person(s)

❏ **1.7** make recommendations to improve the use of resources to the relevant person(s) which clearly show benefits

❏ **1.8** ensure records are accurate, legible and up-to-date.

2. Be able to meet productivity and development targets

❏ **2.1** set, agree and record productivity and development targets with the relevant person(s) to meet the needs of the business

❏ **2.2** actively seek opportunities to meet productivity and development targets

❏ **2.3** make sure that those who assist them with services to clients work effectively and contribute to meeting productivity and development targets

❏ **2.4** regularly review and record progress towards the achievement of productivity and development targets

❏ **2.5** adjust activities to contribute to meeting productivity and development targets

❏ **2.6** meet set productivity and development targets consistently

3. Understand salon procedures and legal requirements

❏ **3.1** explain the salon's requirements and procedures for monitoring the use of resources

❏ **3.2** outline the critical aspects of current legal requirements relevant to hairdressing salons relating to the use of resources

❏ **3.3** describe legal requirements relating to the sale of retail goods

❏ **3.4** explain limits of authority in relation to the use of resources and to whom to report recommendations

4. Understand the use, monitoring and recording of resources

❏ **4.1** explain how effective use of resources contributes to the profitability of the business

❏ **4.2** explain stocking levels and principles of stock control for the salon

❏ **4.3** explain salon ordering systems and how to interpret them

❏ **4.4** explain the importance of keeping accurate records for the use and monitoring of resources

❏ **4.5** explain the resource records for which responsible

❏ **4.6** describe the common problems associated with salon resources and how to resolve them

5. Understand effective methods of communication

❏ **5.1** explain why it is important to communicate effectively

❏ **5.2** explain how to present the benefits of own recommendations in a positive manner to clients

❏ **5.3** explain how to negotiate and agree productivity and development targets

❏ **5.4** explain how to give clear, accurate and timely instructions to those who may be assisting them

❏ **5.5** explain how to encourage others to work effectively on their behalf

❏ **5.6** explain how to respond positively to negative feedback

6. Understand work and time management

❏ **6.1** explain general principles of time management applicable to the delivery of salon services

❏ **6.2** explain how to plan and reschedule own work and that of those who may assist them in order to maximise any opportunities to meet their targets

7. Understand productivity and development targets

❏ **7.1** explain agreed productivity and development targets and the associated timescales for their achievement

❏ **7.2** explain why it is important to meet productivity and development targets

❏ **7.3** explain the potential consequences of failure to meet productivity and development targets

❏ **7.4** describe the types of opportunities that can be used to achieve productivity and development targets

❏ **7.5** explain why targets should be regularly reviewed

❏ **7.6** explain the importance of gaining feedback of own performance and development needs from others

Test yourself

1. The four resources for financial effectiveness are human, stock, tools and equipment and time. Write a statement on what each resource encompasses.

2. How can you ensure positive communication?

3. Why is training important?

4. What two pieces of legislation concerning salon equipment must salons adhere to?

5. Identify two methods of good time management.

6. What does SMART stand for in relation to target setting?

7. What are productivity targets?

8. What are development targets?

9. What opportunities are there to meet targets?

10. Why should you have regular PDRs?

Essential knowledge

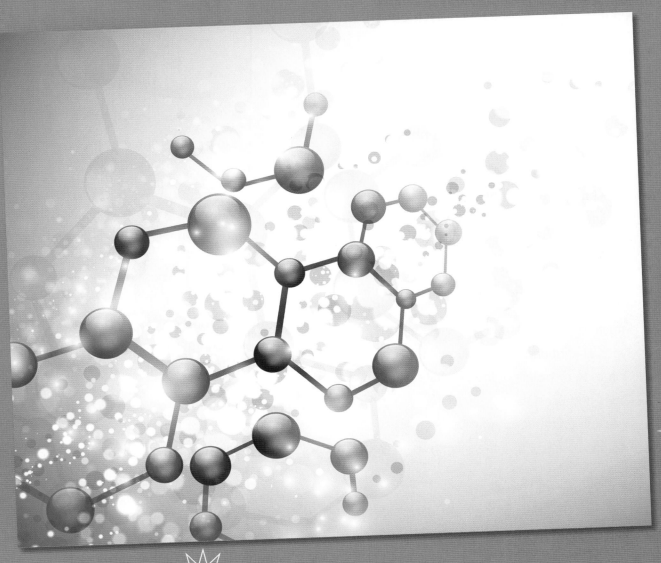

Chapter 4

RELATED ANATOMY AND PHYSIOLOGY

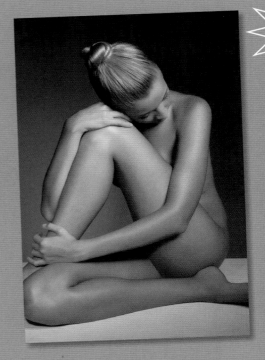

LEARNING OBJECTIVES

In this chapter you will learn about the anatomical systems of the body and how they function and interact with each other to maintain life.

Knowledge of anatomy and physiology is essential in order to understand how beauty therapy treatments affect the body and its tissues. Such knowledge also gives insight into how treatments work and how to perform them safely. The relevant anatomy and physiology knowledge required is shown below.

- Cells and tissues
- Skin structure and function
- Nail structure and nail growth
- Structure of hair and its follicle
- Hair growth cycle and patterns
- Diseases and disorders affecting the skin, nail and hair
- Structure and function of the skeleton
- Types of joint and their position and function
- Common disorders of the skeletal system
- Types of muscle tissue
- Structure and function of muscles
- Position and action of the main muscle groups of the body
- Muscle tone and muscle fatigue
- Common disorders of the muscular system
- Structure and function of the central and autonomic nervous system
- Position and location of the motor points of the body
- Common disorders of the nervous system
- Structure and function of blood and blood vessels
- Location of blood vessels and blood circulation

- Structure and function of the heart
- Blood pressure, pulse and erythema
- Common disorders of the blood circulatory system
- Structure and function of the lymphatic system
- Interaction between the blood and lymph circulatory systems
- Lymph circulation and position of the lymph nodes
- Common disorders of the lymphatic system
- Structure and function of the endocrine system
- Action of key hormones and their circulation in the blood stream
- Common disorders of the endocrine system
- Effects of malfunction of the endocrine system on hair growth
- Structure and function of the respiratory system
- Structure and function of the digestive system
- Common disorders of the digestive system
- Structure and function of the excretory/urinary system
- Common disorders of the urinary system
- Structure and function of the olfactory system
- Position and function of the sinuses
- Structure and function of the eye
- Structure of the male and female genitalia

This table shows the links between the relevant anatomy and physiology and NVQ, VRQ City & Guilds and VRQ VTCT technical units

NVQ units	Cells and tissue	Skin structure and function	Hair and its growth cycle	Nail structure	Skeletal system	Muscular system	Nervous system	Blood circulatory system	Lymph and its circulation	Endocrine system	Respiratory system	Digestive system	Excretory/urinary system	The eye	Olfactory system	Male and female genitalia
B13 Body electrical		✓			✓	✓	✓	✓	✓	✓		✓				
B14 Facial electrical		✓			✓	✓	✓	✓	✓	✓		✓				
B20 Body massage	✓	✓			✓	✓	✓	✓	✓	✓	✓	✓	✓			
B23 Indian head massage		✓			✓	✓	✓	✓	✓	✓	✓				✓	
B24 Pre-blended aroma	✓	✓			✓	✓	✓	✓	✓	✓	✓	✓	✓		✓	
B28 Stone massage	✓	✓				✓	✓	✓	✓	✓	✓	✓	✓			
B29 Epilation		✓	✓					✓	✓	✓						
N6-8 Nail Technology		✓		✓												
C&G VRQ																
305 Body massage		✓			✓	✓	✓	✓	✓	✓		✓	✓			
306 Facial electrotherapy		✓			✓	✓	✓	✓	✓	✓						
307 Body electrotherapy		✓			✓	✓	✓	✓	✓	✓		✓				
308 Epilation		✓	✓				✓	✓	✓							
309 Pre-blended aroma		✓			✓	✓	✓	✓	✓	✓		✓	✓			
311 Indian head massage		✓	✓		✓			✓	✓							
314 Nail enhancements		✓		✓												
321 Microdermabrasion		✓						✓								
322 Stone therapy massage	✓	✓			✓	✓			✓							

NVQ units	Cells and tissue	Skin structure and function	Hair and its growth cycle	Nail structure	Skeletal system	Muscular system	Nervous system	Blood circulatory system	Lymph and its circulation	Endocrine system	Respiratory system	Digestive system	Excretory/ urinary system	The eye	Olfactory system	Male and female genitalia
VTCT VRQ																
UV30403 Facial electrical		✓							✓							
UV30404 Body electrical		✓			✓	✓	✓	✓	✓	✓		✓				
UV30405 Nail enhancements		✓		✓												
UV30424 Body Massage		✓			✓	✓	✓	✓	✓	✓		✓	✓			
UV30425 Pre-blended aroma		✓			✓	✓	✓	✓	✓	✓		✓	✓			
UV30430 Micro-dermabrasion		✓														
UV30474 Epilation		✓			✓			✓	✓	✓						
UV30475 Stone massage					✓	✓		✓	✓							
UV30574 Indian head massage		✓	✓		✓	✓		✓	✓							
Online units																
B15 Lash extensions			✓											✓		
B21 UV tanning		✓														
B25 Self tanning		✓														
B26 Female Intimate waxing		✓	✓													✓
B27 Male intimate waxing		✓	✓													✓
312 UV tanning		✓														
313 Self-tanning		✓														

Online units	Cells and tissue	Skin structure and function	Hair and its growth cycle	Nail structure	Skeletal system	Muscular system	Nervous system	Blood circulatory system	Lymph and its circulation	Endocrine system	Respiratory system	Digestive system	Excretory/ urinary system	The eye	Olfactory system	Male and female genitalia
317 Individual permanent lashes			✓													
318 Intimate male waxing		✓	✓													✓
319 Intimate female waxing		✓	✓													✓
UV30426 permanent lashes			✓													
UV30427 Male intimate waxing		✓	✓													✓
UV30428 Female intimate waxing		✓	✓													✓
UV30450 UV tanning		✓														
UV30451 Self-tanning		✓														

Note: This table only references those units that appear in this publication and online; it does not reference all the units across the suite of the Level 3 qualification.

Introduction

It could be argued that humans are the most successful species on this planet. They have conquered the world in which they live, utilising their environment and the riches the Earth offers and mastering other species to become the dominant animal. But what makes humans so successful?

The human body can be explained more simply by organising its structures into distinct systems which work together in a complex way. This chapter will unravel some of these complexities by exploring the systems of the human body – the main structures within each system and their function, giving examples of common disorders that affect each system and insight into how each works together to form the phenomenon that is the human body.

Cells and tissues

Cells form the building blocks of each system of the human body; that is to say, a cell is the simplest form of life. Cells vary in shape and function but when a group of similar cells clump together, they form a tissue and the tissue itself will take on a specific function. It is as if by grouping together each cell can become more effective in its function.

Different **tissues** with different functions are arranged together to form an organ: a structure that may perform several functions, depending on the types of tissue it is made up of. **Organs** are arranged to form body systems that assist in the working of the body. The figure below explains this arrangement.

> **Key terms**
>
> **Cell** – simplest unit of life that performs a function that assists the maintenance of life.
>
> **Tissue** – a collection of the same type of cells to perform a function.
>
> **Organ** – arrangement of different tissues to perform several or complex functions.

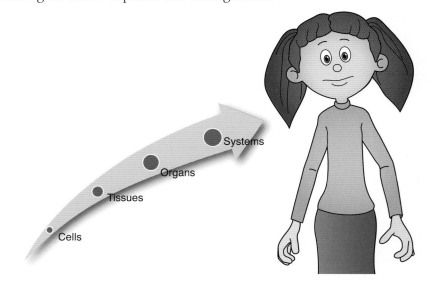

Systems

Organs

Tissues

Cells

△ The arrangements of the units of life

All the cells of the body come from the egg and sperm that join together at conception. At the beginning of life all cells look the same and it is not until later in their development that they take on a particular appearance and function, which is determined by the genetic information contained within them.

A typical cell and the tiny structures contained within it is shown below, but we will see later that cells vary in shape and function from this diagrammatic form and it is these variations that enable cells to perform the different functions that maintain the human body.

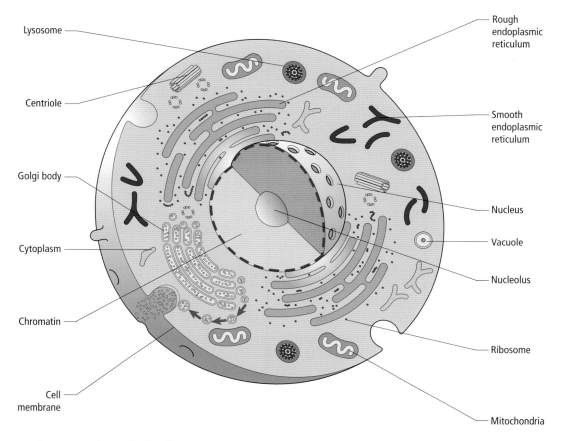

△ Structure of a typical cell

Cell structure and organelles

As you can see from the figure above, the cell contains numerous organelles – little organs – each with a specific function that maintains the life of the cell.

Cell membrane

The cell membrane surrounds the cytoplasm and encloses the cell organelles, giving the cell its shape. The structure of the membrane allows substances to pass in and out of the cell. There are two layers of phospholipids within the membrane consisting of a **hydrophilic** (water-loving) head and a **hydrophobic** (water-repelling) tail, which are arranged so that the tails lie together towards the centre with the

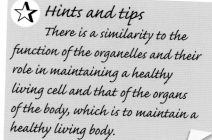

☆ *Hints and tips*
There is a similarity to the function of the organelles and their role in maintaining a healthy living cell and that of the organs of the body, which is to maintain a healthy living body.

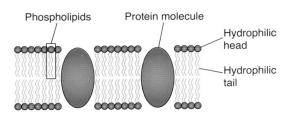

Phospholipids   Protein molecule

Hydrophilic head

Hydrophilic tail

△ Structure of the cell membrane

heads towards the outside. This arrangement facilitates osmosis – the name given to the action of substances crossing the membrane in and out of the cell. Dispersing these phospholipids occasionally are large protein molecules whose functions include acting as a receptor for hormones and other chemical messages, as well as being involved in the effects of the autoimmune system and the transport of substances across the membrane.

Cytoplasm

Cytoplasm is a gel-like substance that is composed of 80 per cent water and contains the cell organelles. The cytoplasm facilitates the storage of nutrients and is where osmosis takes place.

Endoplasmic reticulum (ER) is a series of canals within the cytoplasm, of which there are two types: rough and smooth. Smooth ER produces lipids (fats) and steroid hormones (protein). Rough endoplasmic reticulum is covered with ribosomes and is where the proteins such as enzymes and hormones that are exuded from the cell to be utilised by other cells are made.

Mitochondria are sausage-shaped structures responsible for the metabolism of adenosine triphosphate (ATP) which is used in cellular respiration and energy production by the cell and the tissues to bring about their function. The energy is also used by other organelles to perform their function.

Ribosomes are found in small groups within the cytoplasm or on the surface of rough endoplasmic reticulum. They are responsible for the making of proteins from amino acids using ribonucleic acid (RNA) as a 'template'. The proteins that are made are used within the cell.

The Golgi body or apparatus is involved in the storage of proteins made by the rough ER in readiness to be exuded by the cell. The structure appears as flattened, folded 'sacs' and is only present in cells that make and export proteins. The Golgi apparatus 'packages' the proteins into secretory granules.

Secretory granules or vacuoles are used to store, transport or digest proteins made by the cell until needed or until they are moved to the cell membrane.

Lysosomes are oval-shaped bodies formed by the Golgi apparatus that act as a kind of 'waste disposal system'. They contain enzymes which break down large molecules such as RNA and DNA into smaller ones, which are excreted as waste products through the cell membrane.

Nucleus

The nucleus contains the cell's genetic material in the form of a double chain of DNA (deoxyribonucleic acid) called chromosomes. The sub-units of chromosomes are called genes and are responsible for the generation of proteins that are appropriate for the specific function of the cell. The nucleus consists of an outer wall called the nuclear membrane and contains the DNA and the nucleolus, a dense spherical structure containing ribonucleic acid (RNA), which is used in the making of proteins within the cell.

⭐ *Hints and tips*

Striped muscle cells have a large number of mitochondria. As these organelles are responsible for the utilisation of energy within the cell, striped muscles need a lot of energy readily available for their function, which is contraction to bring about movement.

The nuclear membrane encases the nucleus and separates the nucleus from the cytoplasm. This membrane has small pores, which allow substances to pass from the cytoplasm into the nucleus.

Table 4.1 below shows the characteristics of a cell.

▽ Table 4.1 Characteristics of a cell

Activity	the ability to move to find food
Respiration	the ability to use oxygen
Digestion and absorption	the ability to break down food and prepare it for absorption
Excretion	the ability to rid itself of waste products
Growth and repair	the ability to build up protein from food taken in, to mature during cell division and repair itself if damaged
Irritability	the ability to respond to an outside stimulus and to changes in its environment
Reproduction	the ability to replicate itself to form another identical cell

Cell division

There are two types of cell division: meiosis and mitosis.

Meiosis is the process of cell division of the gametes or reproductive cells. In the female these cells are known as ovum (eggs) and they develop in the ovaries, while the male cells, the spermatozoa, develop in the testes. This type of cell division is specific to these cells only as it results in the 46 pairs of chromosomes being split so that only 23 pairs are found in each cell. As the reproductive cells come together at conception, each brings 23 pairs to the resulting cells to make the full quota of 46 – half from each of the mother and the father. The child inherits some characteristics from the mother and some from the father, such as eye or hair colour, height, facial features and of course, some diseases.

Mitosis is the process of cell division that occurs in all cells except the gametes. It varies from meiosis in that the chromosomes are duplicated before division so that each resulting cell ends up with 46 pairs of chromosomes. There are five phases to cell division:

1 prophase

2 metaphase

3 anaphase

4 telophase

5 interphase.

Prophase

Cell division begins in the nucleus when the genetic material has matured. The thread-like strands of chromosomes become visible and form into strands of chromatids with a central centromere. Outside of the nucleus the centrioles duplicate and separate to either pole of the cell and a spindle begins to form. Prophase ends with the breakdown of the nuclear membrane.

Metaphase

The chromosomes align themselves along the 'equator' of the cell as the nuclear membrane disappears completely. When aligned, the centromere of each chromosome begins to duplicate.

Anaphase

When replication is complete the centromere split apart as if attracted to a particular pole of the cell and particular centrioles separate the attached chromatids as they do so. The cell begins to constrict across the middle.

Telophase

The constriction completes as the nuclear membrane and nucleolus reform at either pole of the cell. The spindle degenerates and the chromatids become new chromosomes. Cell division is complete and there are two identical daughter cells.

Interphase

In this final stage of cell division, the daughter cells mature. The young chromosomes are thread-like and not very visible. As they mature the DNA is replicated and when mature the process may begin again.

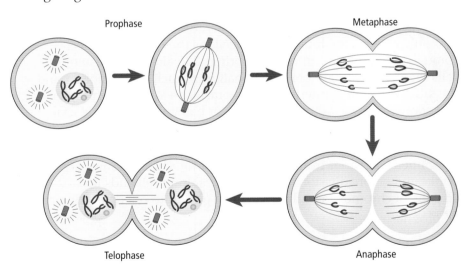

△ Phases of mitosis

Cell growth

Cell growth involves cell metabolism, respiration and reproduction. After reproduction the daughter cell must grow to the size of the parent cell. To do this it uses synthetic chemical reactions to make new structures from molecules present in the cytoplasm. This requires energy provided by cell respiration in the mitochondria.

Cell excretion

During respiration waste products are produced, namely water, carbon dioxide and lactic acid. Water passes through the cell membrane and into the blood where it is taken to the kidneys. If there is excess water, the kidneys will remove the water from the blood and store it in the bladder ready for excretion. Carbon dioxide is passed through the cell membrane into the blood, where it is taken to the lungs and exhaled. Lactic acid is reconverted into sugar when oxygen transported in the blood becomes available to the cell.

Movement in and out of cells

The processes by which substances pass in and out of cells are as follows.

- **Diffusion**: the movement of substances from a region of high concentration to one of a lower concentration, for example oxygen across the cell membrane.

Diffusion

The cell
membrane

| High concentration | Low concentration | | Equal concentration |

△ Process of diffusion

> **Key terms**
>
> **Osmosis** – movement of substances in solution from a low concentration to a higher concentration across a semi-permeable membrane.
>
> **Diffusion** – movement of substances from a region of high concentration to one of lower concentration.

- **Osmosis**: the movement of substances in solution (in water) from a low concentration to a higher concentration across a semi-permeable membrane, for example, sugar across the cell membrane.

Osmosis

The cell
membrane

| Area of low chemical concentration | Area of high chemical concentration | | Equal concentration |

△ Process of osmosis

- Active transport: the movement of substances from a low concentration to a high concentration.

- Phagocytosis and pinocytosis: where the cell engulfs the substance and absorbs it into itself. This action is specific to certain cells, for example white blood cells.

Tissues

The cells made during mitosis are identical and when clustered together form tissues that have the same characteristics laid down by the genetic information of the chromosomes in the nucleus. There are four main tissue types:

1 epithelial tissue

2 connective tissue

3 muscle tissue

4 nervous tissue.

Epithelial tissue

This type of tissue forms the linings of body cavities and tubes, glands and a covering for the body (skin). The function of epithelial tissue is determined by the specialised cells from which it is made and includes:

- protection: for example, it forms smooth surfaces so that organs can 'slide' over the body cavities, while specialised cells of the lining of the respiratory system protect the body from invasion by micro-organisms

- secretion: for example, the cells of the linings of sebaceous glands have special structures that secrete sebum

- absorption: for example, the lining of the small intestine allows the absorption of nutrients.

The cells are seated upon a basement membrane and sit very close together so tissue fluid between the cells is minimal. There are two classifications of epithelial tissue:

- simple: appears as a single layer of cells and shows different degrees of function

- compound: two or more layers of cells that give a high degree of protection.

Simple epithelial tissue

- Squamous (or pavement) epithelial: this arrangement of flat cells one-cell thick on a basement membrane gives the thinnest of linings and allows the exchange of gases, nutrients and waste products. It is found lining the blood and lymph vessels, the heart and alveoli (air sacs) in the lungs.

- Cuboidal epithelial: as the name suggests, the cells are cube-shaped on a basement membrane, giving a slightly thicker lining. It is found in glands and the small tubes of the kidneys. The resulting lining allows the absorption of water and the secretion of small molecules in solution such as sweat.

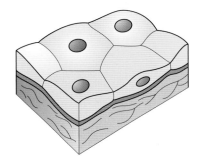

△ Squamous epithelium

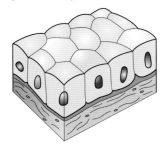

△ Cuboidal epithelium

- Columnar epithelial: the taller cells in columnar epithelial tissue provide some protection but its main function is to absorb the nutrients from food in the digestive system with minimal absorption of unwanted molecules. Specialised goblet columnar cells produce a sticky substance called mucous which aids the digestion process.

- Ciliated epithelial: these columnar cells have hair-like structures called cilia along the free border of the cell. These cells line tubes within the body and the cilia move in a wave-like motion to propel the contents of the tube in one direction along it. This lining epithelial is found in the tubes of the respiratory system, where it removes dust and particles in the air from the lungs and in the uterine tubes, where it moves the released egg into the womb.

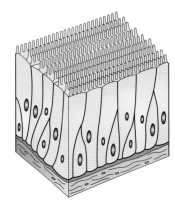

△ Columnar epithelium

Compound epithelial tissue

The main function of compound epithelial tissue is to offer protection for underlying structures and there are two types: stratified (of which there are keratinised and non-keratinised types) and transitional.

- Stratified epithelial: non-keratinised stratified epithelium is found on surfaces that must be kept wet and are prone to wear and tear, such as the conjunctiva of the eye, the lining of the mouth and the oesophagus. Keratinised stratified epithelium is found on dry surfaces (such as the skin, hair and nails) that are also prone to wear and tear.

- Transitional epithelial: this type of tissue allows for stretching of the organ and consists of 'pear-shaped' cells that allow for this unique function. It is found lining the inner surfaces of such organs as the bladder, which fills with urine and so needs to stretch as it does so, rather like a balloon filling with water.

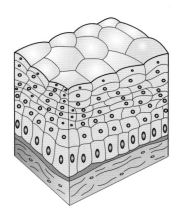

△ Ciliated epithelium

Membranes

Membranes are specialised linings and appear as a very thin, pliable sheath of tissue covering organs and lining cavities. There are three types of membrane:

1. Mucous membranes that cover openings of the body exposed to the external environment, such as those of the respiratory and digestive systems. They offer protection by the secretion of a slippery and sticky substance called mucous.

2. Serous membranes line cavities or cover organs of the body not exposed to the external environment such as the heart, and organs within the abdomen such as the liver. They produce a watery fluid called serous fluid that lubricates the surface to allow the organs to slip over each other without friction.

3. Synovial membranes are found within the cavities of synovial joints only and secrete synovial fluid that acts as a lubricant to protect the surfaces of the bones and prevent them wearing away through constant friction.

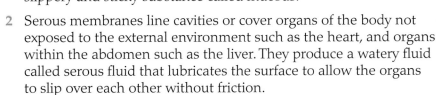

△ Stratified epithelium

Connective tissue

Connective tissue is plentiful and is found in all organs of the human body. Its functions are:

- protection
- transport
- insulation
- binding
- support.

To enable this sort of variety of function, the tissue must also be varied in structure, but characteristically the cells are not as closely packed together as in epithelial tissue. Instead, there is more tissue fluid, or matrix, between the cells. The matrix can be jelly-like in consistency or more solid and dense, depending on the quantity of protein fibres (collagen and elastin) contained within it. There is also the presence of specialised cells for a particular function depending on the type of connective tissue and its role in the body. These specialised cells include the following:

- Fibroblasts: these produce the fibres collagen and elastin.
- Macrophages: specialised cells that engulf cell debris, bacteria and other foreign particles.
- Plasma cells: these produce specific antibodies and release them into the blood stream as a response to exposure to micro-organisms.
- Mast cells: specialised cells that contain heparin, serotonin and histamine which are released when the cells are damaged by disease or injury.
- Fat cells: these group together and vary in shape and size depending on the amount of fat they contain. Adipose tissue has many fat cells and its chief function is insulation.

Areolar connective tissue

This is the most common and useful type of tissue found in the human body and is also known as 'loose connective tissue'. Its structure varies depending on its use but within the jelly-like matrix there can be numerous collagen and elastin fibres which give strength and resilience; these are produced by numerous fibroblasts also present in the matrix. Areolar connective tissue is found almost everywhere in the body, providing support and protection for the organs.

Adipose tissue

Adipose tissue consists of numerous, closely packed fat cells within a matrix of areolar tissue. There are two types: white and brown. White adipose tissue is found under the skin and between muscle fibres and can contribute up to 25 per cent of a normal weight adult. Brown adipose tissue is found in the upper back and in the walls of large

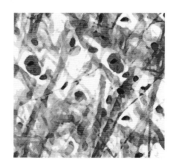

△ Areolar connective tissue

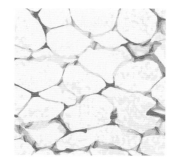

△ Adipose tissue

blood vessels and is involved with the maintenance of body temperature and controlling obesity. When it is metabolised it produces less energy but more heat. The functions of adipose tissue include insulation, protection and as an energy store.

Fibrous connective tissue

There are two types of fibrous tissue: white fibrous tissue and yellow elastic tissue. Both types have considerably more collagen and elastin fibres than areolar tissue with little matrix or other specialised cells except fibroblasts that manufacture the fibres. White fibrous tissue contains of mainly collagen, which provides strength but little elasticity and is found in tendons and ligaments, as a membrane surrounding bones and muscles and as a protective layer of organs such as the kidneys.

Yellow elastic tissue consists of mainly elastin fibres with only a little collagen, which provides a greater ability to stretch and recoil. It is found where the properties of elasticity yet strength are needed, such as in the walls of arteries and within the respiratory system, for example lung tissue.

Cartilage

Cartilage is a specialised form of connective tissue that is firmer and more resilient. This type of connective tissue contains special cells called chondrocytes and these form three types of cartilage, all of which have supportive and protective functions within the body:

1. Hyaline cartilage or smooth cartilage contains small groups of chondrocytes within a smooth and solid matrix. Hyaline is found on the surfaces of bones at the joints in the chest, where it joins the ribs to the sternum and allows movement of the chest. It also enables parts of the respiratory system to remain open when breathing, such as the trachea and bronchi.

2. White fibrocartilage is a tough but slightly flexible tissue with dense white fibres in a solid smooth matrix. It forms the pads of intervertebral discs in the spine, between the surfaces of the knee and hip joints and ligaments that join bones together at joints.

3. Yellow elastic fibrocartilage contains elastin fibres in a solid matrix with the cells lying between the fibres. It forms firm but flexible structures of the body, such as the pinnae of the ears and the epiglottis.

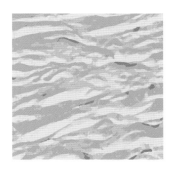

△ White fibrous tissue

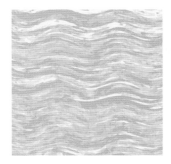

△ Yellow elastic tissue

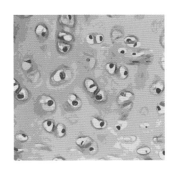

△ Hyaline cartilage

Note: the colours in these pictures are created by dyes used in the photography process to show the structure and are not representative of the colour of the tissue.

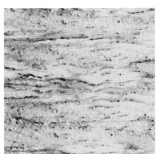

△ White fibrocartilage

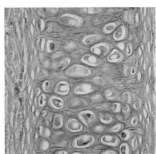

△ Yellow elastic fibrocartilage

Other connective tissues

Bone is a hardened connective tissue that begins as cartilage and has been specialised by the impregnation of the collagen fibres with the mineral calcium by cells called osteoblasts. Its main function is to support body weight and protect delicate organs.

Blood and lymph are more specialised types of connective tissue. At first, they may not appear to be a connective tissue but when considered carefully it can be seen that there is a matrix (fluid), specialised cells (red or white blood cells) and fibroblasts. Due to the different appearance of blood and lymph they cannot provide the same sort of function as other connective tissue but are unique in the function they perform in the body.

The structure and function of these types of tissue and also muscle and nervous tissue will be considered in detail later in this chapter.

We now consider the three similar structures that make up the integumentary system: the skin, nails and hair. Although these structures are distinct in appearance, they perform similar functions.

The skin

The skin forms a hard-wearing outer covering for the whole body. The skin provides a good example of the material on cells and tissues covered so far, because it demonstrates the classification of tissue types and the utilisation of specialised cells to bring about a variety of important functions.

Yet the skin has become important in other ways to humans. To many, it performs a cosmetic and adornment function and provides a means of communication between humans. Blushing and fear are examples of just two emotions that can be portrayed through the skin. It can be an indication of health and diet, age and race, even occupation. Skin is painted, tattooed, pierced and preened to attract the attention of others; it is the human equivalent of a male peacock's tail feathers.

The skin consists of three distinct tissues: keratinised stratified epithelium, areolar connective tissue and adipose tissue. These are arranged into three layers:

- epidermis
- dermis
- subcutaneous layer.

Epidermis

The epidermis is the outermost and visible layer of the skin. 'Epi' means 'a covering for' the 'true skin' (dermis). It is composed of keratinised stratified epithelium and when viewed under a microscope five distinct layers can be seen. Like all stratified epithelia, it begins life at the basement membrane where the cells appear as columnar cells. As the cells divide (mitosis) older ones get pushed towards the skin surface

Activity

In your own words, describe the journey of an epidermal epithelial cell from its beginning to desquamation, making sure you use the correct terminology.

and as they journey upwards they transform and get impregnated with a protein called keratin. This causes the cells to harden, dry out and 'die'. Once at the surface the cells have changed from columnar cells to flat, dead scales which are sloughed off into the environment – a process called desquamation. It takes approximately 30 days for this process to happen, although the process slows as we age. Once a person has reached middle-age this process may have slowed to as long as 45 days, which can result in the skin appearing dull and lifeless as the blood supply is not as easily seen.

Formation of the epidermis

The stratum germinativum (basal layer) is the deepest layer, consisting of live cells that are columnar-shaped, each with a nucleus. These cells are moist and obtain nutrients and oxygen from the tissue fluid that seeps from the blood vessels in the dermis and surrounds them. These nutrients are used for mitosis, where each cell divides to form two identical cells. Star-shaped cells called melanocytes are present at this level and they produce melanin, a pigment which gives the skin its natural colour. When stimulated by exposure to ultra-violet light, the melanocytes produce more pigment to protect the deeper layers and structures within the dermis.

As new cells are formed at the stratum germinativum, old ones are pushed towards the surface, undergoing change as they do so. The cells appear to grow spines or 'prickles', giving rise to the stratum spinosum or prickle layer. It is here in the epidermis that melanin is placed into the cells from the melanocytes. In the lower levels there is still some mitosis taking place and in the upper levels, the keratinisation zone begins where the cells are impregnated with a protein called keratin.

Present at the stratum spinosum level of the epidermis are Langerhan cells – specialised cells that respond to the presence of antigens and help the white blood cells destroy invading micro-organisms, and so form part of the immune system.

As the cells enter the stratum granulosum or granular layer, keratinisation is completed and the cells 'die', losing their moisture and hardening. The nuclei and the cell wall break down as they work upwards towards the surface.

The absence of nuclei and cell walls in the stratum lucidum causes it to appear clear when viewed under a microscope. An enzyme has destroyed the melanin and the keratin has dried the cells, causing them to flatten and giving a transparent appearance. There is also a thick, mucus-like substance present at this area of the epidermis called the Rheims barrier, which forms as the cells of the stratum granulosum expel water and mix with the fatty acids present in the skin. This barrier prevents water, products and micro-organisms penetrating the epidermis into the dermis.

★ **Hints and tips**

The epidermis varies in thickness on different parts of the body and its main function is one of protection. It is often thickest where there is significant wear and tear, such as on the soles of the feet and palms of the hands, and is thinnest on the eyelids and lips.

★ **Hints and tips**

The pigment melanin absorbs ultra-violet light and in doing so darkens and produces a chemical called 7-dehydrocholesterol, a precursor to Vitamin D. The absorption of this light ensures that the collagen and elastin fibres in the dermis are maintained intact, preventing a loss of elasticity and the onset of premature ageing. The darker the skin naturally, the more protection from UV light is provided and the more likely the signs of ageing appearing later in life.

Key terms

Germinative zone – this layer consists of the stratum germinativum and the stratum spinosum.

Keratinisation – the process by which cells are impregnated with keratin, lose their moisture and nucleus and then die.

Keratinisation zone – refers to the upper layers of the stratum spinosum and the stratum granulosum together.

Eventually the cells appear as dry, flat, keratinised flakes of the **stratum corneum** or horny layer. These hardened cells are shed from the surface by natural rubbing from, for example, clothing and by special skin products containing granules that slough off the dead skin. This process is called desquamation.

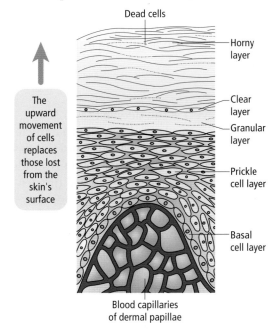

The upward movement of cells replaces those lost from the skin's surface

- Dead cells
- Horny layer
- Clear layer
- Granular layer
- Prickle cell layer
- Basal cell layer
- Blood capillaries of dermal papillae

△ Layers of the epidermis

The dermis or 'true skin'

The dermis is the deeper layer of the skin found directly underneath the epidermis and is also known as the 'true skin' because it contains the structures associated with the skin which perform many of the skin's functions. It is formed from areolar tissue, gives the skin its physical strength and accounts for more than 90 per cent of the skin mass. The fibres, namely collagen and elastin, provide support, strength, elasticity and have moisture retaining properties.

Collagen fibres give the skin its strength, resilience, plumpness and youthful appearance, while elastin fibres give the skin elasticity, enabling it to stretch to accommodate an increase in fat cell distribution in the form of weight gain and/or pregnancy.

The cells of the dermis that connect with the hypodermis underneath form connective tissue made up of two distinct layers:

1 the more superficial papillary layer

2 the deeper reticular layer.

Papillary layer

The papillary layer is the upper most part of the dermis and is in direct contact with the epidermis. It provides vital nourishment to the living layers of the dermis and has irregular protrusions into the epidermis called dermal papillae. These papillae pull the epidermis down towards the dermis and create ridges, which are what give us our unique finger prints. The papillary layer provides the structures within the reticular layer with nutrients and oxygen from its rich blood supply and supports the epidermis above.

The dermal papillae contain nerve endings which allow the skin to be sensitive to extreme temperatures, pain, pressure, irritation and touch. There is also a network of blood and lymphatic capillaries, which enable cellular respiration and metabolism in the strata germinativum and spinosum in the epidermis. The blood vessels can constrict or expand to control the amount of blood that flows through the skin and dictate whether body heat is dispelled when the body is hot or conserved when it is cold; this helps to control body temperature. The lymph capillaries present in the dermal papilla perform a cleansing function by mopping up any foreign bodies that might enter the skin through an opening and micro-organisms that may have invaded the tissues. They also remove waste products from the process of mitosis in the stratum germinativum.

Mast cells are also present at this level of the dermis, which burst when stimulated during inflammation or allergic reactions to release histamine. This allows more blood to flow to the area for assistance.

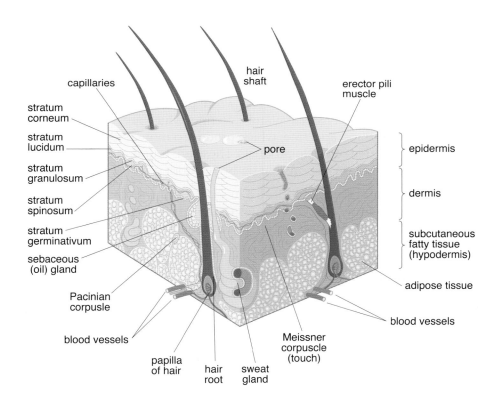

△ Structure of the skin

Reticular layer

Found under the papillary layer, the reticular layer has fewer cells and relatively fewer blood vessels than the papillary layer. It is formed of tough elastic and collagen fibres interwoven with reticular fibres, which provide support for the many structures held within this layer. It is this area which carries most of the physical stress of the skin. The cells present in the reticular layer of the dermis are:

- phagocytic cells: white blood cells that help to defend the body against infection by travelling through the dermis (which is a sterile environment) to destroy foreign matter or harmful micro-organisms

- fibroblast cells: responsible for forming new fibrous tissue. They manufacture collagen and elastin within the dermis.

The dermis also contains structures derived from it:

- Hair follicles: this organ will be discussed in more detail later in this chapter, but this appendage of the skin is responsible for controlling body temperature.

- Arrector pili muscle: attached to the hair follicle, this muscle contracts to pull the hair upright to capture a warming layer of air next to the skin.

- Sensory nerve endings: these alert the brain to outside influences such as changes in temperature, pressure and pain.

- Motor nerves: transmit nerve impulses to the glands and organs of the skin such as the sweat glands and arrector pili muscle.

- Sweat glands: secrete sweat – a fluid that consists mainly of water – to cool the body and excrete waste products such as urea. There are two types of sweat glands: eccrine, which are found all over the body, and apocrine, which produce a more milky fluid with a high degree of waste products. These are found in the groin and axillae and are responsible for body odour.

- Sebaceous glands: produce a lubricant and waterproof natural oil called sebum. This contributes to the flexibility and waterproofing of the skin and provides an acid mantle to fight against disease.

- Blood vessels: bring nutrients and oxygen to the other structures of the skin and remove the waste products produced.

- Lymph vessels: work with the blood vessels to remove waste products but also any foreign particle or micro-organisms. They form part of the body's defence mechanism, i.e. the immune system.

Subcutaneous layer

Under the dermis but overlying the muscular system is a layer of adipose tissue which is a continuation of the reticular layer and its network of collagen and elastin fibres in a gel-like matrix. The fibres are numerous fat cells or adipocytes whose function is to provide insulation, maintain body temperature, protect underlying tissues and organs and act as an energy store.

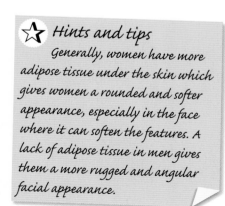

☆ *Hints and tips*
Generally, women have more adipose tissue under the skin which gives women a rounded and softer appearance, especially in the face where it can soften the features. A lack of adipose tissue in men gives them a more rugged and angular facial appearance.

Functions of the skin

The functions of the skin are described below.

Heat regulation

The skin regulates body temperature in a number of ways:

- The blood vessels dilate and constrict to increase or restrict the flow of blood near to the surface of the skin.

- Adipose tissue acts as an insulator, preventing heat loss.

- Sweat glands produce sweat that evaporates from the skin surface, cooling the body as it does so.

- The arrector pili muscle contracts to trap a layer of air near to the skin surface which is heated by the body and prevents further body heat loss.

- The nerve endings in the skin register a drop in temperature which, if severe enough, will instigate the rapid contraction of the body muscles to cause shivering.

Protection

- The epidermis acts as a protective barrier against invasion by micro-organisms. It also thickens in areas of wear and tear to form calluses.

- The skin has a natural acid mantle, which is formed by the mixing of sweat from the sweat glands and sebum from the sebaceous glands on the skin's surface. This protects the skin from invasion by micro-organisms.

- Melanin produced by melanocytes in the epidermis absorbs ultra-violet light, producing a natural tan and protecting the 'true skin' from damage.

- The nerve endings preserve the skin from harm by informing the body of danger, such as burning from a hot surface.

Sensation

- The nerve endings in the skin warn us of pain, cold, heat, pressure and touch and prevent trauma to the skin.

Secretion

- The sebaceous glands produce sebum, which forms part of the acid mantle and a waterproof covering at the skin's surface.

- The sweat glands produce sweat to cool the body as described above.

Absorption

- Although the skin is designed to prevent penetration of substances, some substances such as light, essential oils and some drugs (e.g. nicotine through patches adhered to the skin) are absorbed through the skin.

Excretion

- The sweat glands excrete waste salts and water. The skin is the largest excretory organ of the human body.

Vitamin D Production

- Vitamin D is essential for the health of the body and most is produced by the body rather than being absorbed from our food. The production of Vitamin D is a by-product of the darkening of melanin in the epidermis when exposed to ultra-violet light.

Repair of the skin

Primary healing of the skin follows minor damage when the edges of the wound are close together. When the skin is damaged the area becomes inflamed and blood thickens to block the open wound. The fibres within the blood interweave and blood cells block the wound to form a clot, which then becomes a scab.

Specialised cells within the blood called phagocytes and fibroblasts arrive at the site where the former begin to remove the cell debris (scab) and the fibroblasts begin to produce collagen fibres to bind the broken surfaces together.

The epithelial cells of the epidermis begin to repair the epidermis from the basement layer and upwards to the skin surface. The scab begins to separate from the wound and as this process continues eventually falls off. Meanwhile, the collagen fibres bind the wound more strongly underneath to restore the skin's resilience.

Secondary healing follows the destruction of more substantial tissue, where the edges are a distance from each other and the wound is deep, for example the case of an ulcer.

The area becomes highly inflamed and an area of necrotic (dead) material develops central to the site in the dermis due to the action of phagocytes. New blood capillaries and fibroblasts develop at the base of the site and begin to grow up toward the skin's surface with infection being prevented by the phagocytes. Once at the level of the epidermis, the epithelial cells replicate and grow towards the centre of the wound, before gravitating to the surface until the full thickness and resilience of the skin is restored.

Skin diseases and disorders

The following infectious skin diseases and disorders are described only to enable the therapist to recognise their appearance and to enable her to decide whether any proposed treatment should go ahead, having given due consideration to the safety of the client and others. They are not described in order to enable the therapist to make a diagnosis. A doctor is responsible for accurate diagnosis and he or she will rely on the assistance of a laboratory to confirm the presence of the offending micro-organism.

Knowledge of non-infectious conditions are again to confirm the safety of the client during the treatment but the therapist may, in some cases, be able to suggest treatment that might improve a particular condition or decide upon adaptations of the treatment.

Bacterial infections

Disease/disorder	Cause	Description
Impetigo	Impetigo is caused by two types of bacteria: ● *staphylococcus aureus* ● *streptococcus pyogenes*	Bacteria invade healthy skin through a cut, scratch or insect bite. Appears as fluid filled blisters that rupture and form a yellow crust and may be itchy. Highly contagious and care should be taken not to touch the area. Do not perform treatments if the disease is present. Advise client to see a doctor and return for treatment when the condition has gone.
Furuncle (boil)	Caused by the bacteria *staphylococcus aureus*	Bacteria enter an open hair follicle and/or pore and invade the tissue, causing symptoms of pain, erythema, swelling and formation of pus. Can appear anywhere on the body but are common on the face, neck, axillae, buttocks and thigh, where there can be abrasion by clothing. Do not perform if present in the area being treated. Any fluid or pus from the sore is infectious and should be avoided. Advise client to see a doctor and return for treatment when infection has gone.
Carbuncle	As above	Carbuncles occur when a group of follicles or pores are infected by the bacteria in the same area of the body.
Folliculitis	*Staphylococci* bacteria	Bacteria enter the hair follicle through unhygienic depilatory treatments such as waxing and shaving. Appears as a red rash with small papules and pustules. Common in the beard area of men and underarm or bikini line. Do not treat the area affected and advise the client to see a doctor and to return for treatment when infection has gone.

Viral infections

Disease/disorder	Cause	Description
Herpes simplex	Caused by the herpes simplex virus type 1 (HSV-1)	Causes cold sores and found on and around the lips and nose. Virus is transmitted by direct contact and has periods of inactivity and activity. When triggered, the symptoms of itching or burning are followed by formation of fluid-filled blisters being apparent which burst to form a yellow crust and/or scab. Virus can lay dormant in the body before being stimulated into action again. Common triggers include exposure to sunlight, winds or when the body is run down, such as when infected by the cold virus. Do not perform treatments in areas where the disease is present as it is infectious. Advise the client to see a doctor and to return for treatments when gone.
Herpes zoster	Caused by the varicella zoster virus(VZV)	Same virus that causes chickenpox. Symptoms of the disease begin with pain and/or tingling along the pathway of a sensory nerve and then the breakout of fluid-filled blisters which weep to form crusts. Most common on the back or upper chest wall. Do not perform treatments and advise the client to seek medical advice.
Verrucae or warts	Caused by the human papilloma virus	There are different types of wart caused by this virus that generally are a painless, firm nodule of keratinised cells that is round or oval in shape. Plane warts are smoother with a flat surface and are more common in children; plantar warts or verrucae occur on the feet and can be painful due to the pressure of standing and walking. Common warts appear on the hands. Warts are contagious and the client should seek medical advice.

Fungal infections

Disease/disorder	Cause	Description
Tinea corporis (ringworm)	All fungal infections are caused by the same fungus, dermatophyte, that lives normally on the skin surface. However, given the right conditions of warmth and moisture, they reproduce, living off the dead keratinised cells of the epidermis, nail and hair. Pets can also suffer from the condition and can be responsible for the infection.	Ringworm of the body appears as a ring of red, rash-like pimples, slightly raised and clearer in the centre which may appear scaly. Very contagious through direct contact or through items such as towels. Do not perform treatments. Advise client to seek medical advice and to return when the condition has cleared.
Tinea capitis	Dermatophyte fungus	Ringworm of the scalp is similar in appearance to that of the body, with the addition of broken hairs that are stubbly. Do not perform treatments. Advise client to seek medical advice and to return when the condition has cleared.
Tinea pedis	Dermatophyte fungus	Ringworm of the foot, commonly called athlete's foot. The skin appears flaky, which turns moist and gives off a characteristic smell. Do not perform treatments. Advise client to seek medical advice and to return when the condition has cleared.

Infestations

Disease/disorder	Cause	Description
Scabies	A mite called *acarusscabiei*, commonly known as 'itch mite'	Female mite is responsible for symptoms of this contagious parasitic condition as it burrows into the epidermal layers of the skin to lay eggs. This burrowing leaves red 'tracks' that are extremely itchy and later crusted lesions develop. Common sites are in folds of skin such as between the fingers and toes, the axillary and under the breast, but can appear anywhere. Do not perform treatments. Advise client to seek medical advice and to return when the condition has cleared.

Sebaceous gland disorders

Disease/disorder	Cause	Description
Milia	Activity of the sebaceous gland combined with a fine skin texture	Sebum trapped underneath a layer of epidermal cells gives rise to white or slightly yellow pearl nodules. Found in fine-textured skin, so common around the eye and upper cheek. The epidermis can be broken with a sterile lance and the milia extracted.
Comedones	Hyperactivity of the sebaceous gland	Sebum trapped in an open pore or neck of a follicle, oxidising in the air to give the characteristic black appearance. Comedones should be softened with heat and/or oil before extraction.
Seborrhoea	Hyperactivity of the sebaceous gland due to hormonal influences	Excessive production of sebum gives rise to an excessively shiny, oily skin and scalp. Often leads to the development of acne vulgaris.
Sebaceous cysts	Known as steatocystomas, the neck of the sebaceous glands become blocked with epidermal cells and the sebum builds up within the sebaceous gland	Appear as soft or hard mobile swellings under the skin or scalp, which can be painful depending where they are located. Common on the scalp, ears, back, face and chest where there are numerous sebaceous glands. If they cause the client problems they should be surgically removed by a medical practitioner.
Acne vulgaris	Hyperactivity of the sebaceous gland as a result of hormonal influences	There are the presence of blocked pores, comedones, papules and pustules. Commonly found on the face, back and chest where sebaceous glands are numerous. Severe acne requires medical intervention and the client should be advised to see their doctor.

Sudoriferous gland disorders

Disease/disorder	Cause	Description
Bromidrosis	Activity of the apocrine glands and the action of the bacteria on the skin breaking down the waste products contained within the sweat	Commonly known as body odour. Although there is no risk of cross infection, the salon may wish to refuse treatment on grounds of hygiene and maintenance of reputation.
Anhidrosis	Hypoactivity of the sweat glands caused by dehydration or damage to the sweat glands such as full tissue thickness burns	There is a lack of sweat, particularly noticeabe during exertion. This condition can be life threatening as the body temperature can rise to harmful levels.
Hyperhydrosis	Hyperactivity of the eccrine and apocrine glands associated with nerves/stress	The glands over-produce sweat, resulting in visible beads of sweat appearing on the upper lip or clammy hands and/or sweaty feet. The client is safe to treat if they present with this condition. Botox injections have been found to lessen this condition if it is embarrassing for the client.
Miliariarubra (prickly heat)	Excessive sweating in hot weather	The sweat glands are blocked by occlusive products such as sun creams but also skin cells or other debris and the sweat accumulates under the skin. Gives rise to a red, itchy rash in the affected areas especially under clothing where increased sweating may occur.

Pigmentation disorders

Disease/disorder	Cause	Description
Ephilides	Hyperactivity of the melanocytes in the stratum germinativum	Commonly called freckles, activity of some of the melanocytes gives rise to uneven pigmentation patches which darken in sunlight.
Chloasma	Hyperactivity of the melanocytes through hormonal stimulation	At times when the female body is under hormonal control, such as during puberty, pregnancy, the menopause or when taking the oral contraceptive pill, the melanocytes produce excess melanin in uneven patches which appear darker than the surrounding skin. May appear anywhere on the body but more common on the cheek, forehead and around the eye. The pigment darkens with exposure to UV light but can be avoided by the use of sun protection factor creams.
Vitiligo	Hypoactivity of the melanocytes giving rise to areas lacking pigmentation	Appear as white patches of no pigmentation so more noticeable and stressful for clients with a darker skin colour. The client should avoid exposure to UV light and should use a sun block in the affected areas.

| Albinism | Inactive or absence of melanocytes; normally hereditary | A complete lack of pigment in the skin, hair and eyes which usually appear pink. Sun exposure is dangerous because of the high risk of skin cancer so total sun block should be used on all exposed areas of the body. Skin can be sensitised and so treatment durations and intensities should be considered. |
| Lentigo | Increased number of melanocytes in an area giving rise to pigmentation | Appears as flat, pigmented area with a defined outline that is unaffected by exposure to UV light. |

Vascular disorders

Disease/disorder	Cause	Description
Erythema	Dilation of the blood capillaries superficial to the skin surface	First degree erythema is a healthy reddening of the skin with no distinct outline that dissipates within an hour. It is desirable within a beauty treatment. Second degree erythema is undesirable and appears as a marked reddening of the skin that feels warm to the touch and remains for a couple of hours. Third degree erythema has a defined outline to the reddening and remains visible for days and is painful, e.g. sunburn. Fourth degree appears as third degree but with the addition of swelling.
Telangiecstasis (thread veins)	Persistent dilation of the blood capillaries caused by stimulation, either physical or by extremes in temperature	Blood capillaries are visible under the superficial layers of the epidermis. Commonly found around the nostrils, across the cheek area and areas of the body such as the thighs.
Rosacea	Skin sensitivity that progresses to a chronic inflammatory condition, exacerbated by alcohol, spicy foods or stress	Characterised by the butterfly-shaped flush across the cheeks and nose. Begins as a tendency to blush easily or sensitivity to temperature, touch or products. Develops into a continuous redness that may also develop pustules and resemble acne. As the condition persists, broken capillaries appear and in severe cases there is swelling and growth of the tissues resulting in extended facial features.
Vascular naevi	Vascular birthmark caused by the blood vessels being very close to the skin surface	Irregular-shaped areas of redness that maybe raised or flat. Appears before, during or after birth.
Port wine stain	Deep capillary naevus	Present at birth. Irregular-shaped birthmark that can vary from pale pink to purple in colour but is flat to the skin surface. Can appear anywhere on the body but may be distressing to the client if extensive on the face.

Skin disorders involving abnormal growth

Disease/disorder	Cause	Description
Psoriasis	An inherited non-infectious skin condition. Aggravated by stress and external factors such as products	Irregular-shaped red and scaly patches with a distinct outline. Commonly found on the knees and elbows but in extreme cases on the body, face and even the scalp and eyelids.
Seborrheic or senile warts	Cause is unknown but as the condition is common on sun-exposed areas such as the back, arms, face, and neck, ultraviolet light may play a role	Benign nodular growth that is darker than the surrounding skin. Often referred to as senile warts as common on exposed areas of skin in the elderly.
Skin tags	Overgrowth of the epidermis	Small, extended growths that protrude from the skin that can be flesh-coloured or pigmented from light brown to black. Harmless and can be removed by advanced epilation methods. An experienced therapist may become qualified to do so.
Keloid scarring	Overgrowth of scar tissue	Appears at the site of an injury as a smooth, shiny, raised, irregular-shaped scar. Black skins in particular are prone to keloid scarring.

Malignant tumours

Disease/disorder	Cause	Description
Squamous cell carcinoma	Exposure to sun and UV light, particularly fair skin	Skin cancer affecting the cells of the prickle cell layer (stratum spinosum) of the epidermis. Appears as a raised area of either very dry and scaly or ulcerated skin that has a 'cauliflower' appearance. The cancer can spread to other cells so advise the client to see their doctor immediately.
Basal cell carcinoma	Exposure to sun and UV light; particularly fair skin	Skin cancer affecting the cells of the basal layer (stratum germinativum) of the epidermis. Appears as a flesh-coloured or pink, flat or raised area of skin that often has blood capillaries visible within it. The client should be advised to see a doctor immediately.
Malignant melanoma	Over exposure to UV light particularly fair skin	Blue-black pigmented mole that has recently changed in shape, size or colour. Commonly found on areas of the body frequently exposed without adequate sun protection, such as the face, shoulders and arms. The client should be advised to see a doctor immediately.

Allergies

Disease/disorder	Cause	Description
Dermatitis	Caused by exposure to products such as metals, hair dye, plastics and resins, latex, washing powders, etc.	Mild allergic reaction to an allergen resulting in skin inflammation with a similar appearance to eczema.
Eczema	Internal factors predisposition a person to the condition. Factors that can worsen the condition include dairy products, stress and perfumed products.	There is erythema and itching at the initial stages and this develops into dry flaking, scaling and weeping and the formation of yellow crusts. Often there is a history of asthma and hay fever in the family.
Urticaria (hives)	Caused by external allergens such as nettles and heat or by intake of certain foods and drugs such as penicillin.	Allergic reaction of the skin that appears red and itchy with the formation of raised white or pink wheals that can disappear within moments.

The nail

The function of the nails is to protect the fingertips and toes. The nail also provides an indication of the body's general health. The nail is made of layers of dead cells containing a protein called keratin which is also found in skin and hair. The layers are held together by a substance called lamellae. The nail is divided into three main parts:

1 The free edge: the part that protrudes over the fingertip.

2 The nail plate: forms most of the visible portion of the nail.

3 The nail root: the part of the nail buried into the skin.

The upper part of the nail root forms the nail fold (also known as the mantle) and the lower part forms the matrix. This is part of the germinating layer (stratum germinativum) of the epidermis and is the region from which the nail grows. The matrix receives the nutrients and oxygen for growth from a network of blood vessels in the nail bed.

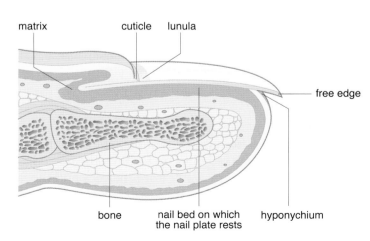

△ Cross-section through the end of the finger and nail

Nail structure

Part of nail	Description	Function
Free edge	The part of the nail plate that protrudes over the fingertip, likened to the claws of an animal	Protects the fingertips from physical harm; improves the nail's appearance when manicured
Hyponychium	A layer of epidermis found under the free edge	Prevents bacteria and dirt from getting under the nail plate and infecting the nail bed
Nail plate	The main part of the nail, made up of layers of dead keratinised cells	Protects the tips of the fingers and toes, which have a network of sensory nerve endings
Lunula	Also known as the half-moon, it is the visible portion of the matrix and appears pale due to a reduced blood supply	As the upper part of the matrix, it is part of the growing area for the nail and the nail bed
Cuticle	A layer of epidermis that overlaps the base of the nail plate	Prevents bacteria and dirt from entering the nail fold
Perionychium	The perimeter of the nail, encompassing the hyponychium and eponychium	Forms the outer border of the nail
Eponychium	Part of the cuticle at the base of the nail over the lunula, which moves forward with the nail plate as it grows	Protects the growing part of the nail
Matrix	Lies beneath the nail fold – an injury to the matrix can cause deformity in the nail plate or the plate can be shed completely from the nail bed	Contains a rich blood supply, which enables it to produce the nail plate and bed
Nail bed	The portion on which the nail plate rests. It has a plentiful blood supply when healthy, giving the nail its pink colour	The blood supply provides the food and oxygen to the matrix and the ridges anchor the nail plate to prevent lifting. Also has a nerve supply making the nail bed sensitive to pain and pressure
Nail wall	The folds of skin running up the sides of the nail plate	Forms the frame to the nail and provides protection from physical harm
Lateral nail fold	Located either side of the nail plate; the skin folds over to enclose the nail plate	Guides the nail to grow straight
Nail grooves	Found either side of the nail and are a vertical ridge in the nail plate	Together with the lateral nail fold, they encourage the nail to grow straight

Nail growth

The nail originates from the cells of the stratum germinativum within the nail fold and the matrix. As the cells divide they push old ones up towards the free edge. The cells keratinise, die and form the nail plate in layers held together by water from the cells and the fatty acids present, called lamellae. The nail bed is formed at the same time but the keratinisation process is not completed so the cells remain living until they reach the hyponychium where they dry out and die to form the protective strip under the free edge.

Normal nail growth for fingernails is 3–4 mm per month and a nail takes 3–6 months to replace itself completely. Toenails grow more slowly at 1–2 mm per month and take 12–18 months to replace themselves.

Healthy nails

Healthy nails appear firm but flexible, smooth and slightly pink in colour. The surrounding cuticle should be unbroken, flexible and should not be stuck to the nail plate.

A healthy nail will grow grow faster in the summer and in children and pregnant women. Children and pregnant women have higher levels of nutrients in the blood. Blood circulation is faster in summer due to the increase in temperature. Toenails grow more slowly than fingernails and are often thicker and harder. To produce healthy nails the vitamins A, B complex and D are needed together with the minerals calcium and iron.

Effects of nail care treatment

Nail treatments such as buffing and massage benefit nail growth by increasing the blood supply to the nail bed. In doing so, more nutrients and oxygen are available for the cells to grow and divide. This means that the nails will grow more quickly and stronger.

Effects of illness

Systemic illness affecting a system of the body can influence the rate of growth and appearance of the nails, as well as the skin and hair. Poor health or poor diet can cause the nails to be brittle with vertical or horizontal ridges in the nail plate or very soft, flexible, pale and discoloured or blue in colour and the cuticles to be dry, split and hardened.

Damage to the nail

Both physical and chemical agents can cause nail damage.

Physical damage

- Nail bed: a knock or blow that is hard enough to damage the nail bed will appear as a bruise under the nail. The blood vessels in the nail bed break, allowing blood to flow out under the nail plate. After a little time the blood vessels mend, leaving some under the nail plate. This dries, sticks to the underside and grows up with the nail plate until it reaches the free edge, where it can be removed.

- Matrix: damage to the matrix can result in temporary loss of the nail or permanent damage to the nail plate. When the matrix is damaged by a severe knock or blow, some of the cells die. This results in a temporary halt in the production of the nail plate and nail bed. This can appear as a ridge in the nail or, if a lot of the matrix is damaged, the loss of the nail plate.

  The dead cells need to be replaced and are made by the matrix itself. When fully healed, the matrix will begin to make the nail plate and nail bed again. If, however, the damage is severe enough, the matrix may not heal completely, leaving scar tissue. This will appear as a permanent condition in the nail such as a vertical ridge or split.

Chemical damage

Strong chemicals: continuous use of detergents or even nail polish remover will cause the nail and cuticle to dry out. The nail may appear brittle, discoloured (usually yellow), flaky and ridged. The cuticle will be dry, white in colour and inflexible.

Nail shapes

Nail shape can be categorised as:

- fan
- narrow
- square
- oval
- concave (also known as spoon or ski jump-shaped)
- convex (also known as hook- or claw-shaped)
- pointed.

(For pictures of different nail shapes, see the online chapter Nail technologies.)

Nail diseases and disorders

Disease/disorder	Cause	Description
Onychia 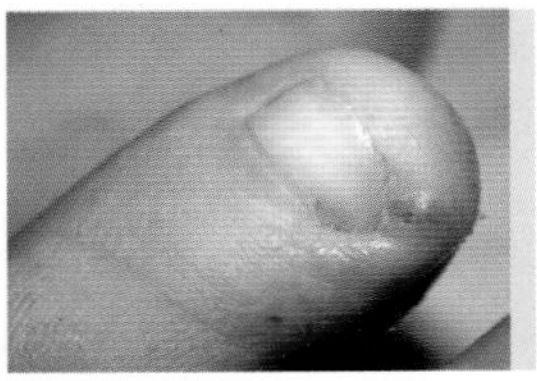	Bacterial infection of the nail tissues	Bacteria invade an open wound and cause the signs of infection of redness, pain, swelling and the formation of pus. Infectious so do not treat. Do not treat the area affected as it is infectious.
Paronychia 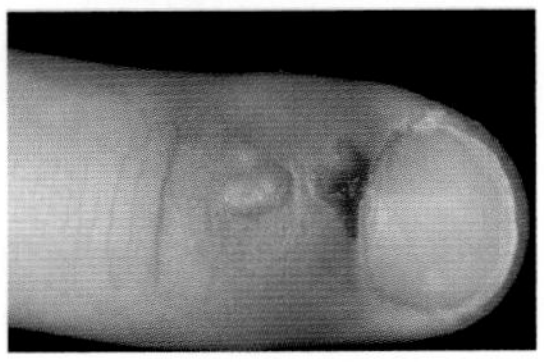	Bacterial infection of the nail wall	Commonly known as whitlow. The nail wall is invaded by bacteria after becoming open, for example from tearing a hangnail.
Tinea ungium 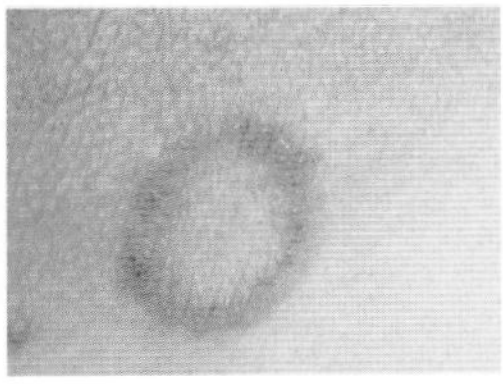	Fungal infection of the nail plate	White or yellow streaks in the nail that invade from the free-edge to the root. The upper layers of the nail become soft and peel to reveal the diseased nail underneath. Often occurs where there is also untreated athlete's foot. Infectious condition so treatment should be avoided.
Beau's lines	Prolonged ill health or damage to the matrix	Deep horizontal ridges in the nail plate.

Hang nails		Dry, split cuticle or skin found at the nail groove.
Koilonychia		Spoon-shaped nails.
Flaking	Dryness of the nail plate	Causes the layers that form the nail plate to separate.
Leuconychia	Minor damage to the nail plate	White spots that grow out as the nail grows.
Longitudinal furrows or corrugations	Can be hereditary; associated with old age but can be a sign of ill health or poor diet	Vertical ridges in the nail plate giving an uneven surface.
Onychophagy	Bitten nails	There is exposure of the hyponychium and/or the nails bed; usually the nail wall and cuticle is also bitten
Onycholysis	Injury, illness or disease such as tinea ungium or as a reaction to drugs	Separation of the nail plate from the nail bed.
Onychocryptosis	Cutting the nails too low at the sides combined with pressure such as that of shoes onto the sides of the nail	In-growing nail.
Pterygium	Hereditary or infrequent care of the nails	Over-growth of cuticle that precedes up the nail plate.
Onychauxis	Associated with disease of the nail, old age or infrequent care of the nails	Thick, curved nails.
Bruised nail	Injury to the matrix and/or the nail bed resulting in the breaking of blood vessels in the nail bed	Discolouration of the nail as the blood leaks out underneath the nail plate which grows up as the nail grows.

Hair and its follicle

Hair is a dead keratinised structure protruding out of an indentation in the skin and can be divided into two sections:

1 Hair shaft: the portion extending above the skin surface.

2 Hair root: the portion below the surface of the skin.

Types of hair

There are three main classifications of hair:

1 Lanugo hair is the soft, downy hair seen on babies while in the womb that is shed before birth or that becomes the terminal hair of the scalp, eyelashes and eyebrows.

2 Vellus hair is the soft, downy colourless hair found all over the body except the eyelids, lips, palms of the hands and soles of the feet. This type of hair often originates from a lobe of a sebaceous gland or a shallow follicle. When the follicle is stimulated, for example by hormonal changes during puberty or when shaving, it is possible for vellus hair to become coarse, dark terminal hair.

Follicle shape determines hair texture

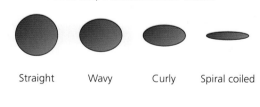

Straight   Wavy   Curly   Spiral coiled

Follicle size determines hair thickness

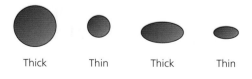

Thick   Thin   Thick   Thin

△ The link between the shape of the hair and straight, wavy and curly hair

3 Terminal hair is deep-seated, strong hair that extends from a deep downward growth of epidermal cells into the dermis called a follicle. It is from the blood supply in the dermis that terminal hair gains the nutrients and oxygen required for growth. Terminal hairs are found on the scalp, underarms, eyebrows, pubic regions, arms and legs. Naturally, terminal hair can be straight, wavy or curly and along with natural colour is a distinguishing feature used to describe ethnic origin. It is the shape of the follicle that moulds the hair and determines its distinguishing feature.

Hair structure

The structure of each hair is divided into three layers:

1 cuticle
2 cortex
3 medulla.

Cuticle

The outermost layer is composed of overlapping transparent scales. The cuticle of hair protects the layers that lie underneath. When substances such as lash tint come into contact with the cuticle, the scales become raised due to the alkalinity of the chemicals. This allows the chemicals to enter into the cortex of the hair.

Cortex

Made of many micro-fibrils arranged into bunches to form elongated cells, the cortex makes up the bulk of the hair and gives it strength and elasticity. It is within the cells of this layer that granules of pigment can be found, giving the hair its colour. Melanin produces the brown-black shades and pheomelanin gives the red-yellow shades.

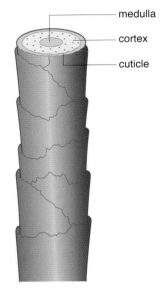

medulla
cortex
cuticle

△ Structure of the hair

Medulla

This layer is not always present, particularly in fine hair. When seen it lies in the centre of the cortex but its function is unclear.

Structure of the hair follicle

The hair follicle is formed by a depression of the epidermis downwards into the dermis to form a tube-like structure. It is from this that the hair grows. The lower portion of the follicle is called the bulb and approximately two-thirds up the follicle are the sebaceous glands which produce sebum, a natural oil. This lubricates the neck of the follicle, the skin surface and the hair.

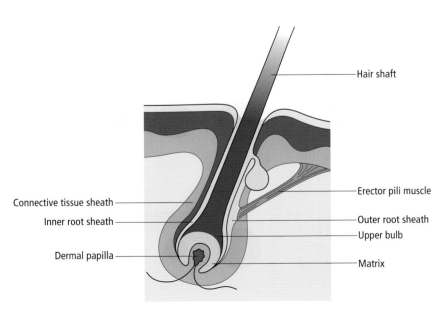

Hair shaft

Connective tissue sheath
Inner root sheath

Dermal papilla

Erector pili muscle
Outer root sheath
Upper bulb
Matrix

△ Structure of the hair follicle

Bulb

The hair bulb is the slightly swollen or 'bulbous' portion of the hair follicle and is the deepest part of the hair follicle into the dermis when the hair is actively growing.

Dermal papilla

The dermal papilla is an elevation into the base of the bulb which contains a rich blood supply. It is from here that the cells receive the nutrients and oxygen necessary for mitosis. While the follicle is in contact with the dermal papilla it will be active, in other words, capable of producing cells to form a growing hair.

Matrix

The matrix is situated at the top of the elevated part of the bulb and is in contact with the dermal papilla. It is a continuation of the germinating layer of the epidermis and is where the cells divide by mitosis and grow or mature. As the new cells mature they are impregnated with melanin from the melanocytes present and are pushed upwards by cells forming underneath. The cells change shape as they do so until they enter the upper bulb or keratinisation zone, where they harden and die to form the layers of the hair or inner root sheath.

Inner root sheath

The inner root sheath is also formed in the matrix and grows up with the hair. It is made of similar cells to the cuticle of the hair, which enables them to 'interlock' to secure the hair in the follicle. This structure is continuous with the hair as it grows up the follicle but discontinues at the level of the sebaceous gland. It can only be seen when the hair is actively growing.

Outer root sheath

The outer root sheath forms part of the follicle wall and is continuous with the stratum germinativum of the epidermis. It enables the follicle to grow and renew cells during its life cycle. The root sheath can be clearly seen as a silver sheath on hairs when they are plucked from the follicle during the active growing stage. It also remains in contact with the dermal papilla during the resting stage of the hair growth cycle and takes an active part in the formation of a new follicle wall during early anagen.

Connective tissue sheath

The connective tissue sheath surrounds the hair follicle and sebaceous gland to form part of the follicle wall. It has a prolific blood and nerve supply and provides the follicle with sensitivity.

Growth cycle of hair

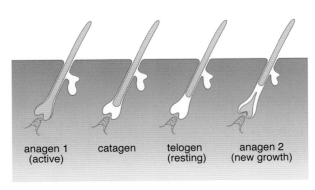

△ Stages of hair growth

A hair follicle actively produces hair for distinct periods of time, before going through stages of change and then rest. A follicle goes through three stages:

1 anagen: the active, growing stage

2 catagen: the changing stage

3 telogen: the resting stage.

Anagen

At the onset of anagen, the hair germ cells in the outer root sheath are stimulated into activity by hormones. This results in the formation of the dermal cord. The cells of the dermal cord undergo mitosis and a new follicle is produced. This grows in length and width, obtaining the food and oxygen for growth from the connective tissue sheath. The newly formed follicle extends downwards to the dermal papilla which enlarges and the bulb is formed around it.

The bulb begins production of new hair cells, receiving the necessary nourishment from the dermal papilla. These new cells become the inner root sheath first and then a new hair. As the new hair grows up the follicle, it may push the old hair out if it has not fallen out already and eventually the new hair appears at the surface. The hair continues to grow while the follicle is active. The time varies according to the area of the body but can be as long as six years. Towards the end of anagen, melanin production begins to slow down and eventually ceases as the follicle enters the next stage.

Catagen

This stage is also known as the transitional stage where the dermal papilla breaks down, the hair detaches itself from the base of the follicle and the bulb shrinks. The hair is now known as a club hair because of its appearance. Initially, a club hair is only attached to the follicle by the inner root sheath but as the hair continues to rise up the follicle to a level just below the sebaceous gland it is no longer attached. The follicle below the hair shrinks and breaks away from the dermal papilla but the remaining cells are already organising themselves to form the new matrix and hair germ cells. All this takes place over a period of a few days.

Telogen

Known as the resting stage, the follicle remains at approximately half of its normal length for a few weeks before anagen begins again. At this time the hair can be removed from the follicle just by brushing. On removal the hair will appear dry and the root often appears rough, giving rise to the name 'brush hair'. Sometimes epidermal cells will grow around the end of the hair, anchoring it in the skin, but when removed appear as a small white ball of cells. The telogen stage may not happen as the follicle can be stimulated to produce a new hair immediately.

Causes of hair growth

The classifications of increased hair growth are:

- Primary causes: these occur as a result of congenital influences or normal changes in hormone levels and so include hereditary causes, ethnic differences, puberty, pregnancy and menopause.

- Secondary causes: these include those brought about by illness and disease such as endocrine disorders, illness and stress.

Hair diseases and disorders

Disease/disorder	Cause	Description
Pediculosis capitis	Pediculosis: a small parasitic louse found in areas where hair grows. (The variations listed in this table relate to the areas of the body where it can be found)	Lice infestation of the scalp. The female clings to the hair with its front legs, which have claw-like structures, and lays her eggs in sacs cemented to the hair shaft, known as nits. The eggs hatch because of the warmth from the scalp. Symptoms include extreme irritation as the adults bite the scalp to feed from the blood supply. Commonly found in the area above and behind the ear. Do not treat. Advise the client to seek medical advice and to return when the condition has cleared.
Pediculosis pubis	The louse in this condition has adapted to become a slightly different shape, looking similar to a crab. This has given rise to the common name for this condition – 'crabs'	The pediculosis condition in the pubic region; it has similar symptoms to that of the scalp. Do not treat. Advise the client to seek medical advice and to return when the condition has cleared.
Pediculosis corporis	The louse's body can be larger in this variation of the condition	This is an infestation of the louse in body hair and is therefore is more common in men.

Skeletal system

Bone tissue

Bone is a hardened connective tissue that begins as cartilage and which has been specialised by cells called osteoblasts that impregnate the collagen fibres with the mineral calcium. Its main function is to support body weight and protect delicate organs. There are two types of bone tissue: compact bone and cancellous bone. All bones have a proportion of the two types. The arrangement of the bone tissue types gives bones their shape and facilitates their specific function.

Key term

Haversian system – formation of compact bone tissue, by which the bone receives nourishment and allows for sensation due to the presence of nerve fibres.

Compact bone

This is the harder of the two types and it forms the outer layer of all bones as well as the shaft of long bones where there may be considerable pressure or weight applied. The tissue is arranged in concentric circles around a central canal, through which nerves and blood capillaries pass. These bring essential nutrients and oxygen needed for growth and repair. This arrangement is known as a 'haversian system'.

Cancellous bone

This has a honey-comb appearance, which gives rise to its more common name of spongy bone. This bone tissue is lighter than but not as strong as compact bone and is found at the ends of long bones and in the centre of others. There are no haversian systems; instead it is penetrated throughout with blood vessels that bring the necessary nutrients and oxygen required for growth and repair.

Bone marrow

This is formed in the cavities created in long bones and in the centre of other bone types; its function is the manufacture of blood cells. Red blood cells are formed in red bone marrow; white blood cells and platelets are formed in yellow bone marrow.

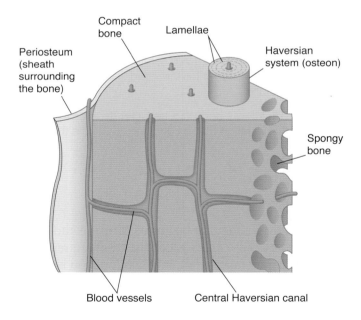

△ Haversian system

Classification of bone tissue

Bones are classified largely by their shape, as shown below.

Type of bone		Where found
Long bones 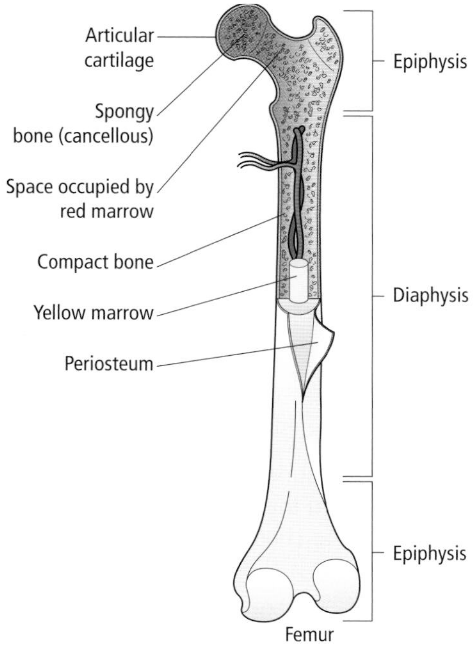	Articular cartilage Spongy bone (cancellous) Space occupied by red marrow Compact bone Yellow marrow Periosteum Epiphysis Diaphysis Epiphysis Femur	Found in the upper and lower limbs
Short bones 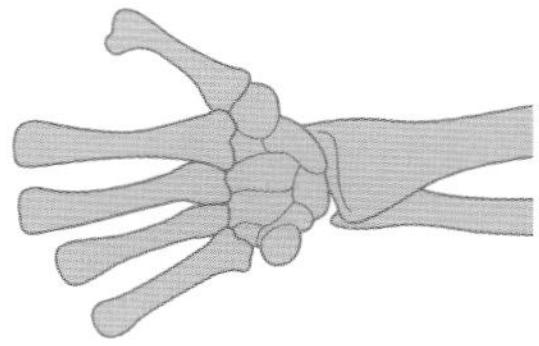		Found in the ankle and wrist. They are strong and compact
Flat bones 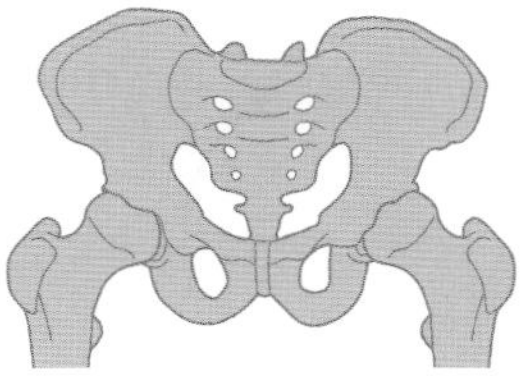		Broad flat bones such as those in the skull, hip and shoulder
Irregular bones 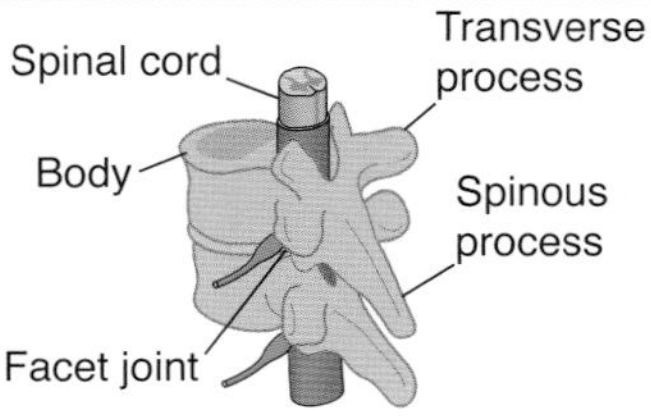	Spinal cord Body Transverse process Spinous process Facet joint	Have no distinct shape and are different in appearance from each other, such as those in the spine
Sesamoid bones 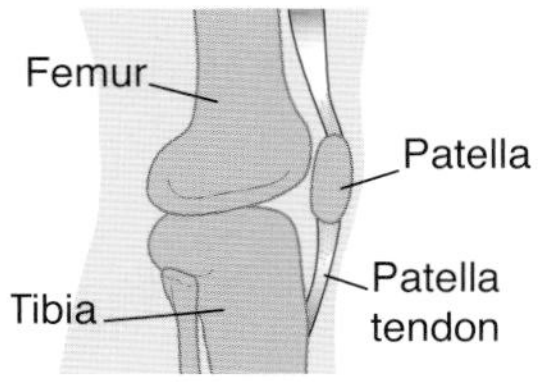	Femur Tibia Patella Patella tendon	Found 'floating' in tendons such as the patella in the knee

The bones shown above, together with another tissue called cartilage (see types of cartilage, page 89) form the skeleton and arranged in the shape of the human body. Where two bones come together joints are formed and are held in place by ligaments.

Types of joint and their range of movement

Joints are formed when two bones meet. The structure and shape of the bones at the joint determines the range of movement at that joint.

Type of joint	Structure	Position	Movement
Fibrous	Also known as fixed joints, the edges of the bones are fused together with strong fibrous connective tissue called sutures	Found between the bony plates of the skull	Little or no movement at this joint
Cartilaginous	These joints contain a pad of cartilage between the articulating surfaces of the bones, also known as semi-moveable joints.	Found at the vertebrae of the spine and at the pubis symphasis	This construction allows each joint of the spine to move a little but collectively allows great flexibility
Synovial	These joints are varied in shape and the movement they allow. The surfaces of the bones are covered in protective hyaline cartilage to minimise wear and tear and the whole joint is held together with strong connective fibre bands called ligaments. It is the shape of the bones at the joints that determines the movement, as described below:		
	Ball and socket joint	There are two main joints of the body, the hip and shoulder 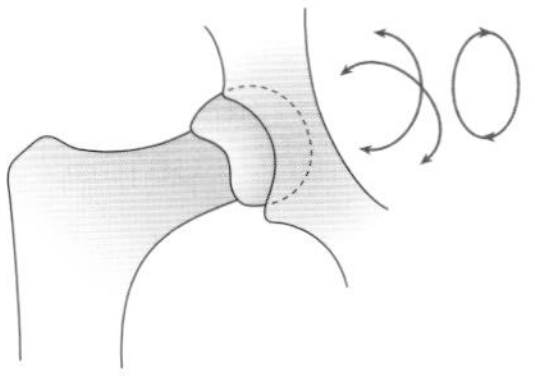	Allow a full range of movement, i.e. flexion, extension, abduction, adduction, circumduction and rotation
	Hinge joint	Found at the elbow, knee and between the phalanges 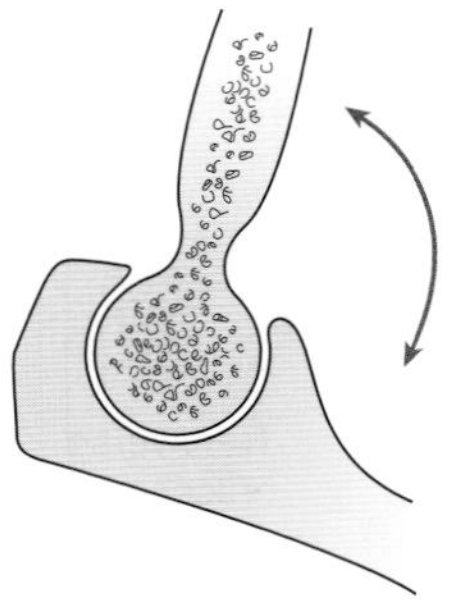	Allow more limited movements – flexion and extension
	Pivot joint	Found between the bones of the forearm and the spine and the skull. 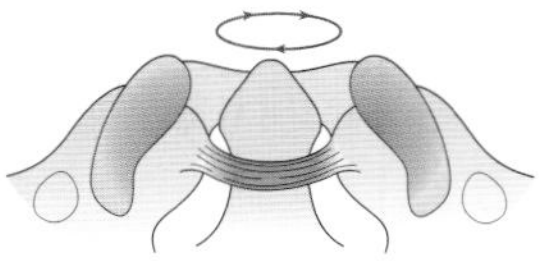	Allows rotation

Synovial	Gliding joint	Found between the bones of the ankle and wrist.		Provides versatility of movement between irregular shaped bones. Each moves in a small way in one direction
	Condyloid joint	Found between the carpals and radius and metacarpals and phalanges		Allows flexion, extension, adduction, abduction and circumduction
	Saddle joint	Found only between the metacarpal of the thumb and its phalanges		Allows flexion, extension, adduction, abduction and circumduction

Structure of a typical joint

A typical joint consists of the following:

- Hyaline cartilage: the surfaces of the two bones forming the joint are covered in a tough fibrous coating of hyaline cartilage which protects the surfaces as they articulate with each other, allowing free movement.

- Capsular ligament: connects the two bones and encases the joint.

- Synovial membrane: lines the inner surface of the capsular ligament and produces synovial fluid. This fluid fills the synovial cavity – the space between the two bones – lubricating the joint and nourishing the hyaline cartilage.

- Accessory ligament: attached to the two bones across the joint; provides it with stability but still allows movement at the joint.

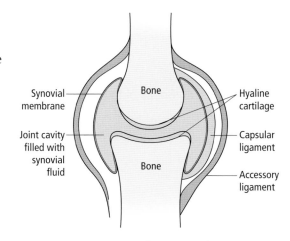

△ Structure of a typical joint

The skeleton

The skeleton is a fairly simple construction that can be seen replicated in many mammals. It has two distinct sections:

- the axial skeleton: consists of the skull, vertebral column, ribcage and sternum. It is this that supports the rest of the skeleton.

- the appendicular skeleton: consists of the bones of the limbs, including the shoulder and hip girdles and the upper and lower limbs.

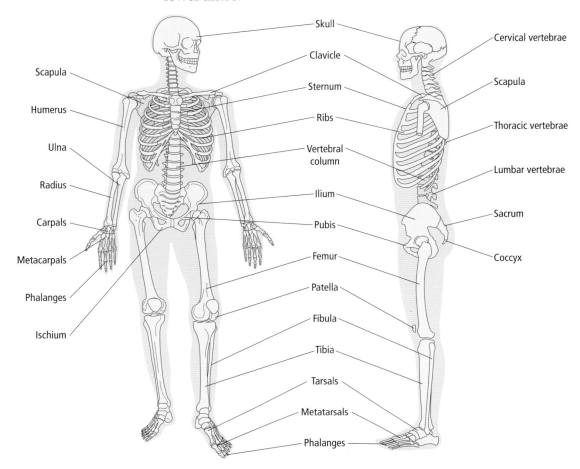

Scapula
Humerus
Ulna
Radius
Carpals
Metacarpals
Phalanges
Ischium

Skull
Clavicle
Sternum
Ribs
Vertebral column
Ilium
Pubis
Femur
Patella
Fibula
Tibia
Tarsals
Metatarsals
Phalanges

Cervical vertebrae
Scapula
Thoracic vertebrae
Lumbar vertebrae
Sacrum
Coccyx

△ Bones of the skeleton

Function of the skeleton

- Shape and support: there is a similarity between the shape of the skeleton and that of the external body, which can also be seen in other animals. The axial skeleton, that is the skull, vertebral column and ribs, supports the limbs of the appendicular skeleton. Together, the skeleton and muscles hold the body upright and give us our posture.

- Protection: the cranium and vertebral column protect the brain and spinal cord respectively, the ribcage protects the heart and lungs, and the pelvis protects the reproductive organs in the female.

- Production of blood cells: the blood brings the required nutrients and oxygen necessary for red blood cell formation, which occurs in the bone marrow of long bones, for example the femur.

- Calcium storage: the blood supply of the bones provides nutrients that are stored and removed depending on the demands of the body, for example calcium, phosphorus and fat.

- Muscle and tendon attachment: there are bony protrusions and rough surfaces of bones that allow for adhesion of muscles and tendons.

- Movement and locomotion: by using joints and with the contraction of muscles the body is able to move.

Skull

The bones of the head are also known as the skull and are divided into two groups: the cranium and the face. Most of the bones of the skull form fixed joints called sutures. The only free-moving joint is that between the mandible (the lower jaw) and the temporal bones, which allow the lower jaw to move up and down when chewing.

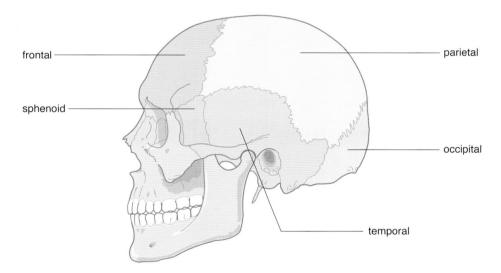

△ Lateral view of the skull

Cranium

There are eight bones that form the cranium, a box-like structure that protects the brain:

Name of bone	Position
Frontal	One bone forming the front of the cranium including the forehead and upper eye sockets
Parietal	Two bones forming the top and sides of the cranium
Occipital	One bone forming the back and floor of the cranium
Temporal	Two bones forming the sides of the cranium, above and around the ears
Sphenoid	One bone forming the floor and the sides of the cranium at the temple region and the back of the eye sockets
Ethmoid	One bone forming the front floor of the cranium, the roof of the nasal cavities and the inner sides of the eye sockets

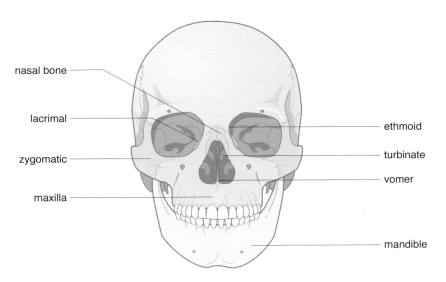

nasal bone

lacrimal

zygomatic

maxilla

ethmoid

turbinate

vomer

mandible

△ Anterior view of the skull showing the bones of the face

Face

There are fourteen bones forming the facial structure and features:

Name of Bone	Position
Zygomatic	Two bones that form the cheekbones and the floor and side wall of the eye sockets
Maxilla(e)	Two bones forming the upper jaw, the front part of the roof of the mouth, the sides of the nose and the floor of the eye sockets. The upper teeth are embedded in the maxillae
Nasal	Two bones forming the bridge of the nose
Mandible	One bone forming the lower jaw in which the lower teeth are embedded
Lachrymal	Two bones forming the inner walls of the eye sockets
Palatine	Two bones forming the back part of the roof of the mouth and sides of the nasal cavities (not shown in illustration)
Vomer	One bone forming the central division of the nasal cavities
Turbinate	Two bones forming the side wall of the nasal cavities
Hyoid	Horseshoe-shaped bone situated in the throat. It is more prominent in men than in women and aids in tongue movement during speech and swallowing

Sinuses

The sinuses are a series of chambers or cavities within the skull that warm and moisten the air we breathe in before it enters the lungs and provide mucous to capture small particles of dust, etc. They are also thought to improve the quality of the sound of the voice by providing resonance.

There are four main sinus cavities in the skull:

1 Maxillary sinuses: found in the upper jaw, they are the largest at around 2.5 cm in diameter.

2 Frontal sinuses: located in the centre of the forehead, they are also large in size.

3 Ethmoid sinuses: located at the bridge of the nose between the eyes.

4 Sphenoid sinuses: also at the bridge of the nose in bones behind the nasal cavity.

The sinuses are lined with mucous-forming membrane tissue and drain into the nose through a small channel called the middle meatus. During cold and flu infections, and when foreign bodies such as pollen enter the nose, the mucous membrane is stimulated to produce more mucous to flush the 'invader' from the respiratory system, leading to the characteristic runny nose. After the invasion the mucous can thicken and block the sinuses, giving rise to headaches and puffy eyes as other fluids such as tears cannot drain away.

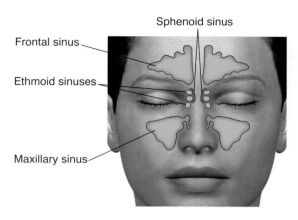

△ Position of the sinuses

Vertebral column

The vertebral column is a series of irregular-shaped bones stacked on top of each other to form a column. Each vertebra is separated from the one above and below it by a disc of cartilage, which prevents the bones rubbing against each other and acts as a cushion or shock absorber for physical stress administered from the upper body to the lower or vice versa.

The spinal cord runs through a channel formed by the arrangement of the bones on top of each other and the vertebral column's function is to protect this important part of the nervous system while allowing a range of movement.

The bones or vertebrae are named after the area in which they are situated, each with a distinctive shape that has adapted to enable it to articulate effectively with the one above it and to allow the passage of the peripheral nervous system through and out from the spinal cord. The vertebrae's spinal processes and shape also allow for muscle attachment.

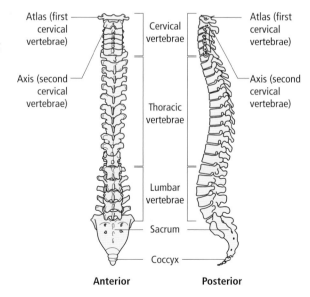

△ Vertebral column

Name of bone	Position
Cervical vertebrae	Seven small vertebrae forming the neck. The top vertebra is attached to the underneath of the occipital bone of the skull and has a hole through which passes the peg-like structure of the second vertebra. This arrangement forms a type of synovial joint called a pivot joint that allows rotation of the head
Thoracic vertebrae	Twelve larger vertebrae, one for each pair of ribs with which they articulate to form the thorax. Together with the ribs they contain and protect the heart and lungs
Lumbar vertebrae	The five largest vertebrae found in the lower back, their size enables the support of the body weight
Sacral vertebrae	Five vertebrae fused together to form a triangular shape within the pelvis
Coccygeal vertebrae	Four smallest vertebrae that are fused together to form the coccyx that equates to an animal's tail. It seems to serve no useful function within the body.

Thorax

The thorax or thoracic cavity is the portion of the trunk that contains and protects the heart and lungs. It is made up of the sternum, ribs and 12 thoracic vertebrae. The arrangement of the ribs and their articulation with the sternum and vertebrae allows for the expansion experienced during inhalation.

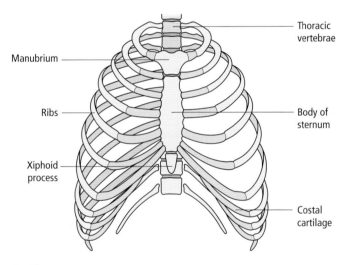

△ Thorax

Name of bone	Position
Sternum	A flat bone found centrally in the chest, commonly called the breast bone. It has three distinct parts: the manubrium at the top, the largest part in the middle called the body and at the bottom the xiphoid. It articulates with the ribs via the costal cartilages and protects the heart from physical damage
Ribs	There are twelve pairs of ribs that form a cage around the heart and lungs for protection. Their arrangement with the intercostal and diaphragm muscles brings about inhalation and exhalation for the respiratory system. The first seven pairs articulate directly with the sternum and are known as 'true ribs'; three pairs articulate indirectly and are known as 'false ribs' and two pairs attach at only one end and are known as 'floating ribs'.

Shoulder girdle

The shoulder girdle is made up of the clavicle, scapula and humerus bones. The clavicle or collarbone is situated at the front of the body and forms a joint with the sternum or breastbone. The scapula is commonly called the shoulder blade and is situated at the back of the body, forming a ball-and-socket joint with the humerus, the upper bone of the arm.

Name of bone	Position
Clavicle	Two long bones, a left and a right, found at the front of the body from the shoulder to the sternum
Scapula	Two flat bones, a left and a right, found in the upper back of the body at the shoulder
Humerus	Two long bones, a left and a right, forming the upper arm with a ball and socket joint at the shoulder at one end and a hinge joint at the elbow at the other.

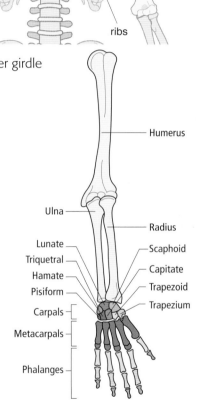

clavicle (collar bone)

scapula (shoulder blade)

sternum

humerus

ribs

△ Shoulder girdle

Humerus

Ulna

Radius

Lunate

Scaphoid

Triquetral

Capitate

Hamate

Trapezoid

Pisiform

Trapezium

Carpals

Metacarpals

Phalanges

△ Upper limb

Upper limb

The humerus bone extends from the shoulder to form the upper arm. The lower end of the humerus forms a hinge joint at the elbow with the lower arm bones called the ulna and radius. The ulna is the stronger of the two bones, is weight bearing and allows for the attachment of the muscles that move the wrist and hand. The radius carries little weight and is mainly for muscle attachment. These bones extend from the elbow to form the lower arm and at the lower end form joints with the wrist or carpal bones – eight irregular-shaped bones arranged loosely in two rows of four. The carpals form joints with the metacarpals of the hand or palm and these in turn articulate with the small bones of the fingers and thumb known as the phalanges.

Name of bone	Position
Ulna	Runs down the little finger side of the lower arm
Radius	Runs down the thumb side of the lower arm
Scaphoid	Found in the top row of carpals and articulates with the radius on the thumb side
Trapezium	Found in the lower row of carpals and articulates with the thumb metacarpal
Lunate	Top row, next to the scaphoid
Triquetral	Top row, next to the lunate
Pisiform	Top row of the carpals overlapping the triquetral on the little finger side
Trapezoid	Bottom row, next to the trapezium
Capitate	Bottom row, next to the trapezoid

★ *Hints and tips*
The ulna and radius articulate with each other to form pivot joints that allow the palm of the hand to turn forwards, a movement known as supination and backwards known as pronation.

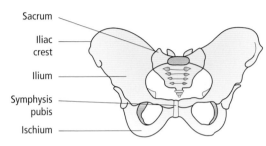

△ Pelvic girdle

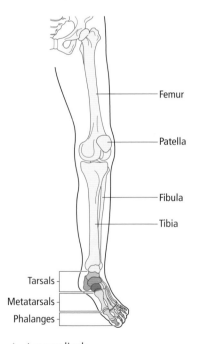

△ Lower limb

Hamate	Bottom row, next to the capitate
Metacarpals	Five long bones of the palm of the hand, one for each of the digits
Phalanges	Fourteen small bones in each hand that make up the digits, arranged with three to each finger and two to the thumb

Pelvic girdle

The pelvic girdle or hips is made up of the ilium, ischium and pubis bones and together they are called the innominate bones. The arrangement of the bones forms a protective ring around the delicate lower abdominal organs, in particular the reproductive organs in women.

Name of bone	Position
Ilium	Two bones, a left and a right. They are flat and wing-shaped and form the hips. They articulate with the sacrum at the back and their shape allows for the attachment of the large muscles of the abdomen
Ischium	Two irregular-shaped bones that articulate with the lower borders of the ilium at the back of the pelvis and are fused to the two pubic bones towards the front of the pelvis. It is upon these bones that the body weight is placed during sitting and they are also used for the attachment of muscles originating from the back of the thighs
Pubis	Two pubic bones make up the pubis; they are fused to the ischium at one end and come together in the lower centre of the pelvis separated by a pad of cartilage called the pubic symphysis. It is this arrangement that facilitates the act of childbirth in women.

Lower limb

The femur extends down from the hip to the knee where it articulates with the tibia to form a hinge joint. 'Floating' over the knee is the kneecap or patella, which is embedded in the tendon of the front thigh muscles, the quadriceps.

The tibia forms the main bone of the lower leg and supports the weight of the body. Running parallel to it on the lateral side of the body is the fibula which has largely a muscle attachment function.

The seven bones making up the ankle are collectively known as the tarsals. These support and distribute the body weight from the feet throughout the body. The calcaneus forms the heel and attaches the strong muscles of the calf to the foot and enables walking and running, etc.

Name of bone	Position
Tibia	To the medial side of the lower leg, from knee to ankle
Fibula	To the lateral side of the lower leg, from knee to ankle
Patella	At the knee joint, commonly called the kneecap
Calcaneus	Forms the heel at the lower back of the ankle
Talus	Found at the top front of the ankle
Navicular	Forms part of the top of the foot at the ankle
Cuboid	Lies to the outside of the foot at the ankle
Outer cuneiform	Lies between the cuboid and the middle cuneiform
Middle cuneiform	Lies between the outer and inner cuneiform
Inner cuneiform	Lies next to the middle cuneiform to the medial side of the foot
Metatarsals	Five long bones making up the length of the foot, one for each of the toes
Phalanges	Fourteen small bones of the toes in each foot. Two in the big toe and three in the other toes. Can be fused together in the little toe

★ *Hints and tips*
The bones of the feet are not flat but form transverse arches, one across the ball of the foot and another towards the heel, and two longitudinal arches, one to the inside of the foot and the other to the outside. The four arches support the weight of the body, aid posture and fully utilise energy to propel the body forward when walking and running.

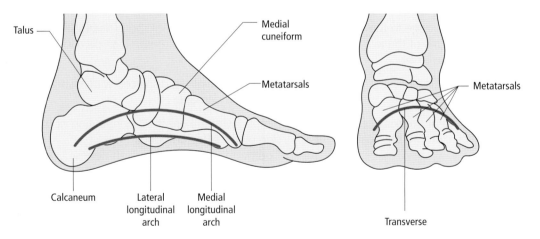

△ Arches of the foot

Disorders of the skeletal system

Disease/disorder	Cause	Description
Arthritis	Osteoarthritis is the wear and tear of the bones at the joints caused by use, so common in the elderly. Rheumatoid arthritis is an inflammatory condition that can affect anyone at any age	Joints are often swollen, sometimes misshapen and very painful
Gout	The deposit of sodium urate in the joints caused by high levels of uric acid in the blood	Swollen, painful joints
Bursitis	Inflammation of the bursae – sac-like structures filled with synovial fluid found in some joints	Pain with movement at the joint; reduced mobility at the affected joint
Synovitis	Inflammation of the lining of a synovial joint	Sufferer exhibits pain, swelling and a reduction in movement of that joint; associated with rheumatoid arthritis
Torn cartilage	Physical trauma to the cartilage of a joint caused by excessive force	Pain with movement of the joint, particular if it mimics the action by which it was caused
Tendonitis	Inflammation of a tendon after overuse or injury	Pain and a reduction in the mobility of the affected joint
Sprain	Soft tissue damage to the ligaments and/or tendons of the joint caused by an injury or overuse	Pain with movement of the joint initially and if repair is incomplete there can be a loss of range of movement
Dislocation	Physical trauma	Bones of a joint are displaced with associated soft tissue damage
Fractures	The cracking or breaking of bones caused by extreme physical trauma	Simple: where there is no penetration of the skin by the affected bones Compound: where the broken bones penetrate the skin Comminute: greenstick; impacted; complicated
Osteoporosis	Reduction of bone tissue associated with age or repeated impact on hard surfaces	The bones become brittle and break very easily
Rickets	Vitamin D deficiency	Vitamin D facilitates the absorption of calcium from the diet and without it the bones become soft, causing the characteristic 'bowing' of the long bones of the legs due to body weight

Paget's disease	Hyperactivity of the osteoblasts and osteoclasts resulting in soft bone tissue	The bones appear thick and enlarged and 'bow' under the body weight
Scleroderma	Connective tissue disorder where it thickens under the influence of the immune system	Localised scleroderma only affects the skin and the tissues immediately beneath, but systemic sclerosis can affect the other connective tissues in the body such as the lungs with more damaging consequences
Bunions	Deformity of the joint of the big toe caused by pressure on the joint by shoes, etc.	Pain, swelling and inflammation can be seen and there is displacement of the big toe laterally
Hammer toes	Deformity of the proximal joint of the toes causing the proximal phalange to bend	The second, third or fourth toes can be affected and the toe resembles a hammer
Scoliosis	Can be present at birth but in this case usually corrected at an early age while the bones are still relatively soft. Mild cases can be seen due to overuse of one shoulder and the associated upper limb	Sideways curvature of the spine resulting in a loss of flexibility and movement
Kyphosis	Can be present at birth but more commonly through poor posture and everyday activity using the arms. A lack of exercise of the appropriate anti-gravity muscles will exacerbate the condition	Exaggerated curvature of the spine in the thoracic region, resulting in drooped breasts, round shoulders and forward head tilt
Lordosis	Can be present at birth but can develop during or after pregnancy or with obesity as a result of the extra weight in the abdominal area and an associated lack of tone in the abdominal muscles	Exaggerated curvature of the spine in the lumbar region resulting in protruding abdomen, forward hip tilt and lower back pain
Cervical spondylitis	Wear and tear on the neck vertebrae through repetitive action or acute injury such as whiplash	The vertebrae show signs of degeneration and there is associated pain and discomfort
Herniated (slipped) disc	Pressure on the cartilage discs between the vertebrae of the spine	A 'bulge' appears that displaces and may put pressure on nerves, giving rise to the associated pain

For more information and images of the spinal curvatures and their associated postural faults see Chapter 7 Skin and body analysis.

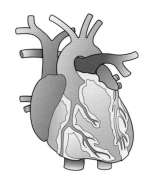

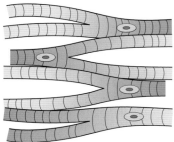

△ Cardiac muscle tissue

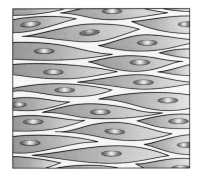

△ Smooth muscle tissue

Muscular system

The muscular system is made up of contractile tissue called muscle and tendons and facia.

There are three types of muscle tissue:

1 Cardiac muscle

2 Smooth, non-striated, visceral or involuntary muscle

3 Skeletal, striated or voluntary muscle.

Each has a different appearance and function but with a unique feature: the ability to contract in response to a nervous stimuli and then to return to its original shape.

Cardiac muscle

Cardiac muscle is only found in the heart and when contracted forms the heartbeat. Its function is to pump blood around our bodies. It is a form of involuntary muscle tissue but its structure resembles skeletal muscle in that it is striped in appearance, with fewer nuclei and mitochondria.

Smooth muscle

As indicated by the name, smooth muscle tissue appears smooth under an electron microscope, without a striped appearance. This type of muscle tissue is present in the walls of blood vessels and the intestines to assist the passage of blood or digested food along the vessels. The cells are spindle in shape and have few nuclei. The muscles are under sub-conscious control and contract without our knowledge and consequently are also known as involuntary muscle tissue.

Skeletal muscle

As the name suggests, this is the type of muscle attached to the bones of the skeletal system and when contracted brings about movement of the skeleton at the joints. It is also known as striated or striped muscle due to its appearance under a microscope. Within the cells there appears alternative darker and lighter bands, which are the overlap of the two proteins from which it is made, actin and myosin. Another name for this type of muscle is voluntary muscle tissue as the tissue is under conscious control from the central nervous system.

There are over 600 individual skeletal muscles in the human body, the superficial of which will be discussed later in this chapter. Each will be discussed in terms of its individual position and function.

Structure of skeletal muscle

Skeletal muscles are made up of bundles of muscle cells or fibres that run alongside each other in groups along the length of the muscle. When each muscle fibre contracts, the result is a shortening of the whole muscle, which pulls on the bones and movement occurs at the joints.

Under an electron microscope, the muscle appears striated or striped. Skeletal muscle tissue is described as 'multi-nucleate' (more than one nucleus per cell), shown as darker areas between the cells and there are many mitochondria to provide the vast energy requirements of the muscle fibres to contract.

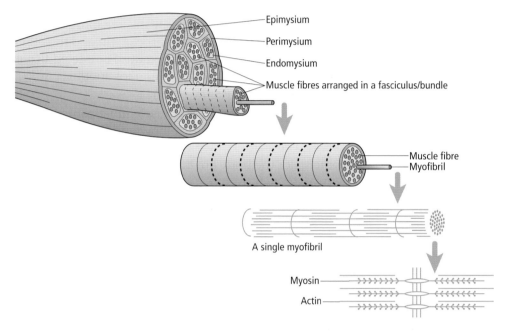

△ Skeletal muscle tissue

Muscle contraction

The striped appearance of skeletal muscle comes about through the overlap of two proteins, actin and myosin. It is this arrangement that allows the shortening of the cell during contraction. Responding to stimulation from the nervous system, these proteins slide over each other along their length in one direction, determined by their attachment to bones. The energy for such contraction is obtained from the numerous mitochondria present and involves the metabolism of adenosine triphosphate (ATP) during the utilisation of oxygen.

Skeletal muscle contraction is brought about by a series of events. First, the central nervous system, the brain and spinal cord, sends a message in the form of an electrical impulse along a motor nerve to the muscle. When it reaches the muscle the nerve divides so that a nerve fibre serves each muscle fibre. This area is called the motor point. The message is passed from the nerve to the muscle fibres and the muscle contracts.

The ends of the muscles are attached to bones via tendons across a joint and bring about movement at that joint. In the face the muscles can be connected to bone at one end and skin or another muscle at the other. This allows the skin to move and create facial expressions. The fixed end of the muscle is called the origin and during a specific movement will remain stationary, while the other end moves towards it, known as the insertion. For some muscles within the body this remains so during contraction of that muscle, the same end being the origin and the other the insertion, but for other muscles this can alternate. For one particular movement, one end of the muscle is the origin and for another movement the opposite end becomes the origin.

To reverse a particular movement another muscle must contract. For example, the biceps muscle bends the elbow and the triceps straightens the elbow. These are known as antagonistic pairs and virtually all movements of the body are brought about in this way.

During such contraction, the muscles surrounding a joint may perform different roles for a particular movement and swap roles during another. The muscle that is responsible for bringing about the movement is known as the prime mover and this muscle can be assisted by another called the synergist. During the contraction the joint may need to be stabilised, either to prevent injury or to give strength to the movement, and the muscle or group of muscles that perform that function are called fixators.

Normally during contraction the origin and insertion of a muscle will get closer together and there is shortening of the muscle fibres; this sort of contraction is called concentric contraction. Sometimes, however, the same muscle may contract when the origin and insertion are moving away from each other and there is lengthening of the muscle fibres; usually as a result of weight or force and the action of gravity on the muscle. This type of contraction is called eccentric contraction and the action of the biceps in everyday use is a good example of this.

The functions of skeletal muscle are:

- to facilitate movement

- raise body temperature

- maintain the posture of the body (anti-gravity muscles)

- assist in the return of the blood in the veins.

Muscle tone

Muscle tone is described as the tension felt in a muscle when it is not actively contracting. This condition is brought about by a few of the muscle fibres remaining in a contractile state and is important in maintaining the correct body posture. A muscle with good muscle tone is ready to contract so the body is able to respond effectively in an emergency. There will be increased blood supply to the toned muscle with the benefit of increased nutrients and oxygen supply and the muscle is unlikely to attract the laying down of body fat among its fibres.

Muscle tone varies with use; the more use the better the muscle tone and this leads to a variation of muscle tone throughout the body. For example, the biceps in the anterior aspect of the upper arm is used concentrically and eccentrically in all everyday movements involving the arm and has good muscle tone. However, its antagonistic pair, the triceps, is not effectively used and this results in poor muscle tone in this muscle. Muscle tone naturally diminishes with age unless the muscles are placed under stress in the form of exercise.

Muscle fatigue

Muscle fatigue is a condition caused by prolonged or acute activity of the muscle, resulting in a lack of readily supplied energy. During normal activity the mitochondria provide instant energy by the metabolism of adenosine triphosphate (ATP) in the presence of oxygen but the chemical reaction takes time to do so as the supply of oxygen may not be readily available. During continuous work the energy from this source can run out very quickly.

Where instant or prolonged energy is needed for contraction the muscle uses ATP anaerobically, resulting in the formation of 'lactic acid', a toxin that causes the muscle cells to fatigue and therefore the muscle too. The result is a weak muscle contraction or one that causes rapid contraction of the muscle fibres and 'trembling' of the muscle can be seen. Lactic acid, however, is readily returned to ATP in the presence of oxygen and so with time the levels of ATP are returned to normal. However, if lactic acid is allowed to accumulate in the muscle, cramp may occur and it is this build-up of lactic acid that is the cause of muscle stiffness sometimes felt in muscles after abnormal work levels.

> ☆ **Hints and tips**
>
> Often during body analysis a client will complain of being unhappy with their figure but on further investigation the client's weight is considered normal. In this instance it is often a lack of muscle tone that is the cause of the client's concern, as a general lack of tone throughout the body's main muscle groups can give rise to a general overweight appearance: protruding abdomen, sagging breasts, flabby thighs and arms and drooping buttocks. Exercise is the answer, not dieting.

Muscles of the head and face

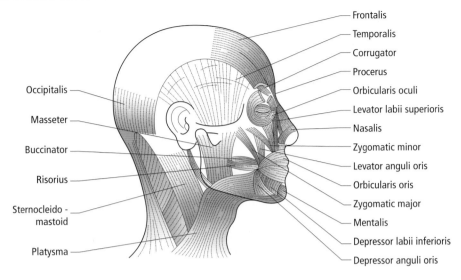

Frontalis
Temporalis
Corrugator
Procerus
Orbicularis oculi
Levator labii superioris
Nasalis
Zygomatic minor
Levator anguli oris
Orbicularis oris
Zygomatic major
Mentalis
Depressor labii inferioris
Depressor anguli oris

Occipitalis
Masseter
Buccinator
Risorius
Sternocleido-mastoid
Platysma

△ Muscles of the head and neck

Name of muscle	Position/location	Action
Occipitalis	Found at the back of the head; attached to the occipital bone and attached to the scalp	To move the scalp backwards towards the occipital bone
Frontalis	At the forehead across its width; attached to the skin of the eyebrows and the skin of the scalp	Wrinkles the skin of the forehead and raises the eyebrows creating a surprised expression
Occipito-frontalis	The two muscles described above together with the epicranialaponeurosis or scalp; covers the skull	Moves the scalp backwards and wrinkles the skin of the forehead to raise the eyebrows.
Temporalis	Surrounds the ear and lies over the temporal bone, passing under the zygomatic arch to attach to the lower jaw	Raises the jaw when chewing
Corrugator	Between the eyebrows; attached to the frontalis muscle and the frontal bone	Brings the eyebrows together creating frowning
Procerus	Between the eyebrows; attached to the nasal bones and the frontalis muscle	Draws the eyebrows inwards, creating a puzzled expression
Nasalis	At the sides of the nose; attached to the maxillae bones and the nostrils	Dilates and compresses the nostrils
Orbicularis oculi	Surrounds the opening of the eye socket; attached to the bones at its outer edge and the skin of the eyelids at the inner	To close the eyes as in sleeping, winking, squinting and blinking
Orbicularis oris	Surrounds the opening of the mouth occupying the entire width of the lips	Closes or narrows the lips, used to press the teeth against the lips and to purse the lips as in whistling
Quadratuslabii superioris (levator labii superioris)	Located towards the inner cheek beside the nose; attached to the maxillae and the skin of the corners of the mouth and upper lip	Raises the corner of the mouth to create a snarling expression

Buccinator	Main muscle of the cheek, attached to both the maxilla and mandible. Forms a muscular plate between the teeth	Keeps the cheek stretched during all phases of opening and closing the mouth. Also to compress the cheeks when blowing
Depressor labii inferioris	Located under the mouth and lower lip, from the mandible to the skin of the lip	Turns the lower lip outwards in an expression of doubt or sorrow
Triangularis (depressor angulioris)	Found at outer aspects of the mouth from the mandible to the corners of the mouth	Draws down the corners of the mouth to give a sad expression
Mentalis	Located at the point of the chin, attached to the mandible and the skin of the lower lip	Lifts and wrinkles the skin of the chin and turns the lower lip outwards, creating a pouting expression
Masseter	Found at the outer cheek in front of the ear attached to the zygomatic arch and the mandible	Raises the lower jaw, exerting pressure on the teeth when chewing
Risorius	Lies above the buccinator, attached to the angle of the mandible and the skin at the corner of the mouth	Pulls the corner of the mouth sideways to create a grinning expression
Zygomaticus (major and minor)	Lies across the inner cheek, attached to the zygomatic bone and the corners of the mouth	Lifts the corners of the mouth upwards and sideways to create a smiling expression
Sternocleidomastoid	Lies across the side of the neck; attached to the clavicle and sternum and the mastoid process of the temporal bone	Contraction of one muscle turns the head in the opposite direction and when contracted together the chin is pulled down towards the chest
Platysma	Extends down the front of the neck from the sides of the chin across the mandible to the clavicle, either side of the throat	Draws down the mandible and lower lip causing wrinkling in the skin of the neck
Digastrics (not shown)	Located under the mandible; attached to the mastoid process and the lateral aspects of the hyoid bone in the throat.	Elevates the hyoid bone during speech and swallowing
Pterygoids (not shown)	Located under the masseter muscle, extending from the maxilla to the mandible	Elevates the mandible and assists the masseter in mastication

Muscles of the back

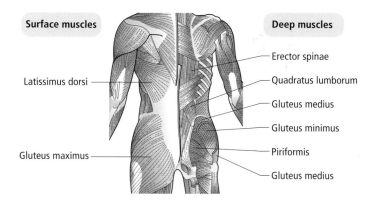

△ Muscles of the back

Name of muscle	Position	Action
Trapezius	Diamond-shaped muscle at the upper back, neck and shoulder, attached to the occipital bone and the vertebrae of the neck and thorax to the scapula and outer end of the clavicle	Raises the shoulder to the ear, holds the scapula and shoulder still during arm movements and extends the neck
Erector spinae (sacro-spinalis)	Extends the length of the back next to the spine; attached to the crest of the ilium to the occipital bone, sending out attachments to the vertebrae along the length of the spine	Extends the spine and is an anti-gravity muscle so important in maintaining body posture
Latissimusdorsi	Large muscle that covers almost the entire back, extending from the lumbar region of the spine across and upwards to the shoulder joint	Extends, adducts and rotates the arm
Quadratuslumborum	Deep muscle found in the lower back, either side of the lumbar vertebrae	Lateral flexion and extension of the trunk

Deep muscles of the upper back

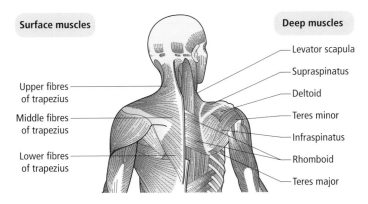

△ Deep muscles of the upper back

Name of muscle	Position	Action
Levator scapulae	Deep muscle underlying the trapezius, attached from to the upper borders of the scapula to the cervical vertebrae	Raises and adducts the scapula
Splenius capitis	Found in the back of the neck under the trapezius; there is a right and left and they extend from the cervical vertebrae to the mastoid process of the temporal bone	Extension of the neck when they work together; when working separately each flexes the neck laterally
Supraspinatus	Attached to the bony ridge (spine) of the scapula at the top and the humerus bone in the upper arm across the shoulder joint	Abducts the upper arm, assisting the deltoid muscle
Infraspinatus	Deep muscle attached under the spine of the scapula; covers the lower portion of the scapula as it extends out to the top of the humerus bone	Rotates the upper arm laterally
Rhomboids	Found between the scapula; attached to the medial edge of the scapula at one end and the thoracic vertebrae at the other	Adducts the scapula and keeps it steady during movements of the arm

Subscapularis (not shown)	Located beneath the scapula; attached to its underside and the top of the humerus	Rotates the upper arm medially
Teres major	Attached to the side edge of the scapula and the back of the humerus	Adducts and medially rotates the upper arm
Teres minor	Located above the teres major; attached from the side edge of the scapula to the back of the humerus	Rotates the upper arm laterally

Muscles of the anterior aspect of the trunk

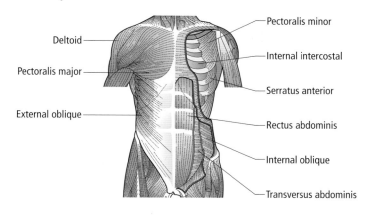

△ Anterior muscles of the trunk

Name of muscle	Position	Action
Pectoralis major	Large muscle covering the chest and lying underneath the breast in women; attached to the sternum and clavicle at one end and the top of the anterior humerus at the other	Adducts and medially rotates the upper arm; used when pushing
Pectoralis minor	Lies beneath the pectoralis major; attached to the ribs and the scapula	Pulls the shoulder forwards
Serratus anterior	Lies at the side of the chest wall; attached to the medial edge of the scapula	Rotates the scapula and pulls the shoulder forwards
Internal and external intercostals	Located between the ribs	Raise the ribs during respiration and maintain the shape of the thorax
Diaphragm	Dome-shaped muscle under the ribs; separates the thorax and the abdominal cavities	Used in respiration; it flattens on contraction, increasing the thorax cavity in inhalation
Rectus abdominis	Lies along the length of the abdomen from the ribs to the pubis	Flexes the trunk forwards and supports the organs of the abdomen
External and internal obliques	Lies to the side of the abdomen from the ribs to the iliac crest	Flexes and rotates the trunk and supports the organs of the abdomen
Transversus abdominis	Lies at the front and sides of the abdomen at the waist; attached to the bottom of the ribs, the iliac crest and the pubis	Supports and contains the organs of the abdomen

Muscles of the upper limb

The muscles that bring about movement of the lower arm at the elbow are situated in the upper arm and those that bring about movement in the wrist and hand are located in the forearm. The tendons that attach these muscles to the bones of the lower arm and hand are long and need to be held in place by ligaments at the wrist. This formation gives strength and power to the hands and wrist.

Anterior aspect

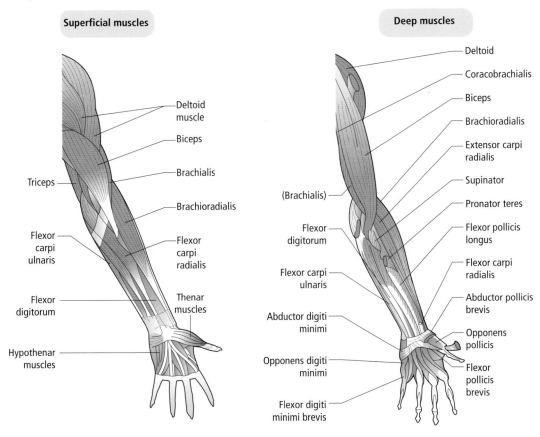

Superficial muscles

Deltoid muscle
Biceps
Brachialis
Brachioradialis
Triceps
Flexor carpi ulnaris
Flexor carpi radialis
Flexor digitorum
Thenar muscles
Hypothenar muscles

Deep muscles

Deltoid
Coracobrachialis
Biceps
Brachioradialis
Extensor carpi radialis
Supinator
Pronator teres
(Brachialis)
Flexor pollicis longus
Flexor digitorum
Flexor carpi radialis
Flexor carpi ulnaris
Abductor pollicis brevis
Abductor digiti minimi
Opponens pollicis
Opponens digiti minimi
Flexor pollicis brevis
Flexor digiti minimi brevis

△ Muscles of the upper limb – anterior aspect

Name of muscle	Position	Action
Deltoid	Forms a cap over the shoulder. The front is attached to the clavicle and the back to the scapula and the two meet to attach to the humerus	The front portion brings the arm forward, the back takes it backwards and together they take the arm out to the side
Biceps	Anterior aspect of the upper arm; attaches to the scapula at the shoulder at one end and the radius in the forearm, crossing the two joints	Flexes the elbow and supinates the forearm and hand
Brachialis	Attached from the shaft of the humerus to the ulna at the bony process of the elbow	Flexes the elbow
Brachioradialis	Anterior aspect of the forearm across the elbow; attached to the humerus and the radius bones	Flexes the elbow
Coracobrachialis (not shown)	Runs from the scapula to the shaft of the humerus	Brings the arm forward (flexion) and over towards the middle of the body
Flexor carpi ulnaris	Runs along the ulna side of the forearm from the lower end of the humerus across the wrist to the fifth metacarpal	Flexes the wrist
Flexor carpi radialis	Runs the radial side of the forearm from the lower end of the humerus across the wrist to the second and third metacarpal	Flexes the wrist
Flexor carpi digitorum	Runs from the lower end of the humerus; attached to the ulna and radius to the second to fifth fingers	Flexes the fingers
Pronator Teres (not shown)	Anterior aspect of the lower humerus and the radius	Pronates the forearm and hand
Flexors	Medial aspect of the forearm; attached to the lower humerus, radius and ulna and the metacarpals and phalanges of the fingers	Flexes the wrist, fingers and thumb
Hypothenar eminence	Located in the palm of the hand below the little finger; attached to the carpals, metacarpals and phalanges of the little finger	Abducts, adducts and flexes the little finger
Thenar eminence	Located in the palm below the thumb; attached to the carpals, metacarpals and phalanges of the thumb	Abducts, adducts and flexes the thumb and draws it towards the palm
Mid-palm group	Located in the centre of the palm below the middle three fingers; attached to the carpals, metacarpals and phalanges of those fingers	Abducts, adducts and flexes the middle three fingers

Posterior aspect

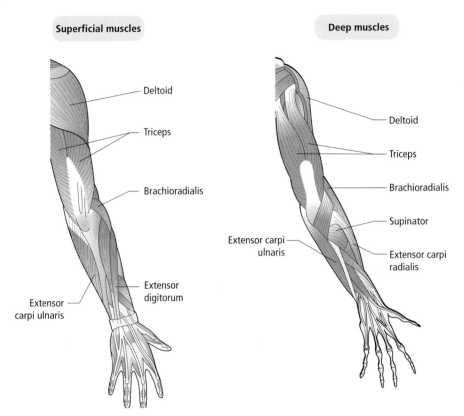

Superficial muscles

- Deltoid
- Triceps
- Brachioradialis
- Extensor digitorum
- Extensor carpi ulnaris

Deep muscles

- Deltoid
- Triceps
- Brachioradialis
- Supinator
- Extensor carpi radialis
- Extensor carpi ulnaris

△ Muscles of the upper limb – posterior aspect

Name of muscle	Position	Action
Triceps	Posterior aspect to the upper arm; from the scapula and humerus to the ulna	Extends the elbow; taking the forearm away from the upper arm
Extensor carpi radialis	Radial aspect of the back of the forearm; from the lower portion of the humerus to the second metacarpal	Extension of the wrist
Extensor carpi ulnaris	Ulna aspect of the back of the forearm; from the lower portion of the humerus to the fifth metacarpal	Extension of the wrist
Extensor carpi digitorum (not shown)	Medial aspect of the back of the forearm; from the lower portion of the humerus to the second to fifth fingers	Extension of the fingers
Supinator radii brevis	Lateral aspect of the back of the forearm; from the humerus to the radius	Supinates the forearm

Muscles of the lower limb

The muscles that bring about movement of the lower leg at the knee are situated in the thigh or upper leg and those that bring about movement in the ankle and toes are located in the lower leg. These muscles have long tendons that attach the muscles to the bones of the lower leg and foot.

Anterior aspect

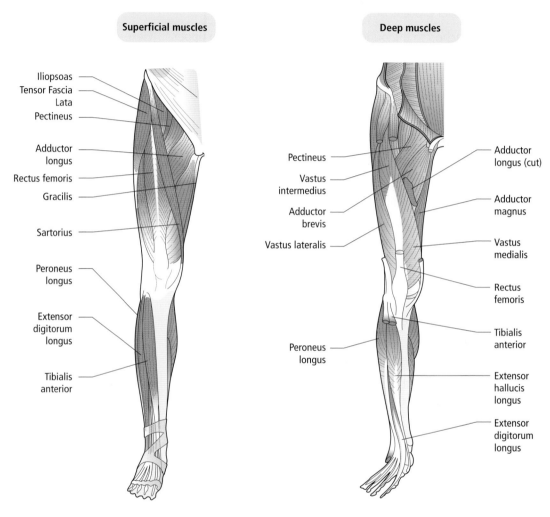

Superficial muscles

Iliopsoas
Tensor Fascia Lata
Pectineus
Adductor longus
Rectus femoris
Gracilis
Sartorius
Peroneus longus
Extensor digitorum longus
Tibialis anterior

Deep muscles

Pectineus
Vastus intermedius
Adductor brevis
Vastus lateralis
Peroneus longus

Adductor longus (cut)
Adductor magnus
Vastus medialis
Rectus femoris
Tibialis anterior
Extensor hallucis longus
Extensor digitorum longus

△ Muscles of the lower limb – anterior aspect

Name of muscle	Position	Action
Tensor facia lata	Found at the outside of the thigh; attaches to the ilium of the hip and runs down into a tendon that attaches to the lateral aspect of the tibia	Flexes, abducts and medially rotates the lower limb
Iliopsoas	Situated within the hip cavity; attached to the lower thoracic and lumbar vertebrae at one end and the smaller process of the femur	Rotates the lower limb medially and flexes the hip
Rectus femoris	Attached to the pubis bones at one end and the upper portion of the tibia via a large tendon, crossing both the hip and knee joints	Flexes the hip and extends the knee
Vastuslateralis	Attached to the large process of the femur at one end and the upper portion of the tibia via a large tendon at the other end	Extend the knee
Vastusmedialis	Attached to the femur at one end and the upper portion of the tibia via a large tendon at the other end	Extend the knee
Vastusintermedius	Attached to the shaft of the femur and the upper portion of the tibia via a large tendon at the other end	Extend the knee
Adductor longus	Found in the inner thigh; attached to the pubis and ischium bones and the shaft of the femur	Adducts and laterally rotates the lower limb; assist in flexing the hip
Adductor brevis	Found in the inner thigh; attached to the pubis and ischium bones and the shaft of the femur	Adducts and laterally rotates the lower limb; assist in flexing the hip
Adductor magnus	Found in the inner thigh; attached to the pubis and ischium bones and the shaft of the femur	Adducts and laterally rotates the lower limb; assist in flexing the hip
Pectinius	Found in the inner thigh; attached to the pubis and ischium bones and the shaft of the femur	Adducts and laterally rotates the lower limb; assist in flexing the hip
Gracilis	Attached to the pubis and ischium bones at one end and the medial bony process of the tibia at the other end	Adducts and rotates the lower limb medially and flexes the knee
Sartorius	Attached to the lateral anterior aspect of the ilium at one end and the medial process of the tibia at the other end	Flexes both the hip and the knee; also abducts and rotates the lower limb laterally
Tibialis anterior	Anterior aspect of the lower leg; attached to the tibia and the middle cuneiform and first metatarsal	Dorsi-flexes the ankle and inverts the foot
Extensor digitorumlongus	Anterior and lateral aspect of the lower leg; attached to the tibia and fibula and the phalanges of the toes	Extend the toes and help dorsi flex the ankle
Extensor hallucislongus	Anterior aspect of the lower leg; attached to the fibula and the phalanges of the big toe	Extend the big toe; dorsi-flexes and inverts the foot

Posterior aspect

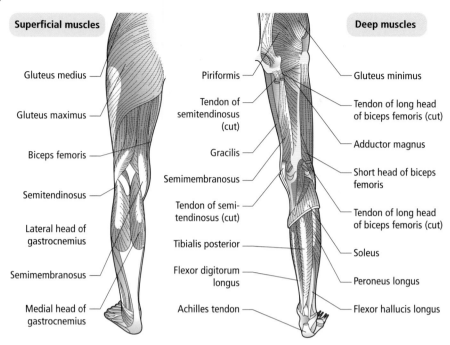

Superficial muscles

- Gluteus medius
- Gluteus maximus
- Biceps femoris
- Semitendinosus
- Lateral head of gastrocnemius
- Semimembranosus
- Medial head of gastrocnemius

- Piriformis
- Tendon of semitendinosus (cut)
- Gracilis
- Semimembranosus
- Tendon of semi-tendinosus (cut)
- Tibialis posterior
- Flexor digitorum longus
- Achilles tendon

Deep muscles

- Gluteus minimus
- Tendon of long head of biceps femoris (cut)
- Adductor magnus
- Short head of biceps femoris
- Tendon of long head of biceps femoris (cut)
- Soleus
- Peroneus longus
- Flexor hallucis longus

△ Muscles of the lower limb – posterior aspect

Name of muscle	Position	Action
Gluteus maximus	Large muscle forming the buttocks; attached to the ilium, sacrum and coccyx at one end and the upper portion of the femur at the other	Extends the hip
Gluteus medius	Attached to the ilium and the femur	Abducts the lower limb
Gluteus minimus	Attached to the ilium and the femur	Abducts the lower limb
Piriformis	Attached to the sacrum at one end and the large process of the femur at the other end	Rotates the lower limb laterally
Biceps femoris	Attached to the ischium at one end and the upper portion of the tibia and fibula at the other end, crossing the hip and the knee	Extends the hip and flexes the knee
Semitendinosus	Attached to the ischium and the tibia	Extends the hip and flexes the knee
Semimembranosus	Attached to the ischium and the tibia	Extends the hip and flexes the knee
Gastrocnemius	Posterior aspect of the lower leg, main muscle forming the calf. Attached to the lower part of the femur across the back of the knee and ankle to the calcaneum	Flexes the knee and plantar-flexes the ankle
Soleus	Located under the gastrocnemius; attached to the tibia and fibula across the ankle to the calcaneum	Plantar-flexes the ankle, an important action for propelling the body forward in walking and running
Tibialis posterior	Located very deep in the calf; attached to the tibia and fibula across the ankle to the navicular bone in the ankle	Assists in plantar-flexion of the ankle and inverts the foot

Name of muscle	Position	Action
Peroneus longus	Found laterally and posterior in the calf; attached to the fibula across the ankle to the underneath of the first and fifth metatarsals	Plantar flexes and everts the foot
Flexor digitorumlongus	Located deep in the posterior aspect of the lower leg; attached to the tibia and fibula and the phalanges of the toes	Flexes the toes and plantar-flexes and inverts the foot
Flexor hallucislongus	Located deep in the posterior aspect of the lower leg attached to the tibia and fibula and the phalanges of the big toe	Flexes the big toe and helps to plantar-flex and invert the foot

Disorders of the muscular system

Disease/disorder	Cause	Description
Fibrositis	A general term used by doctors to describe pain and stiffness in the muscles that have no apparent cause	Tenderness and stiffness in the muscles
Fibromyalgia	Caused by reduced energy production in the affected muscles and the inability of the fibres to relax	Pain in the muscle fibres that can be widespread throughout the body; varies in severity and can be made worse by cold and stress
Frozen shoulder	Cause is unknown but thought to be related to an injury or trauma to the area	Inflammation of the connective tissue surrounding the structures of the shoulder joint, resulting in pain and restricted movement of the joint
Lumbago	Caused by muscles or soft tissue sprain or strain after heavy work such as digging the garden	General term used to describe non-specific lower back pain
Muscular dystrophy	Inherited condition passed down through generations	Progressive condition that worsens over time. Causes muscle wasting, weakness, and degeneration, leading to immobility and reduced activity depending on the muscles affected
Myositis	Caused by a heightened autoimmune response or an infection	General term used to describe inflammation of the muscle tissue
Tendonitis (tendinitis)	Injury to the tendon; usually referred to by the specific tendon affected, e.g. achilles tendinitis	Literally means inflammation of the tendon; tendinitis is inflammation as a result of an injury to the affected tendon
Tennis/golfers elbow	Overuse of the muscles that affect the elbow joint such as the extensor carpi ulnaris or radialis during activity such as golf or tennis	Tendonitis of the elbow
Shin splints	Overwork of the muscles during a sport such as running or gymnastics, but can be caused by any sudden increase in intensity and duration of an activity in a person who is usually less active; the tendons and muscles become fatigued	Pain along the medial border of the tibia where the anterior muscles of the lower leg attach

Whiplash	Most whiplash injuries are caused by a rear-end motor car collision but are not exclusively associated. Any sudden distortion of the neck will give rise to the symptoms	A non-medical term used to describe an injury to the neck involving extreme displacement and extension in particular. Symptoms include pain in the neck and/or shoulders, headaches and sensory disturbances in the arm
Torticollis	Can be congenital when there is trauma to the neck during birth, resulting in excessive shortening of the sternocleidomastoid muscle on one side. Other non-congenital causes include infection of the ear, trauma and tumours in the area	Also known as wryneck, there is lateral flexion and the head is tilted to one side
Tetanus	Infection by the tetanus bacteria through a wound such as a cut or deep puncture wound	Prolonged contraction of the muscle fibres leading to muscle spasm
Sprain	Caused by trauma or exerted force to extend the range of the joint	Injury to the ligaments of a joint where they are stretched beyond their normal capacity
Strain	Overwork during activity or trauma	Injury to the muscle fibres, which tear as a result of over-stretching

Nervous system

The nervous system, together with the endocrine system, forms the body's internal communication system. The endocrine system uses a chemical message and the nervous system an electrical one (impulse).

The nervous system can be described in terms of reacting to external stimuli, such as sound, light, smell, taste and touch, all of which give the brain vital information in order to react to survive. The brain processes the information and decides on the appropriate action. These reactions can be in the form of muscle contraction in order to move away from danger, blinking for example closes the eye against foreign bodies, or may be an internal reaction such as the stimulation of a gland to produce a product, for example, the sweat glands may be stimulated to produce more sweat to cool the body as a result of the skin registering an increase in temperature. The functions of the nervous system are to:

- sense change in the external environment outside of the body, for example temperature
- relay information from the external environment via sensory organs, for example sight and sounds
- sense change within the internal environment of the body
- interpret and respond to these changes and information in order to maintain the body's homeostasis (i.e. the ability of the body to adjust its physiological processes in order to maintain its eternal equilibrium).

The nervous system is organised into three major parts:

- the central nervous system (CNS): the brain and spinal cord
- the peripheral nervous system (PNS): made up of motor sensory and autonomic nerves
- the autonomic nervous system (ANS): made up of the autonomic nerves which have two functions – sympathetic and parasympathetic.

These systems are made from nerve tissue and nerve cells and are specialised for the transmission of electrical type messages or impulses.

Nerve tissue

Nerve tissue is made up of nerve cells, known as **neurones**, which are capable of transmitting impulses which are like an electrical message. These impulses are created when there is a chemical change within the cell body caused by pressure, temperature change or other stimuli. Within the cell body are negatively charged potassium ions and outside the cell are positively charged sodium ions; when the chemical change occurs the membrane becomes permeable and the sodium ions leak into the cell body. The mix of the negatively and positively charged ions creates an electrical charge known as an impulse. Sodium and potassium ions are therefore known as neurotransmitters.

Each neurone joins along its length with the next, forming a junction or synapse, but one individual nerve cell can be up to a metre in length. The impulses are passed from one cell to the next from the brain and spinal cord to muscles to instigate contraction and to glands where they are stimulated to increase their activity, producing sweat for example. However, the most important function of the neurones is to take information from the external environment to the brain where it is considered and acted upon. There are three types of neurone, defined by their function:

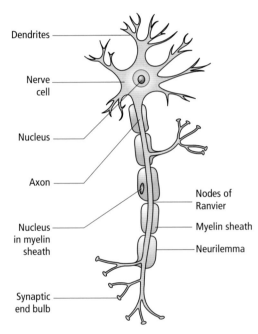

Dendrites

Nerve cell

Nucleus

Axon

Nodes of Ranvier

Nucleus in myelin sheath

Myelin sheath

Neurilemma

Synaptic end bulb

△ Structure of a typical nerve cell

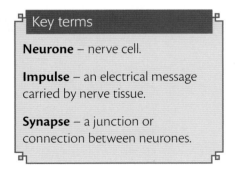

Key terms

Neurone – nerve cell.

Impulse – an electrical message carried by nerve tissue.

Synapse – a junction or connection between neurones.

- **Sensory or afferent neurones** receive stimuli and take the impulses to the spinal cord and brain.
- **Motor or efferent neurones** carry impulses away from the spinal cord and brain to muscles and glands.
- **Association or internuncial neurones** bring about the distribution of the incoming and outgoing impulses.

Structures associated with nerve cells

- Nerve cell body: contains the components of a typical cell such as the nucleus and mitochondria (see page 55 earlier in this chapter).
- Axon: carries impulses away from the cell body and can vary greatly in length from 1mm to over 1m.
- Dendrites: carry impulses to the cell body.

- Myelin sheath: a membrane that covers the axon of a nerve cell, it is made from fatty substances that insulate the nerve cell, ensuring the conduction of the impulse and increasing its speed.

- Nodes of Ranvier: gaps within the myelin sheath about 2–3mm in length that increase the rate of conduction of the impulse.

- Schwann cells: specialised **neuroglial** cells that exist outside of the CNS and are associated with sensory neurones. They wrap around the axon at intervals to protect and support the neurone.

- Neurilemma: the membrane that covers the Schwann cell.

Central nervous system (CNS)

The CNS consists of the brain and the spinal cord and is vital to the life and continued functioning of the body. It is considered to be the central area responsible for the assimilation and transmission of impulses to and from the external and internal body environments. It is protected by the skull (brain) and vertebrae of the spine (spinal cord) of the skeletal system.

Brain

The brain is the 'control centre' of the nervous system. Different areas of the brain specialise in the assimilation of different stimuli as shown in the diagram.

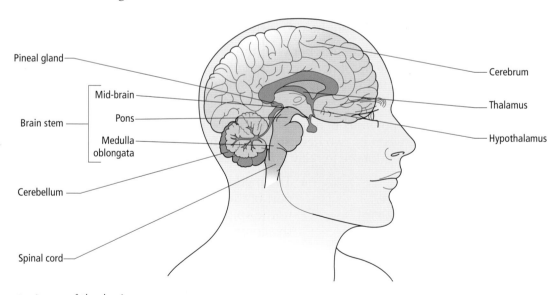

△ Areas of the brain

The brain is divided into three parts:
1 The cerebrum, which is divided into two hemispheres, which are further divided into lobes named after the skull bones under which they lie.
2 The cerebellum, or 'small brain', positioned under the cerebrum.
3 The brain stem, consisting of the hypothalamus, midbrain, pons and the medulla oblongata.

Cerebrum

The structure of the cerebrum has an outer layer made of folds of 'grey matter' consisting of nerve cell bodies. The inner layer of the cerebrum is made of 'white matter' or nerve fibres and it is these fibres that link the areas of the brain together so that the separate sections work together. This structure of the brain is responsible for controlling voluntary muscle contraction in movement and locomotion, the assimilation of conscious sensations such as pain, heat and cold and the control of mental activity such as reasoning and memory.

Cerebellum

The cerebellum sits under the cerebrum at the back of the skull and is divided into a left and right hemisphere; it has a similar structure with white matter on the inside surrounded by grey matter.

The functions of the cerebellum are more subconscious and include the coordination of muscular activity for the maintenance of muscle tone, posture and balance.

Brain stem

- The hypothalamus forms the uppermost part of the brain stem and is situated within the hemispheres of the cerebrum. Its function is to control the body's metabolism, water balance and body temperature. Emotions such as thirst, sex drive, pain and pleasure are elicited here and it is in close contact with the pituitary gland, the master gland of the endocrine system, forming a link between the two systems.

- The midbrain lies between the cerebrum and cerebellum and is made up of nerve cells and fibres. Its function is to relay information to and from the spinal cord and cerebrum and cerebellum.

- The pons sits in front of the cerebellum and bridges the gap between its two hemispheres. Its function is the same as that of the midbrain, to relay information.

- The medulla oblongata forms the lower part of the brain stem and is connected to the spinal cord. It forms a major role in the control of the body's functions. There are four control centres: 1) the cardiac centre, which controls the rate and force of the heart contractions, 2) the respiratory centre, which controls the rate and depth of breathing, 3) the vasomotor centre, which controls the constriction and dilation of the blood vessels and 4) the reflex centre, which controls vomiting, coughing, sneezing and swallowing.

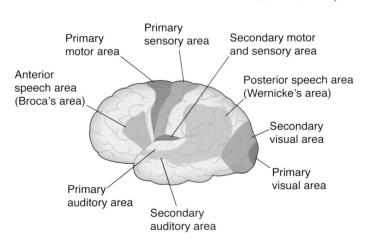

Primary motor area
Primary sensory area
Secondary motor and sensory area
Anterior speech area (Broca's area)
Posterior speech area (Wernicke's area)
Secondary visual area
Primary visual area
Primary auditory area
Secondary auditory area

△ Areas of the brain in terms of their function

Spinal cord

In connection and in continuation with the medulla oblongata, the spinal cord forms part of the central nervous system, stretching down the central back from the brain to the lumbar vertebrae. It is encased within the vertebrae of the spine and the arrangement of these bones allow for flexibility and protection. The spinal cord is made of grey matter encased by white matter with the nerve fibres running along its length. Its function is to relay messages sent to and from the peripheral nervous system and the brain.

Cerebrospinal fluid

This is a clear, colourless fluid that resembles blood plasma and is formed by specialist cells within the CNS. Its function is to:

● protect the brain and spinal cord by acting as a 'shock absorber' between these delicate organs and the bony structures that surround them

● maintain a constant pressure around the brain and spinal cord

● act as 'tissue fluid' in that it allows the flow of nutrients and the removal of waste products in and out of the CNS.

Meninges

The CNS is surrounded by three membranes or meninges which have a protective function. They are called:

● The dura mater – outermost layer

● The arachnoid mater – situated immediately below the dura mater.

● The pia mater – a vascular membrane which closely covers the brain and along the length of the spinal cord.

Peripheral nervous system (PNS)

The PNS is a network of sensory and motor nerve fibres that relay the electrical impulses to and from the CNS to the extremities and organs of the body. Sensory nerve fibres carry messages from the external environment to the CNS for assimilation and recognition. This gives the body details of its surroundings so that it can react in an appropriate or possibly even life-saving manner. The responses to these stimuli are transmitted to muscles, organs and glands via the motor nerves to bring about the necessary action. The PNS consists of pairs of nerves, one from the left and the other from the right side of the body:

● Twelve pairs of cranial nerves that emanate from the brain. Many of these have a purely sensory function, such as the optic nerve, or a purely motor function, such as the facial nerve that provides stimulus for the movement of facial muscles for expression, while others are a mix of both sensory and motor functions.

● Thirty-one pairs of spinal nerves that emanate from the spinal cord, eight from the cervical region of the spine, twelve from the thoracic, five each from the lumbar and sacral regions and one pair from the coccygeal. The spinal nerves are mixed with both sensory and motor functions and serve the specific areas of the body associated with the particular area of the spinal cord from which they leave through channels within the vertebrae.

Reflex arc

A reflex arc or action is the quick response to stimuli that could endanger or harm the body and serves as a means of protection. An example of this is when an object such as a flying insect comes too close to the eye. On seeing the insect, or at least being aware of it, the eye will blink and the muscles of the neck contract to move the head away quickly. This and other reflexes rely on the coordination of the sensory and motor neurones to and from the spinal cord with no impulse taken to the brain for assimilation and response. Instead the response is immediate, requiring no thought, and in this way the quickness of the response avoids the danger.

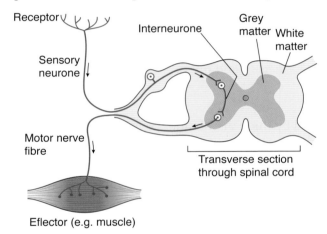

△ Typical reflex arc

Autonomic nervous system

The autonomic nervous system forms part of the peripheral nervous system but has an involuntary function. It is controlled by the hypothalamus within the brain and the nerve fibres arising from the medulla oblongata. The autonomic system is divided into two parts: the sympathetic and the parasympathetic.

Sympathetic

The function of the sympathetic part of the autonomic nervous system is to prepare the body for stressful situations, either excitement or 'fight or flight'. The nerve fibres arise from the thoracic and lumbar region of the spine and the neurones (nerve cells) release chemicals called hormones that bring about the following effects on the body:

- increased heart rate and force
- vasodilation of blood vessels in the heart and skeletal muscles
- vasoconstriction of blood vessels within the digestive system
- dilation of the bronchioles in the lungs, increasing lung capacity
- dilation of the pupils to increase the use of available light
- stimulation of the sweat glands to increase activity
- contraction of the arrector pili muscles in the skin to make hair 'stand on end'.

The nerve fibres arise from the brain and sacral region of the spine and their function is to maintain the body's normal functioning in non-stressful situations. The effects on the body are:

- decreased heart rate
- vasoconstriction of the coronary arteries of the heart
- vasodilation of the blood vessels in the digestive and urinary systems
- constriction of the bronchioles decreasing lung capacity.

Disorders of the nervous system

Disease/disorder	Cause	Description
Bell's palsy	Compression of the facial nerve as it runs through the temporal foramen leading to inflammation and swelling of the nerve	Paralysis of the muscles on the affected side of the face leading to a visual drooping of the features. The condition is temporary but recovery can take up to several months
Cerebral palsy	Damage to the CNS during pregnancy, birth or soon after as a result of bleeding or lack of oxygen	Signs and symptoms vary according to the part of the brain affected but include impaired speech, hearing or sight, muscle spasticity and poor coordination, muscle weakness and associated postural faults
Epilepsy	Reccurring seizures (fits) caused by abnormal and excessive neurological activity in the brain; causes are varied but can include trauma and/ or infection	There are several grades of seizure, from a simple loss of awareness or recollection to unconscious, violent fitting
Multiple sclerosis (MS)	Degeneration of the myelin sheath that leads to the nerve tissue being exposed in the CNS. Cause is unknown but factors thought to contribute to its development include changes in environment and climate in particular, genetically abnormal myelin or viral infection	Symptoms vary depending on the affected site but usually muscle weakness, lack of coordination and disturbed sensations such as burning or 'pins and needles'

Disease/disorder	Cause	Description
Parkinson's disease	Destruction of neurones and lack of neurotransmitters; specific causes are as yet unknown, but may be a result of environmental factors, misuse of drugs and repeated trauma to the head such as occurs in boxing	Symptoms include lack of muscle coordination, fixed muscle tone, muscle tremor and progressive disability with no effect on the intellect
Meningitis	Inflammation of the meninges, the protective membranes covering the brain and spinal cord due to infection with bacteria, virus or other micro-organisms	Symptoms include headache, stiff neck, vomiting, fever, confusion and drowsiness; sometimes a rash is also seen
Migraine	Cause is unknown but common triggers have been identified including stress, hunger or thirst, fatigue, hormone disturbances during menstruation, pregnancy or menopause. Some attribute the condition to foodstuffs such as cheese and red wine but there is no confirmed evidence that this is so	Severe headache affecting usually one side of the head with accompanied visual disturbances, increased sensitivity to light and sometimes to sound, nausea and vomiting
Sciatica	Pressure or damage to the sciatic nerve as it appears from the lumbar region and travels down the back of the leg	Pain, weakness, tingling or numbness in the affected leg
Carpal tunnel	Pressure to the median nerve in the forearm and wrist	Leads to numbness, tingling, weakness or muscle damage in the hand and fingers

Cardiovascular system

The cardiovascular system is the name given to the system by which blood is circulated around the body and it includes the heart, blood and blood vessels.

Heart

The heart is the centre of the cardiovascular system and is the driving force of the blood circulatory system because it is responsible for pumping the blood around the body. It is situated in the thoracic cavity between the lungs contained within a membrane called the pericardial sac and protected by the sternum. The centre of the heart lies centrally in the body but slightly angled to the left; in addition, the left-hand side of the heart is larger, leading to the misconception that the heart is on the left-hand side of the chest.

The heart is made of cardiac muscle tissue and contains four hollow chambers through which the blood is pumped by the contraction of the cardiac muscle tissue. The blood flow is controlled by the opening and closing of valves contained within the organ and it is the sound of these valves closing that give rise to the heart beat.

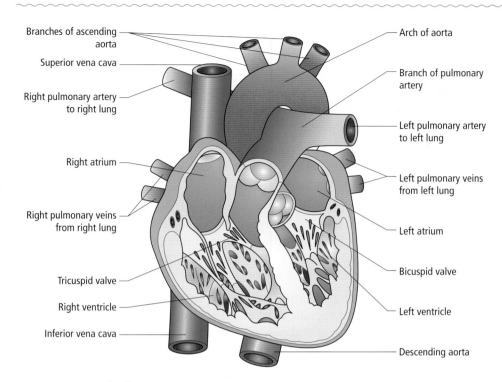

Branches of ascending aorta

Superior vena cava

Right pulmonary artery to right lung

Right atrium

Right pulmonary veins from right lung

Tricuspid valve

Right ventricle

Inferior vena cava

Arch of aorta

Branch of pulmonary artery

Left pulmonary artery to left lung

Left pulmonary veins from left lung

Left atrium

Bicuspid valve

Left ventricle

Descending aorta

△ Structure of the heart

Blood circulation

As mentioned previously, blood is moved along the vessels by the pumping action of the heart. The heart has four chambers: right atrium, right ventricle, left atrium and left ventricle. A wall separates the left and right sides and valves that open and close separate the top chambers from the bottom. The tricuspid valve separates the right atrium from the right ventricle; the bicuspid or mitral valve separates the left atrium and ventricle.

The valves allow blood to flow from the top atria into the bottom ventricles. When the heart contracts or beats, the right side beats just before the left and this pushes blood out of the ventricles into the blood vessels. The aortic valve and pulmonary valve in the vessels prevent the blood from reversing back into the heart so that when it relaxes blood is drawn into the atrium. The vessels from the lower right ventricle carry blood to the lungs where it gives up carbon dioxide and takes on fresh oxygen. It then returns to the heart, entering the top left atrium. The blood passes through the mitral valve into the bottom left ventricle where it is pumped out along a large vessel called the aorta, which supplies the whole body with blood. To complete the journey, blood returns from the areas of the body through the inferior and superior vena cava to the top right chamber to begin the cycle again.

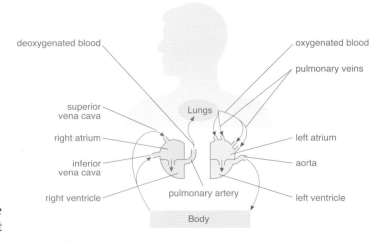

deoxygenated blood

oxygenated blood

pulmonary veins

superior vena cava

right atrium

inferior vena cava

right ventricle

Lungs

left atrium

aorta

pulmonary artery

left ventricle

Body

△ Simplified diagram of the blood circulation

Blood circulatory systems

There are a number of blood circulatory systems throughout the body:

- The pulmonary circulation system is the blood supply between the lungs and the right atrium of the heart, carrying deoxygenated blood which is then replaced with oxygenated blood by an interchange of gases within the lungs.

- Systemic (general) circulation system is the oxygenated blood supply to the body from the left ventricle of the heart omitting the pulmonary circulation.

- Coronary circulation system is the circulation concerned with the heart itself as a working organ. Blood vessels called the coronary arteries branch off the aorta almost immediately as it leaves the heart to supply freshly oxygenated blood to the cardiac muscle of the heart in order for it to contract.

- Portal/hepatic circulation system is part of the general blood circulation but specific from the digestive system to the liver where the latter metabolises and maintains safe levels of glucose, fats and protein in the blood before it is returned to the heart.

Blood

Blood is a liquid that is pumped by the heart through the blood vessels. There are approximately 5–6 litres of blood in an average-sized adult. Around 55 per cent of blood is made up of a yellowish/clear liquid called plasma, which consists of mainly water (90–92 per cent) in which mineral salts such as sodium chloride, nutrients from digestion such as amino acids and waste products are dissolved. Blood also transports hormones, antibodies, enzymes and proteins around the body. The other 45 per cent of blood is made up of red and white blood cells or corpuscles and thrombocytes.

Red blood cells (erythrocytes)

These are small biconcave discs with no nucleus which contain a protein called haemoglobin. They are capable of combining with oxygen to make oxy-haemoglobin, for which iron and vitamin B12 are required. Arterial blood containing a high percentage of oxygen will appear bright red in colour; whereas venous blood is a much darker red.

White blood cells (leucocytes)

Leucocytes are large, irregular-shaped cells that fight infection. They are produced in bone marrow and lymph nodes. They fight against disease and infection by destroying micro-organisms and ingesting bacteria, dead tissues and foreign bodies that may enter the body.

Thrombocytes (platelets)

Thrombocytes are responsible for blood clotting, preventing entry of micro-organisms into the body.

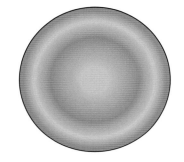

△ Erythrocyte

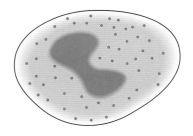

△ Leucocyte

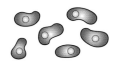

△ Thrombocyte

Functions of blood

Transport:

- Oxygen is carried from the lungs to all living tissues.

- Carbon dioxide is carried from the tissues to the lungs to be exhaled.

- Nutrients from the digestive system are carried to the tissues.

- Excess water is taken from the tissues to the kidneys for excretion.

- Waste products from cell activity are taken to the kidneys or skin for excretion.

- Hormones released from endocrine glands are carried to their target organs.

Defence:

- White blood cells are taken to a site of injury to fight invading bacteria and so stop infection.

- Other white blood cells produce antibodies that fight diseases that have entered the bloodstream.

- Blood proteins and platelets combine at the site of injury or damage to form a clot that plugs the wound, preventing blood loss and the invasion of bacteria. The clot hardens to form a scab, which protects the area while new tissue grows underneath.

Heat distribution and regulation:

- Body heat produced in the organs and muscles of the body is distributed around the body to maintain a temperature of 37°C.

- The dilation of the blood capillaries in the skin allows excess heat to be lost to the atmosphere. When the temperature of the body needs to be maintained, the blood capillaries constrict, preventing blood from nearing the surface of the skin.

Blood vessels

Blood is transported in a continuous network of vessels around the body. Blood is carried away from the heart in arteries and returns to the heart in veins.

The circulation away from the heart is very successful as the blood is under the most pressure in the arteries but there comes a problem when the blood tries to return to the heart. This is because there is reduced pressure in veins and, in the case of the legs, the blood needs to travel against the force of gravity. The blood circulation needs help from the contraction of nearby muscles to force the blood upwards. The important muscles in this are the gastrocnemius and the soleus. Blood is also further pushed upward when the diaphragm contracts and flattens during inhalation. This pushes the abdominal organs down, reducing the size of the cavity and causing blood to be pumped upward. As well as this, a suction pressure within the chest is created by inhaling and this draws blood from the lower parts of the body to the heart.

Structure and function of blood vessels

There are several types of blood vessels:

- Arteries: thick-walled blood vessels which transport blood away from the heart, carrying oxygen and nutrients to the cells and tissues. They vary in size but all have the same structure, with the walls consisting of involuntary muscle tissue that expands as blood is pumped into the artery. The artery then recoils, pushing the blood further on its way round the body, helping the blood to circulate around the body. The pulse or heart beat can be felt within the walls of these vessels and they assist in the maintenance of blood pressure.

- Arterioles: these are smaller arteries that extend from arteries and are formed mainly from muscular tissue, which are controlled by adrenaline from the sympathetic nervous system. These vessels are able to close off the supply of blood to some extent, for example from the skin tissues in order to conserve heat within the centre of the body. The arterioles open up again in conditions of warmth to allow heat from the centre of the body to reach the skin, where cooling will take place.

- Capillaries: the arterioles split up into a number of minute vessels known as capillaries. They are very fine vessels with walls that are one cell thick, which allows for the exchange of food and waste material, oxygen and carbon dioxide to and from the body cells. This is the only part of the circulation where exchange can take place. The dilation and contraction of these minute vessels help to regulate the body temperature and control the passage of blood in different parts of the body according to need.

- Veins: these are thinner-walled, muscular tubes which take blood away from the tissues and back to the heart. They have valves which prevent back-flow of blood. There is usually more blood than the amount needed for the circulation and the larger veins store this blood.

- Venules: these are small venous vessels which carry blood from capillaries to veins.

Blood vessels of the head, neck and face

Oxygenated blood leaves the heart through the aorta. This large vessel stretches upwards in front of the heart and then arches over to run down behind it. As it does so, two smaller arteries branch off and travel upwards on either side of the neck. Once in the neck area they are called the common carotid arteries and as they near the head they divide to form the external and internal carotid arteries. At the level of the ear, the internal carotid disappears through a hole in the skull to supply blood to the brain and eyes. The external carotid artery splits further to supply blood to the skin and muscles of the face and scalp. There are three main branches, called the facial artery, the temporal artery and the occipital artery and they supply blood to the areas after which they are named.

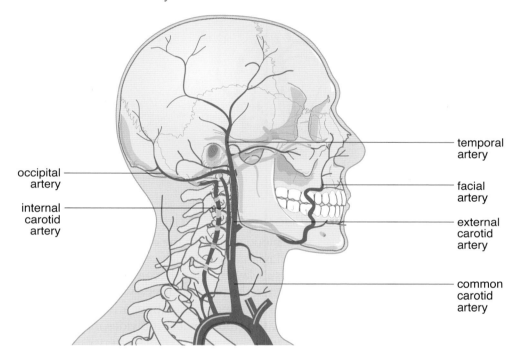

△ Arteries of the head, neck and face

Once the exchange of nutrients for waste products and oxygen for carbon dioxide has occurred in the capillaries the blood begins its journey back to the heart. The veins returning the blood back to the heart from the head and neck are called the internal and external jugular veins. The former exits the skull through a hole near the ear as before and the external jugular vein drains blood from the facial, temporal and occipital veins.

The internal and external jugular veins do not join together but run down the neck independently to join a large vein called the superior vena cava, which eventually returns the blood to the heart.

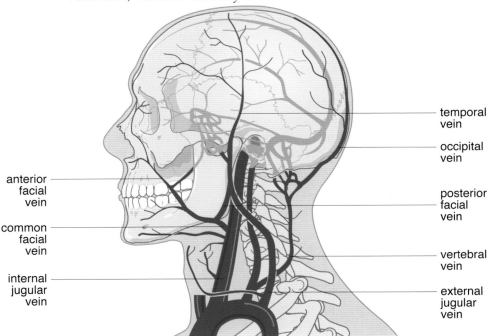

temporal vein

occipital vein

posterior facial vein

vertebral vein

external jugular vein

anterior facial vein

common facial vein

internal jugular vein

△ Veins of the head, neck and face

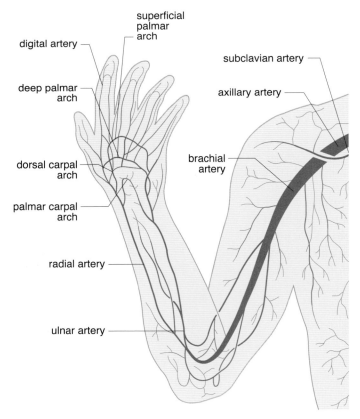

superficial palmar arch

digital artery

deep palmar arch

dorsal carpal arch

palmar carpal arch

radial artery

ulnar artery

subclavian artery

axillary artery

brachial artery

△ Arteries of the arm and hand

Blood vessels of the arm and hand

The blood supply to the arm begins with the subclavian artery, which branches off the aorta. The subclavian artery becomes the axillary artery and then the brachial artery, which runs down the inner aspect of the upper arm to about 1cm below the elbow, where it divides into the radial and ulnar arteries. The radial artery runs down the forearm next to the radius bone to the wrist, where it nears the surface and can be felt as the radial pulse. It continues over the carpals to pass between the first and second metacarpals into the palm. The ulnar artery runs down the forearm next to the ulna bone, across the carpals into the palm of the hand. Together they form two arches in the hand – the deep and superficial palmar arches. From all these arteries branch others to supply blood to the structures of the upper arm, forearm, hand and fingers.

The venous return of blood from the hand begins with the palmar arch and plexus, which is a network of capillaries present in the palm. Three veins carry the deoxygenated blood up the forearm: the radial vein, the ulnar vein and the median vein. The former two run parallel to the bones of the same name, the latter runs up the middle. Just above the elbow, the radial and ulnar veins join to become the brachial vein, and the median vein joins the basilic vein, which originates just below the elbow along with the cephalic vein. As the veins continue over the elbow they link to form a network that eventually divides, with the basilic vein joining the brachial vein, which then becomes the axillary vein. The cephalic vein travels up the arm separately and becomes the subclavian vein in the upper chest.

Blood vessels of the leg and foot

The aorta travels down the length of the trunk to the lower abdomen where it divides into two arteries which supply either leg. The artery in the thigh is called the femoral artery, named after the bone of the thigh. At the knee the femoral artery becomes the popliteal artery, which divides into two below the knee. One of these arteries runs down the front of the lower leg and is called the anterior tibial artery, while the other runs down the back and is known as the posterior tibial artery. This artery divides at the inside of the ankle, becoming the medial plantar artery on the inside of the foot and the plantar arch on the sole of the foot. The anterior tibial artery becomes the dorsal metatarsal artery on top of the foot.

There is a network of veins in the foot that become the dorsal venous arch on top of the foot. This travels the inside of the foot to the ankle, where it becomes the small saphenous vein. It continues up the back of the whole leg to the thigh, where it is known as the great saphenous vein. Two small veins called the anterior tibial veins travel up the front of the lower leg while two veins, the posterior tibial veins, run up the back. These four veins converge just below the knee to become the popliteal vein at the back of the knee and then eventually the femoral vein in the thigh. The great saphenous vein and the femoral vein join at the groin and return to the heart via the iliac vein inferior vena cava.

Blood pressure

Blood pressure is the force which is exerted on the walls of the blood vessels by the blood. It varies between the types of vessel, the highest being within arteries and the lowest in capillaries.

Blood pressure is measured using a sphygmomanometer and for medical purposes is measured in an artery, commonly the brachial artery in the arm. The pressure is measured by inflating a cuff placed around the arm which temporarily prevents the blood from flowing. The pressure is represented by two figures, one when the heart muscle contracts – systolic pressure – and the other when the heart is relaxing – diastolic pressure. A healthy adult will have a blood pressure of 120/80 mmHg (or millimetres of mercury).

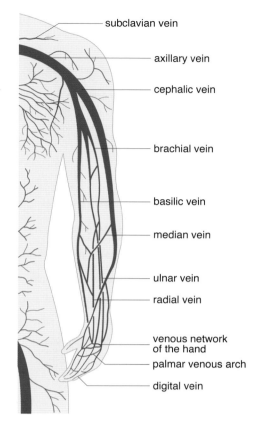

△ Veins of the arm and hand

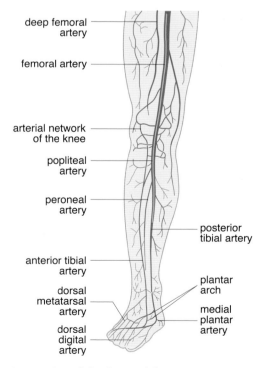

△ Arteries of the leg and foot

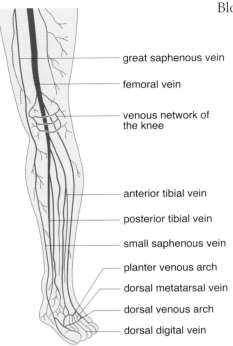

- great saphenous vein
- femoral vein
- venous network of the knee
- anterior tibial vein
- posterior tibial vein
- small saphenous vein
- planter venous arch
- dorsal metatarsal vein
- dorsal venous arch
- dorsal digital vein

△ Veins of the leg and foot

Blood pressure is affected by:

- cardiac output: blood pressure increases with exercise
- vasoconstriction: hormones such as adrenaline will cause the blood vessels to constrict, increasing blood pressure
- blood volume: during extensive blood loss, blood pressure is lost. The opposite is true of oedema because swelling increases blood pressure
- viscosity of the blood: the thicker the blood the higher the blood pressure; sitting still for several hours, such as when on an aeroplane, will cause the blood pressure to rise
- elasticity of the vessel walls: a loss of elasticity in blood vessels causes hardening of the artery walls and an increase in blood pressure.

Changes in blood pressure can be caused by:

- a decrease in the volume of blood caused by excessive blood loss, resulting in a drop in blood pressure
- an increase in volume such as that caused by fluid retention will cause a rise in blood pressure
- an increase in body temperature and increased activity and exercise. Stress will also cause an increase in blood pressure as the blood vessels constrict
- a period of inactivity such as relaxing and during treatments such as massage, both of which will cause blood pressure to drop.

Other systems connected to the cardiovascular system

The liver has numerous functions but its connection to the cardiovascular system is that it:

- breaks down worn out blood cells and destroys micro-organisms
- stores iron from broken down red blood cells.

The spleen assists the cardiovascular system by:

- destroying old and abnormal erythrocytes, leucocytes, platelets and microbes
- producing lymphocytes, namely B- and T-lymphocytes, in response to invasion of the body by disease-forming micro-organisms
- producing blood cells when needed.

Disorders of the cardiovascular system

Disease/disorder	Cause	Description
Angina	Obstruction within the coronary arteries	Chest pain associated with a lack of oxygen to the heart. The sufferer experiences pressure, heaviness, tightness, squeezing, burning or choking sensations
Hypertension (high blood pressure)	Sedentary lifestyle, obesity, smoking and stress all contribute to hypertension	Heart is placed under exertion as it is more difficult to pump blood around the body
Hypotension (low blood pressure)	Shock, blood loss; can indicate serious heart, endocrine or neurological disorder	Symptoms include dizziness and fainting. In someone who exercises frequently it can be a sign of good health
Stroke	Inadequate supply of blood to the brain because of a blockage in the blood vessels such as a clot or when a blood vessel in the brain bursts	Symptoms vary depending on the part of the brain affected but typically there is loss of sensation and movement to one side of the face and/or body
Deep vein thrombosis (DVT)	Blood clot in the deep veins of the leg normally but can affect the arm. Can occur after surgery and long periods of immobilisation, associated with obesity, injury or advanced age and on long haul flights	Affected limb will be painful, swollen, red and warm to the touch
Varicose veins	Can be hereditary but contributing factors are obesity, pregnancy, ageing, prolonged standing, leg injury, abdominal straining, and crossing legs at the knees or ankles	Condition affecting the superficial veins of the legs, although can affect any vein. As the walls are thinner, they stretch and the valves in the veins no longer meet, allowing blood returning up the leg to accumulate and stagnate in the vein. The thin walls then balloon, giving rise to the appearance of enlarged and bulbous blue/purple veins

Lymphatic system

The lymphatic system is a secondary circulation system that runs alongside the blood circulatory system. The lymphatic system defends the body from infection and works as a waste disposal system by removing waste products and toxins from the tissues by a network of fine tubes and larger vessels.

The functions of the lymphatic are to:

- transport waste products and foreign particles, including micro-organisms, away from the tissues

- return nutrients and blood proteins to the blood circulatory system

- prevent oedema by draining excess tissue fluid

- transport lymphocytes to the blood circulatory system

- produce lymphocytes that destroy waste products and toxins

- fight infection through the development of antibodies

- transport fats from the digestive system to the blood circulatory system.

Structures of the lymphatic system

The lymphatic system is made up of the following structures:

- lymph capillaries
- lymph vessels
- lymph nodes or glands
- lymph ducts
- lymphatic organs, such as the tonsils.

These structures together are responsible for lymph drainage where fluid within the body tissues is removed, cleansed and deposited back into the blood stream at the subclavian veins.

Lymph capillaries

These are fine, blind-ended tubes about the size of a blood capillary or a human hair; they have thin walls only one cell thick and are permeable to most substances. They are present between the cells of all tissues but are found in large numbers in the areas of the body most likely to become infected or where micro-organisms can enter easily, such as the toes, fingers, around the stomach and small intestine, the mouth, ears, eyes and nose. The tissue fluid enters the capillary by osmosis; the fluid, now known as lymph, contains waste products from cell metabolism and foreign particles and/or micro-organisms. The capillaries link to form larger lymph vessels.

Lymph vessels

The lymph capillaries form a network that join to form larger lymph vessels. These are similar to veins in structure in that they follow the venous return of blood to the heart. They have thin, weak, muscular walls and valves to prevent the backflow of lymph, again similar to veins.

The lymphatic system relies on the pumping action of surrounding muscles to move the lymph along these vessels. As the muscles contract they become shorter and fatter, which squeezes the lymph vessels and pushes the lymph along, with the valves preventing its return. This causes a vacuum below the valve, which is filled from lymph further down the vessel, causing more tissue fluid to be drawn into the lymph capillaries. In this way the lymph is transported through the vessels to the lymph nodes.

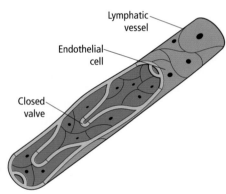

Lymphatic vessel

Endothelial cell

Closed valve

△ Structure of a lymph vessel

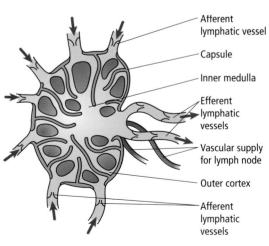

Afferent lymphatic vessel

Capsule

Inner medulla

Efferent lymphatic vessels

Vascular supply for lymph node

Outer cortex

Afferent lymphatic vessels

△ Structure of a lymph node

Lymph nodes

Lymph nodes are swellings along the lymph vessels that vary in size from a pinhead to a small nut such as an almond and are found all over the body. Here the lymph is cleansed by first being filtered and then by the action of special white blood cells. These cells destroy micro-organisms and other unwanted material so that when the lymph leaves the node it consists of mainly white blood cells and food materials. The nodes are found in groups so the lymph is forced to pass through several nodes to be cleansed before being deposited back in the bloodstream at the chest.

Lymph ducts

Once the lymph has been cleansed it travels along vessels to the chest area where it is deposited back into the bloodstream through large vessels called lymph ducts. Lymph collected from the right side of the head, chest and the right arm drains into the right lymphatic duct while lymph from the rest of the body drains into the thoracic duct. These ducts deposit the lymph into the subclavian veins. The cisterna chyli is a specific duct that drains fat-laden lymph from the digestive system.

These structures form the main lymphatic drainage system for the tissues of the body and their arrangement can be seen in the illustration below.

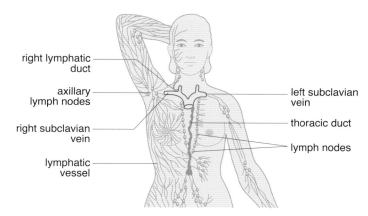

△ Position of the lymph ducts

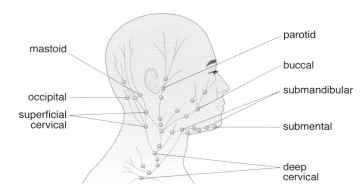

△ Lymphatic system of the head and neck

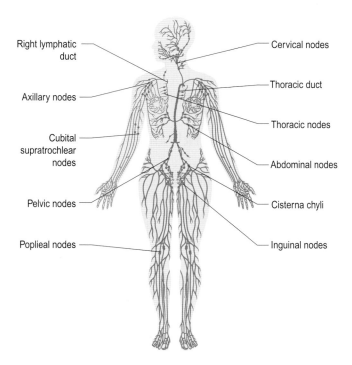

△ Lymphatic system of the body

Lymphatic organs

Other organs that make up the lymphatic system are described below.

● Tonsils: these lie at the back of the throat and protect this entrance to the body from invasion by bacteria.

● Small intestine: the lining of the ileum contains areas of lymphoid tissue called Peyer's patches, which protect the ileum from infection. Projecting into the small intestine are the villi containing the lacteals, which transport emulsified fats from the intestine and communicate directly with the lymph vessels. The transport of fats to the bloodstream is one of the main functions of the lymph system.

● Spleen: this is a red/purple organ or gland which lies on the left of the abdomen, under the 9th–11th ribs and is the largest of the lymphatic organs. It lies between the stomach and the kidney, just under the diaphragm. The inner capsule is divided by trabeculae and contains lymphoid tissue. The cells of the spleen come into direct contact with the blood and are bathed in blood and lymph. The spleen forms red blood corpuscles in the foetus (baby in the womb) and works with the bone marrow to produce extra red cells after blood loss due to severe injury or due to impairment of the bone marrow. It separates worn-out red cells from the bloodstream and manufactures lymphocytes.

● Thymus: this lies behind the sternum at the base of neck. It consists of two lobes joined by areolar tissue and its role is to mature T-lymphocyte cells.

● Pharynx: the posterior wall of the pharynx contains small masses of lymphoid tissue which form the pharyngeal tonsils or adenoids; like the tonsils, their role is to filter bacteria.

● Appendix: this is a fine tube, closed at one end, which leads from the colon. It is usually about 13 cm long and contains lymph tissue. Its role is to deal with foreign particles and micro-organisms in the digestive system.

△ Relationship between blood and lymph

Arteriole   Capillary   Venule

Plasma escapes capillary to bathe tissue cells

Waste products pass out of cell into capillary

Nutrients pass into cells

Tissue fluid

Excess fluid drains into lymph vessels

Filtered lymph re-enters bloodstream

Lymphatic vessel (blind-ended tube)

Lymph node

Origin and composition of lymph

Lymph is very similar in composition to that of blood plasma but it contains no erythrocytes, so appears straw-coloured rather than red. Lymph also contains fewer blood proteins and nutrients but does contain blood plasma substances such as fibrinogen, serum albumin and globulin and of course water. It also has a higher percentage of lymphocytes, fats and waste materials than blood plasma.

Lymph is derived from blood, leaking out of the blood capillaries by osmosis and capillary filtration and surrounding the cells. At this stage the fluid is known as tissue fluid and it bathes the cells, allowing the exchange of nutrients for waste products as the cells perform their function. The fluid is only known as lymph once it is taken up by the lymph capillaries.

Lymphatic system and immunity

The lymphatic system plays an important role within the body's defence system known as the immune system. Lymphatic tissue contains large numbers of white blood cells called lymphocytes. There are three types of lymphocytes that contribute to the immune responses: B-cells, T-cells and phagocytes:

- B-cells: develop into plasma cells that protect us against disease by producing antibodies that destroy or disarm antigens – the foreign cells and microbes invading the body. These antibodies remain in the blood stream for many years in some cases, providing protection from a particular disease for that time. Immunisation against disease is a treatment that has developed with this knowledge and involves inoculation with a vaccine. The vaccine contains a weakened version of the disease but the body still produces antibodies against it, protecting the body from the disease when exposed to it.

- T-cells: protect us against disease by attacking and destroying foreign cells and microbes directly.

- Phagocytes: this is a group of immune cells specialised in finding and engulfing bacteria, viruses and dead or injured body cells.

A sensitive immune system is often responsible for allergic reactions that can be experienced when in contact with everyday objects or particles. When exposed to the allergen, the body's defence system comes into action, bringing about an allergic response that may include sneezing and watery eyes (as with hay fever) and wheezing and tightness of the chest (as with asthma) and swelling, erythema, itching and irritation (as with a skin allergy). Autoimmunity is when the body fails to recognise its own constituent parts as self, seeing them instead as an antigen or allergen, and triggers the immune system into a response.

Disorders of the lymphatic system

Disease/disorder	Cause	Description
Cancer	Specific causes of a specific cancer are unknown but many things are known to increase the risk of cancer, including tobacco use, infection, radiation, lack of physical activity, poor diet and obesity and environmental pollutants	Normal cells control their own growth and destroy themselves if they are abnormal. In cancer the cells do not do this, allowing abnormal cells to grow into malignant tumours. These abnormal cells can easily be spread by the normal functioning of the lymphatic system as it places them into the blood stream
HIV/AIDS	Invasion by the body of the human immunodeficiency virus	Acquired immune deficiency syndrome is the result of the invasion by HIV; the virus interferes with the immune system, making the sufferer susceptible to infections which can be fatal
Lymphoedema	Localised fluid retention due to the lymphatic system being compromised, e.g. blocked or damaged	There is considerable swelling and pain or burning

Disease/disorder	Cause	Description
Mastitis	Inflammation of the breast tissue as a result of breast feeding	The tissues become sensitive and painful, with localised swelling and warmth and maybe erythema
Oedema	Can be of a systemic nature associated with heart, kidney, lung or endocrine disorders or can be temporary due to an obstruction in the lymph vessels or as a result of an injury	Medical term for fluid retention; there is swelling in the affected area and also maybe pain, burning sensation, joint stiffness, aching limbs and raised blood pressure

Endocrine system

The endocrine is a message-relaying system and works with the nervous system to control the functions of the body. Unlike the nervous system there are no structures along which these messages are carried and instead the messages are carried in the blood circulatory system. The messages concerned are chemical messages called hormones and are produced by ductless glands called endocrine glands. The messages are deposited directly into the blood for transportation.

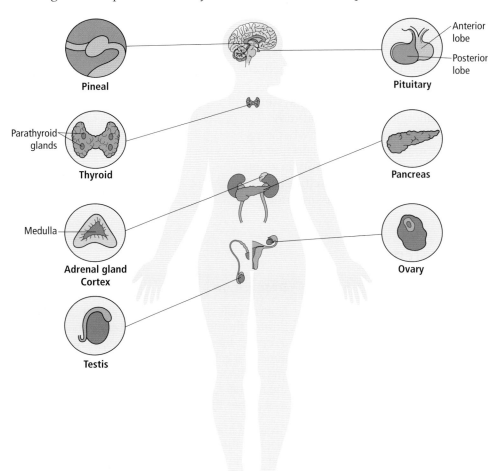

Hormones control the following functions of the body:

- emotions
- appetite
- sexual activity
- metabolism
- water balance.

The main glands that make up the endocrine system are:

- pituitary (anterior and posterior)
- pineal
- thyroid
- parathyroids
- thymus
- adrenals
- pancreas (Islets of Langerhan)
- gonads (ovaries and testes).

△ Position of the endocrine glands

Glands of the endocrine system and the hormones they produce

Endocrine gland	Hormone secreted	Target site for the hormone	Function of the hormone
Hypothalamus: ● Found in the brain ● Often called the 'master' gland ● Forms an attachment with the pituitary gland allowing two-way communication to take place between the endocrine and nervous systems			Detects the level of hormones in the blood and secretes hormones into the pituitary glands
Anterior pituitary: ● Is about the size of a pea ● Situated at the base of the brain behind the nose ● Linked to the hypothalamus ● Its hormones control the other endocrine glands	Thyroid stimulating hormone (TSH)	Thyroid	Regulates the body's metabolism
	Adrenocorticotropic hormone (ACTH)	Suprarenal glands	Stimulates the adrenal cortex to produce hormones such as cortisol
	Somatotrophic or growth hormone	Bones and other hard tissue	Increases rate of growth in adolescents and maintains size in adults
	Follicle stimulating hormone (FSH)	Sex organs	Increases production of oestrogen and the maturation of ovarian follicles as part of the menstrual cycle in women and stimulates sperm production in men
	Luteinising hormone (LH)	Sex organs	Prepares breasts for lactation during pregnancy and the production of progesterone in women and testosterone in men
	Lactogenic hormone (prolactin or PRL)	Mammary glands	Stimulates the production of milk
Posterior pituitary	Antidiuretic hormone (vasopressin or ADH)	Kidneys and arteries	Decreases urine production
	Oxytocin	Uterus and breasts	Stimulates labour and ejects milk from the breast
Pineal	Melatonin	Brain	Regulates the body clock
Thyroid: ● Consists of two lobes which take the shape of a butterfly ● Situated just below the larynx and in front of the trachea in the neck	Thyroxine	Throughout the body	Controls basal metabolic rate
	Calcitonin	Bones and kidneys	Regulates calcium levels in the blood

Endocrine gland	Hormone secreted	Target site for the hormone	Function of the hormone
Parathyroids: • Four parathyroid glands arranged in pairs • Each pair is embedded on the back of the lobes of the thyroid gland	Parathormone (PTH)	Bones	Regulates calcium and phosphorus levels; increases blood calcium levels and activates vitamin D
Adrenals: • Situated on top of each kidney • Each gland is composed of an outer cortex and inner medulla	Mineralocorticoids, e.g. aldosterone	Kidneys	Regulates the mineral content of body fluids, salt and water balance and therefore blood pressure
	Glucocorticoids e.g. cortisol	Liver	Regulates metabolism of carbohydrates in response to stress
	Sex hormones (oestrogen and androgens)	Reproductive organs	Development and functioning of the sex glands and gives rise to the secondary sexual characteristics associated with puberty
	Adrenaline	Several target organs including muscles, eyes, skin, digestive system, etc.	Controls the 'fight or flight' mechanism
	Noradrenalin	Blood vessels	Causes blood vessels to constrict and so responsible for an increase in blood pressure
Pancreas: Elongated flat organ Situated within the abdomen	Insulin	Blood sugar	Controls the metabolism of carbohydrates and lowers blood sugar levels
	Glucagon	Blood sugar	
	Somatostatin	Several organs	Controls the levels of other hormones such as growth hormone and insulin

Note: The pancreas also has a digestive function to secrete pancreatic juice for the digestion of proteins.

Ovaries	Oestrogen	Female reproductive organs and breasts	Responsible for the secondary sexual characteristics of girls during puberty; regulates the menstrual cycle
	Progesterone	Female reproductive organs and breasts	Active during pregnancy, the development of the placenta and the preparation of the breasts for lactation
Testes	Androgens	Male reproductive organs	Development of the secondary sexual characteristics of boys: development of the genitalia, male hair growth patterns, increase in muscle bulk and deepening of the voice
	Testosterone	Male reproductive organs	Promotes the development of the sperm in the testes

Disorders of the endocrine system

Disease/disorder	Cause	Description
Goitre	Inflammation of the thyroid gland	Swelling of the thyroid gland resulting in swelling of the neck and voice box
Hyperthyroidism: Graves' disease	Hyper (excessive) secretion of thyroxine	Symptoms are weight loss, insomnia, hyperactivity, palpitations and increased blood pressure, bulging eyes, muscle weakness and moist, warm skin
Hypothyroidism: Cretinism	Hypo (inadequate) secretion of thyroxine in children	Small stature but with fat deposits and impaired mental ability
Myxoedema	Hypo secretion of thyroxine in adults	Lethargy, slow metabolism, slow mental and physical activity, brittle hair and nails, dry and coarse skin
Polycystic ovaries	Hyper secretion of testosterone and other male sex hormones	Cysts on the ovaries that cause menstruation to cease, hair growth in a male pattern, development of obesity
Cushing's syndrome	Hyper secretion of glucocorticoids	Weight gain, excess growth of facial and body hair, raised blood pressure and bone softening
Addison's disease	Hyper secretion of adrenocorticosteroids	Loss of appetite and weight loss, low blood sugar and blood pressure, tiredness and muscle weakness
Acromegaly	Hyper secretion of growth hormone in adults	Thickening of the bones, most apparent in the face, hands and feet
Dwarfism	Hypo secretion of growth hormone	Stunted growth
Gigantism	Hyper secretion of growth hormone in children	Rapid growth with abnormally large hands and feet with coarse features
Diabetes mellitus	Deficiency or absence of insulin	Increased thirst and urine output, weight loss
Diabetes insipidus	Lack of the vasopressin hormone	Dehydration, increased thirst and urine output
Amenorrhoea	Hormonal disturbances associated with the hypothalamus or the pituitary glands; a symptom of anorexia	Absence of menstrual cycle and no periods
Gynaecomastia	Hyper secretion of oestrogen and progesterone in males	Development of large breasts in males and muscle atrophy
Hirsutism	Over-production of androgens in women	Hair growth in a male sexual pattern
Seasonal Affective Disorder (SAD)	Hypo secretion of melatonin	Depression, slow mental and physical activity, excessive sleeping and overeating
Virilism	Hyper secretion of testosterone in women	Masculinisation occurs, e.g. deepening of the voice

Respiratory system

The respiratory system is responsible for the process by which vital oxygen is extracted from the air and made available for use by every cell of the human body. The air that we breathe contains only 21 per cent oxygen and of that, only 4 per cent is utilised by the respiratory system. Without oxygen the body's cells die within two or three minutes, with the brain cells being most sensitive to a lack of oxygen resulting in brain damage.

The respiratory system is the most important excretory system in the human body as it removes the waste product produced by this process – carbon dioxide – and expels it into the external environment. If carbon dioxide is allowed to accumulate in the body, it becomes poisonous and therefore dangerous.

Most of the organs of the respiratory system lie within the thoracic cavity (chest) of the body, with the openings of the mouth and nose providing the link to the external environment.

The rates at which oxygen is inhaled and carbon dioxide exhaled are determined within the respiratory centre situated in the medulla oblongata of the brain stem.

Structures of the respiratory system

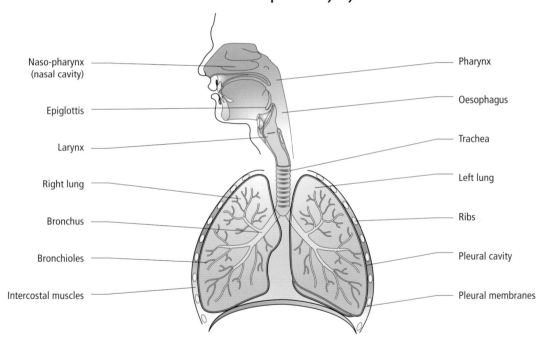

Naso-pharynx (nasal cavity)
Epiglottis
Larynx
Right lung
Bronchus
Bronchioles
Intercostal muscles

Pharynx
Oesophagus
Trachea
Left lung
Ribs
Pleural cavity
Pleural membranes

△ Structures of the respiratory system

- Nose: consists of two nasal cavities; moistens, warms and filters air.
- Pharynx: two distinct areas – the back of the nose and back of the throat. The air continues to be warmed in the pharynx.
- Larynx (voice box): when air passes over the vocal chords the voice is created; during swallowing the larynx is closed off by the epiglottis.

- Trachea: the main airway from the nose and mouth to the lungs. Rings of cartilage hold the trachea open during breathing.

- Bronchi: two tubes derived from the trachea, one into each lung.

- Bronchioles: smaller tubes which branch from the bronchi within the lung tissue and divide into even smaller tubes that lead to the alveoli. There are no cartilage rings present.

- Alveoli: small sacs where gaseous exchange takes place (external respiration). Surrounded by numerous blood capillaries.

- Lungs: two lungs that lie in the thoracic cavity.

- Pleura: a membrane that lines the outer surface of each lung and the inside of the thoracic cavity; between is a space called the pleura cavity.

- Diaphragm: a thin sheet of muscle that separates the thoracic and abdominal cavities; when it lowers it increases the chest cavity and causes air to be drawn into the lungs.

Stages of respiration

There are two stages of respiration that deliver vital oxygen and remove carbon dioxide from the tissues:

- external respiration: the exchange of oxygen and carbon dioxide with the external environment, the air.

- internal respiration: the exchange between the internal environment at the tissues known as gaseous exchange.

External respiration

The thoracic cavity exists within a 'vacuum' and when the volume of this cavity increases by the lowering of the diaphragm and the raising of the ribs, the lungs inflate and air is drawn into the body (as long as either the nose or mouth is open).

The oxygen in the air diffuses through the wall of the alveoli into the blood and carbon dioxide diffuses from the blood through the wall into the alveoli.

Internal respiration

This is the diffusion of oxygen from the blood into any of the tissues for use by the body's cells and the waste product carbon dioxide produced by the cells during metabolism into the blood.

Principles of gaseous exchange

Internal and external respiration relies on the process of diffusion, which is defined as:

'Gases diffuse from a higher pressure to a lower pressure until equal pressure is achieved.'

Disorders of the respiratory system

Disease/disorder	Cause	Description
Asthma	Allergen/antigen such as a micro-organism or cold air	Lining of the airway becomes inflamed and swells and the muscles within the walls of the airway tighten; together there is a narrowing of the airway and the person has difficulty breathing, as well as coughing, wheezing and a tight feeling in the chest
Hay fever	Allergen is usually pollen or spores from plants	When the pollen enters the airway the linings release histamine, which brings about the allergic reaction of sneezing, runny nose, watery and itchy eyes
Bronchitis	Acute bronchitis is caused by a respiratory viral infection, e.g. cold or flu	Structures of the respiratory system become inflamed, starting with the nose, sinuses and throat and spreading to the lungs. Symptoms are chest pain, cough with mucous, wheezing, shortness of breath and fatigue
Pneumonia	Infection of the lungs caused by viruses, bacteria or fungi	Susceptible people are the young and the elderly where there is a chance of death if left untreated. Other risk factors are smoking, recent cold or flu, heart disease. Symptoms include cough, fever, shortness of breath, sharp or stabbing chest pain
Pleurisy	Pneumonia or other chest infections can lead to pleurisy	Inflammation of the lining of the lungs, leading to sharp chest pain during breathing and coughing
Emphysema	Prolonged bouts of other respiratory conditions such as bronchitis. Caused by smoking or exposure to gases and smoke, e.g. while at work	Destruction of the lung tissue, resulting in permanent narrowing of the airways leading to breathing difficulties
Sinusitis	Inflammation of the linings of the sinuses caused by a bacterial or viral infection	Symptoms are runny or blocked nose, pain or tenderness in the face, headache, pressure problems with the ears and loss of taste and smell
Rhinitis	Can be caused by a viral infection such as a cold but also as a response to an allergen such as smoke, perfumes, paint fumes, etc.	Inflammation of the lining of the nose temporarily giving rise to cold-like symptoms

Digestive system

The digestive system consists of a number of organs and structures that are involved with the process of taking in food and making it available to the body for absorption. The digestion system is coordinated by the hypothalamus of the brain, hormones and nerves.

All the energy the body needs and the raw materials for growth and repair of body structures come from the ingestion of food and drink. The food and fluids are processed by the digestive organs into small nutrient molecules that can be absorbed from the intestine and circulated around the body for use by the organs, tissues and cells to perform their individual functions. Any materials left after absorption that cannot be ingested become waste material or faeces and are eliminated from the body by defecation.

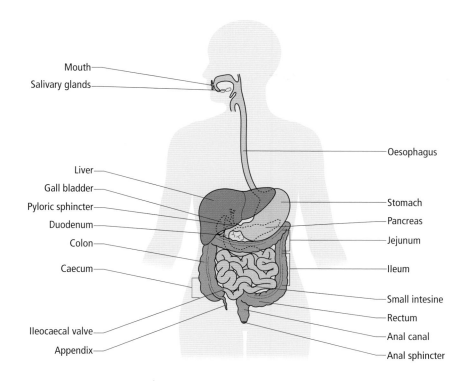

Mouth
Salivary glands
Liver
Gall bladder
Pyloric sphincter
Duodenum
Colon
Caecum
Ileocaecal valve
Appendix
Oesophagus
Stomach
Pancreas
Jejunum
Ileum
Small intesine
Rectum
Anal canal
Anal sphincter

△ Structures of the digestive system

Process of digestion

The process of digestion can be divided into the following stages:

- Ingestion: the journey of food along the alimentary canal begins in the mouth. Here, mechanical digestion takes place with the food being broken into small pieces by mastication (chewing). Chemical digestion also begins by the action of saliva which wets and softens the food ready for swallowing.

- Digestion: once in the stomach, digestion begins and involves both the mechanical and chemical breakdown of the food stuffs ready for absorption. The stomach and accessory organs produce juices which contain enzymes that break down the food into its constituent parts, while churning the contents to ensure that the food stuffs and juices are thoroughly mixed.

- Absorption: the contents of the stomach are periodically released into the small intestine so that the digested food can pass through the walls into the surrounding blood and lymph capillaries for circulation round the body to be used by cells and tissues.

- Elimination: food substances which have been eaten but cannot be digested and absorbed are excreted by the bowel.

Structures of the digestive system

The structures of the digestive system can be divided into two parts – the alimentary canal and the accessory organs. The alimentary canal is made up of:

- mouth
- pharynx
- oesophagus
- stomach
- small intestine
- large intestine.

The accessory organs involved with digestion are:

- liver
- gall bladder
- pancreas.

Mouth

The tongue, teeth and salivary glands all have a part to play in the digestive processes that occur in the mouth. The tongue is used to move and mix the food, presenting it to the teeth for mastication.

The teeth perform the tearing off and breaking down of the food into smaller particles that are easier to swallow and are assisted by the muscles of mastication that provide the force needed. There are different types of teeth, each performing different functions within this mechanical digestion process.

The incisor and canine teeth are used for biting off pieces of food and have sharp edges for this purpose. The premolars and molars have broad, flat surfaces and are used for grinding and chewing the food into smaller pieces.

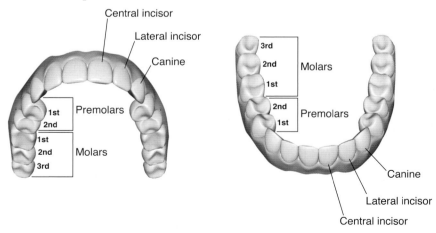

△ Different types of permanent teeth

The saliva glands in the mouth provide the chemical digestion part of the process. The glands produce saliva, which serves two functions: first, it moistens the food, making it easier to swallow and then it begins the breakdown of carbohydrates (mainly starch).

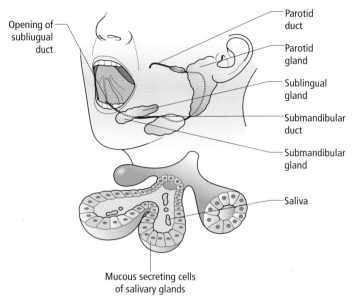

Opening of subliugual duct

Parotid duct

Parotid gland

Sublingual gland

Submandibular duct

Submandibular gland

Saliva

Mucous secreting cells of salivary glands

△ Salivary glands

Pharynx

After sufficient chewing and mixing with saliva the ball of food is forced to the back of the mouth by the tongue into the pharynx or throat, where it is swallowed by the action of the muscles of the pharynx.

Oesophagus

The oesophagus is a tube that links the mouth and throat to the stomach. Involuntary muscle tissue within the walls of the oesophagus contract in a wave-like motion called peristalsis to move the ball of food into the stomach.

Stomach

The stomach is positioned to the left-hand side of the abdominal cavity underneath the diaphragm and is a strong muscular hollow structure into which the ball of food from the mouth enters via the cardiac sphincter. The inner lining of the stomach is made of specialised epithelial cells that secrete gastric juices that break down the food ball into its chemical constituent parts, namely the enzyme pepsin, which acts upon proteins in the food and hydrochloric acid, which is needed to activate the pepsin. The latter also destroys the micro-organisms present in and on food. The muscular walls of the stomach contract to churn and mix the gastric juices and the food together to ensure thorough break down into its chemical parts so that they can be absorbed by the body. Alcohol and water are absorbed through the stomach wall into the blood stream. Food can remain in the stomach for 4–5 hours and is released in phases into the small intestine via the pyloric sphincter.

Liver

The liver has several important functions within the body and assisting in the digestion of food is just one. It is a large organ situated in the upper abdominal cavity to the right of the stomach and produces an alkaline substance called bile. Bile is stored in the gall bladder and released into the small intestine to neutralise the acidic contents of the stomach. The other functions of the liver include:

- storage of vitamins A, B and D, iron and other minerals

- detoxification of the blood, e.g. removal of drugs, including alcohol

- conversion of carbohydrates into fats to be stored elsewhere in the body.

Gall bladder

The gall bladder is a small organ connected to the liver and the small intestine and stores the bile until it is needed.

Pancreas

The pancreas is situated behind the stomach and serves a digestive and endocrine function. To aid digestion, it produces pancreatic juice containing several enzymes which act upon fats, carbohydrates and proteins in the food to break them down into their chemical components so they can be absorbed.

Small intestine

The small intestine is a hollow tube about 7 metres long that winds around to fill the abdominal cavity. It has numerous folds or projections into the centre of the tube called villi which increase its surface area and facilitate the absorption of the chemical parts of the food ball being broken down by the action of enzymes. It has three distinct parts:

- Duodenum: the first part of the small intestine and is about 25–30cm long. The bile and pancreatic ducts open out into the duodenum and intestinal juice is produced by special cells in the lining to digest the food, further acting upon fats, carbohydrates and proteins.

- Jejunum: about 2.5 metres long and follows on from the duodenum.

- Ilium: about 4.2 metres long and follows on from the jejunum. It empties into the large intestine via the ileo-caecal sphincter. Absorption of the nutrients from the food has mostly been completed, including the re-absorption of water, and what remains is a hardened mass of undigested material. Present also at the junction of the ilium with the large intestine is the appendix, a small projection about 8cm long made of lymphatic tissue.

Large intestine

The large intestine is about 1.5 metres long and is often called the colon. It has three parts

- Ascending colon: runs from the lower right-hand side of the abdomen upwards towards the ribs.

- Transverse colon: runs across the upper abdominal cavity from right to left.

- Descending colon: runs down the left-hand side of the abdominal cavity.

The hardened undigested material or faeces is pushed through the large intestine by the action of its muscular walls into the rectum and finally excreted out of the anus.

Dietary components

The foods we eat are a complex and varied mix of the following dietary components and it is the job of the digestive system to break these down into chemical components that are small enough to be absorbed and utilised by the body. The main dietary components are:

- carbohydrates

- fats

- proteins

- vitamins

- minerals

- fibre

- water.

Dietary component	Common food sources	Chemical components	Use in the body
Carbohydrates including starch, sugar and cellulose	Cereals, confectionary, potatoes, pasta and rice, fruit and milk and milk products	Glucose; fructose; sucrose; lactose	Prime source of energy in the body but can be converted into body fat when eaten in excess
Fats	Meat, milk and milk products, crisps and peanuts, biscuits and chocolate	Fatty acids	Used for energy and insulation to maintain body temperature but stored when eaten in excess
Proteins	Meat, chicken, fish, pulses	Amino acids	Growth and repair of body tissues; can be used for energy if carbohydrates and fats are not available
Vitamins A, B, C, D, E and K	Variety of fresh foods such as meat and fish, fruit and vegetables	N/A	Healthy functioning of the body's organs
Minerals such as calcium, sodium, iron, etc.	Meat and fish, cereals and grains, fruit and vegetables	N/A	Healthy functioning of the body's organs
Fibre	Wholegrain cereals, pulses, fruit and vegetables	Unchanged by digestion	Insoluble fibre adds bulk to the faeces; soluble fibre reduces blood cholesterol levels
Water	Found in many of our foods as well as in the fluids we drink	Unchanged by digestion	Essential for life; needed by many of the body's processes

Disorders of the digestive system

Disease/disorder	Cause	Description
Crohn's disease	Caused by a genetic disposition to the immune system reacting to its environment. Foods, stress and some drugs including cigarette smoking are thought to be aggravating factors	Inflammation of the digestive tract with a variety of symptoms from abdominal pain, diarrhoea, vomiting and weight loss
Gall stones	Deposits such as cholesterol accumulate in the gall bladder; exacerbated by diabetes, liver dysfunction, organ transplant or rapid weight loss associated with 'crash' dieting	Hard, stone-like accumulations found within the gall bladder, varying in size from as small as a grain of sand to a table-tennis ball. Symptoms include pain in the abdomen, fever and jaundice
Hiatus hernia	Obesity, pregnancy, heavy lifting, excessive coughing or sneezing, constipation	A weakness in the diaphragm allows a part of the stomach to protrude through into the thoracic cavity, leading to dull pain in the chest, shortness of breath and heart palpitations
Irritable bowel syndrome (IBS)	Cause is unknown but stress is thought to be a contributing factor; also certain foods can aggravate the condition	Symptoms include pain and discomfort, bloating and bouts of diarrhoea and constipation

Excretory/urinary system

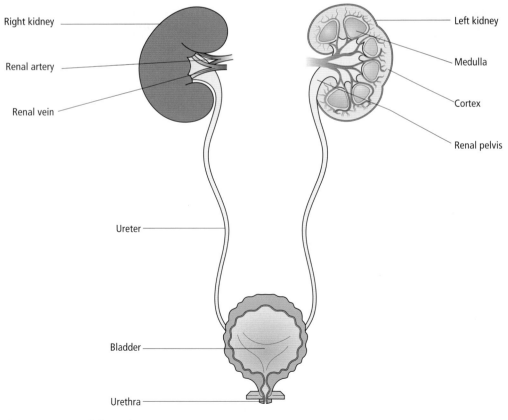

△ Structures of the urinary system

The organs of the urinary system form part of the body's excretory system, the others being the skin and the respiratory system. The urinary system is involved with the regulation and balance of water levels within the body and the elimination of water soluble waste products. Its functions are to:

- filter the blood, removing waste products
- balance fluid intake with the elimination of excess fluid in the form of urine
- distribute tissue fluid throughout the body
- balance the body's salts needed for cellular function
- maintain safe levels of pH within the body's fluids and therefore assist in cellular processes such as osmosis
- regulate blood pressure.

Structure of the urinary system

The urinary system includes the following organs:

- kidneys
- ureters
- bladder
- urethra.

Kidneys

The kidneys are two bean-shaped organs fixed to the inner back wall of the abdominal cavity behind the liver and the stomach. They are supplied with blood by the renal arteries which have branched off the descending aorta as it travels down the body and before it splits to form the femoral arteries. Blood is filtered as it is taken through the intricate structure of the kidney, removing the toxic nitrogen-enriched waste from the blood plasma to produce urine. This process occurs within millions of tiny structures within the kidney called nephrons and can be explained as follows:

1. The increase in pressure of the blood entering the fine blood capillaries within the kidney forces the blood plasma out of the capillaries and is captured by the nephrons – a process called filtration.

2. The captured fluid is taken through a series of winding tubes where substances such as body salts, vitamins, amino acids and glucose within the fluid are reabsorbed by osmosis back into the blood stream and are taken away from the kidney by the renal vein, leaving the harmful substances and excess water. This process is called selective reabsorption.

This excess water and waste product is now called urine and is collected at the core of the kidney and passed into the ureters.

Ureters

The ureters are two tubes, one from each kidney, that run down the back wall of the abdomen and curve forward to the bladder, situated in the pelvis.

Bladder

The bladder is a flexible, sac-like structure with muscular walls into which the urine is passed and stored. The walls are able to stretch as the bladder fills with urine until, in the average adult, 200ml of urine is collected. Stretch receptors in the bladder walls then stimulate the desire to pass urine. The bladder can hold as much as 800ml of urine if this desire is ignored voluntarily but eventually the urine will be forced into the urethra by the contraction of the muscular walls of the bladder, the relaxation of a sphincter muscle at the neck of the urethra and the action of the abdominal muscles including the diaphragm.

Urethra

The urethra carries the urine from the bladder to the outside of the body. In women it is about 4cm long and opens out to the external body in front of the vagina. In men it is about 20cm long and is shared by the reproductive system, opening at the tip of the penis.

Disorders of the urinary system

Disease/ disorder	Cause	Description
Cystitis	Commonly caused by a bacterial infection	Symptoms include pain when passing urine, increased desire to urinate, lower abdominal pain and possibly blood in the urine
Nephritis	Caused by infections or toxins, either in the blood or being passed from the bladder up the ureters to the kidney	Inflammation of the kidney; pain in the lower back and trouble passing urine. Can be life threatening if very severe
Urinary tract infection (UTI)	Bacterial infection	Any part of the urinary tract can be affected; has similar symptoms to cystitis (which is also a type of UTI)
Renal colic	Abdominal pain caused by kidney stones	Severe abdominal pain depending on the size of the stone
Kidney stones	Solid mass of nitrogen-based crystals found in the kidney or ureters	Symptoms include severe pain in the abdomen or side of the back that may move to groin area. Other symptoms can include abnormal urine colour, fever, and nausea

Reproductive system

The reproductive system in both males and females is concerned with the continuation of the human race rather than forming part of the necessities for health or life. They are very different from each other as males and females play a different role in this process.

The primary sexual characteristics, i.e. male or female, are decided at conception, but the organs and structures are not able to perform their functionary role until puberty. At puberty the organs begin readying themselves for their function by producing hormones that provide the secondary sexual characteristics of adulthood.

During female adulthood the reproductive system undergoes ovulation – the release of an egg for fertilisation once a month. If the egg is not fertilised, the system undergoes a series of changes brought about by hormones and there is a menstrual flow. If the egg is fertilised the system maintains the pregnancy under the control of hormonal influence and assists in the birth process.

At menopause the female reproductive system has served its function. The organs stop producing the hormones needed to maintain their reproductive function and the female body undergoes changes.

Female genitalia

The structures of internal female genitalia are as follows:

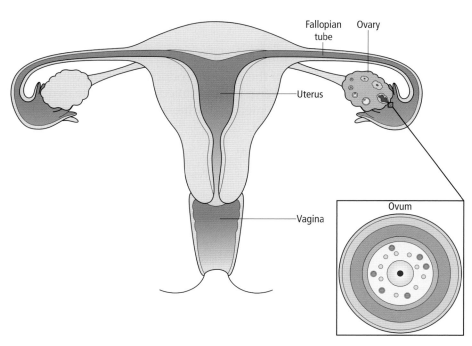

△ Structures of the internal female genitalia

- Ovaries: are oval-shaped organs that produce the ova or egg, usually one per month. They also produce hormones to control the menstrual cycle and maintain pregnancy in its early stages.

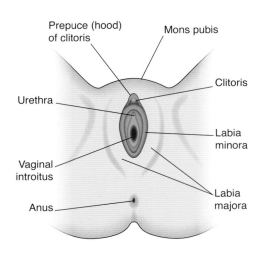

△ Structures of the external female genitalia

- Fallopian tubes: lay either side of the uterus and capture the ovum as it is released from the ovary and carry it to the uterus. It is here where the fertilisation of the egg by the sperm occurs.

- Uterus: a pear-shaped hollow organ, commonly called the womb. It has a thick, blood-enriched, muscular wall which receives the fertilised egg and is where the embryo will grow safely into a baby. It is the muscular walls of the uterus that contract during childbirth to deliver the baby.

- Cervix: the neck of the womb through which the sperm pass to fertilise the ovum and the baby must pass during child birth.

- Vagina: a strong muscular tube that connects the internal and external structures of the female reproductive system.

The external female genitalia structures are the:

- clitoris

- labia minora

- labia majora.

Male genitalia

The structures of the male reproductive system are as follows:

Testes: two egg-shaped organs of the male reproductive system that produce sperm.

Scrotum: a sac-like structure that contains the testes.

Penis: the external organ of the male reproductive system whose function is to deliver the sperm in fluid called semen to the ovum for fertilisation to occur. Both semen and urine are conveyed along a narrow tube called the urethra.

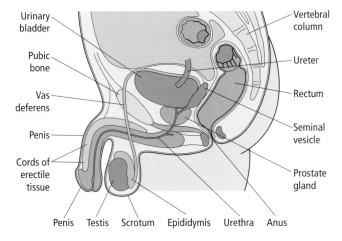
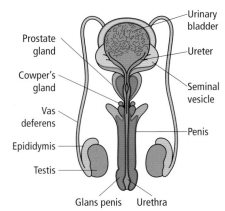
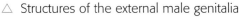

△ Structures of the external male genitalia

Olfactory system

The olfactory system is concerned with our sense of smell, an important sense that evokes memories and essential bodily instincts such as hunger. The olfactory nerves culminate at the olfactory bulb where the nerve cell bodies can be found. Other nerve fibres from the bulb extend backwards along the olfactory tract towards the temporal lobe of the cerebrum where the sense of smell is perceived.

Structure and function of the olfactory system

The structures of the olfactory system are as follows:

- Nose: the external organ of the olfactory and respiratory systems, through which the chemicals that we perceive as smell are delivered.

- Mucous membrane: the lining of the nose that is made up of ciliated epithelial cells and contains a rich blood supply; air is warmed as it passes over the lining.

- Cilia: tiny, hair-like structures that filter larger particles from the air before it enters the other structures of the respiratory system. Specialised versions in the roof of the mucous membrane in the uppermost portion of the nasal cavities become the dendrites of the olfactory nerve cells and are stimulated by the chemicals or odour to register the sense of smell.

- Olfactory cells: situated in the lining of the mucous membrane in the upper nasal cavity. The axon of these cells passes upwards through the ethmoid bone to a portion of the brain called the olfactory bulb.

- Olfactory bulb: the area of the brain where the sense of smell is perceived. It is connected via nerve cells to the limbic system or area where the odour can evoke an emotion, memory or more a more basic instinct such as hunger.

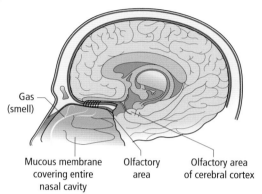

Gas (smell)

Mucous membrane covering entire nasal cavity
Olfactory area
Olfactory area of cerebral cortex

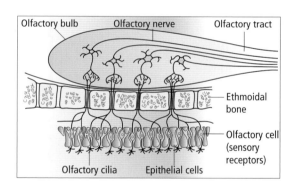

Olfactory bulb   Olfactory nerve   Olfactory tract

Ethmoidal bone

Olfactory cell (sensory receptors)

Olfactory cilia   Epithelial cells

△ Structures and position of the olfactory system

The eye

The eye is a sensory organ that is sensitive to light and is responsible for the sense of sight.

The external structures of the eye are as follows:

- Eyelids: the upper and lower eyelids are thin flaps of skin containing muscle fibres that enable them to open and close over the surface of the eyeball. The lids contain hairs called eyelashes which form protective filters to prevent particles from entering the eye. The lashes are replaced, on average, every 4–6 weeks.

- Eyeball: the eyeball sits within a bony structure surrounding the eye called the eye socket which protects it from physical harm. It is held in place by many small muscles that are able to move the eyeball to make full use of the light available and to focus the light from a specific object.

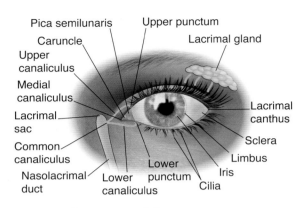

Pica semilunaris
Caruncle
Upper canaliculus
Medial canaliculus
Lacrimal sac
Common canaliculus
Nasolacrimal duct
Upper punctum
Lacrimal gland
Lacrimal canthus
Sclera
Limbus
Iris
Cilia
Lower punctum
Lower canaliculus

△ External structures of the eye

- Iris: the coloured portion of the eye. It contains circular muscles which control the diameter of the pupil and therefore the amount of light that is permitted to enter.

- Pupil: light passes through the pupil and through a lens immediately behind it and onto the light sensitive cells of the retina at the back of the eyeball. The stimulation is then conveyed to the brain by the optic nerve.

- Conjunctiva: a thin transparent membrane that covers the surface of the eye and lines the eyelids.

- Lacrimal glands and ducts: the glands produce a fluid secreted through the ducts that bathes and disinfects the outer surface of the eyeball and eyelids to keep them moist and allows the eyelids to move freely over the surface of the eyeball. Excess fluid is commonly called tears.

Disorders associated with the eye

Disease/disorder	Cause	Description
Conjunctivitis	Bacterial infection of the conjunctiva of the eye	Redness of the conjunctiva with a gritty feeling and with a yellowy discharge. Can easily spread to both eyes
Stye (hordeolum)	Bacterial infection of the hair follicle of the eyelashes	Red, painful swelling of the eyelid; there maybe weeping and pus formation
Pink eye	Viral rather than bacterial	Similar symptoms to conjunctivitis, but usually only affects one eye and there is no yellowy discharge

Test yourself

1. Explain the difference between mitosis and meiosis.

2. Describe the following processes:

   a) Diffusion
   b) Osmosis
   c) Active transport

3. 'Adipocytes' can be found in which structure of the skin?

   a) The epidermis
   b) The papillary layer
   c) The reticular layer
   d) The subcutaneous layer

4. Which type of joint allows a free range of movement?

5. What structures make up the axial skeleton?

6. Name the bones responsible for the facial features.

7. Name the five sections of the vertebral column.

8. Name the three types of muscle tissue.

9. What is the action of the Zygomaticus muscle?

   a) Chewing
   b) Snarling
   c) Grinning
   d) Smiling

10. Which muscle adducts the scapula and keeps it steady during movements of the arm?

    a) Rhomboids
    b) Latissimus dorsi
    c) Pectoralis major
    d) Deltoid

11. What is the name given to nerve cells?

12. Name the three types of neurone defined by their function.

13. Which two structures make-up the central nervous aystem?

14. Briefly describe the peripheral nervous system.

15. Name three types of blood cell or corpuscle.

16. What are the functions of blood?

17. State whether each of these statements is true or false.

    a) Arteries carry blood away from the heart
    b) Blood from the left ventricle is pumped to the lungs
    c) The left atrium accepts oxygenated blood from the lungs
    d) The vena cava empties deoxygenated blood into the right atrium

18. Which structure of the lymphatic system is primarily responsible for the formation of leucocytes?

19. Which gland of the endocrine system is known as the master gland?

20. Which glands are responsible for the development of the secondary sexual characteristics in males and females?

21. Define the following terms:

    a) External respiration
    b) Internal respiration

22. Name the four stages of digestion.

23. Give four functions of the liver.

24. Where can the kidneys be located in the body?

25. Briefly describe the structure of the bladder.

Chapter 5
PRINCIPLES OF ELECTRICITY AND LIGHT

This chapter provides knowledge for the following technical units:

NVQ unit B13 Provide body electrical treatments

NVQ unit B14 Provide facial electrical treatments

NVQ unit B20 Provide body massage treatments

NVQ unit B21 Provide UV tanning treatments

NVQ unit B29 Provide electrical epilation treatments

City & Guilds VRQ unit 305 Provide body massage

City & Guilds VRQ unit 306 Provide facial electrotherapy treatments

City & Guilds VRQ unit 307 Provide body electrotherapy treatments

City & Guilds VRQ unit 308 Provide electrical epilation

City & Guilds VRQ unit 312 Provide UV tanning

VTCT VRQ unit UV30403 Provide facial electrotherapy treatments

VTCT VRQ unit UV30403 Provide body electrotherapy treatments

VTCT VRQ unit UV30424 Provide body massage

VTCT VRQ unit UV30430 Apply micro dermabrasion

VTCT VRQ unit UV30450 Provide UV tanning

VTCT VRQ unit UV30474 Provide electrical epilation

LEARNING OBJECTIVES

In this chapter you will learn about the use of electricity and light in beauty therapy treatments and the working practices required to use them safely.

In this chapter we will look at:

1 Types and structure of matter
2 Electricity and types of current
3 Conductors and insulators
4 Uses of electrical currents in beauty therapy
5 Electrical safety
6 Light and its uses in beauty therapy

NVQ evidence requirements

You will need to show that you can:

- ask your client questions to identify if they have any contraindications to electrical treatments and record their answers accurately
- correctly carry out thermal and tactile tests to accurately determine the client's skin response to heat and pressure stimuli
- carry out a patch test, if necessary, to determine skin sensitivity and to avoid adverse reactions

- clearly explain the sensation created by the electrical equipment being used
- safely use the correct treatment settings, applicators and accessories
- adjust the intensities and duration of the treatment to suit the client
- safely use electrical treatments to bring about the beneficial effects of the treatment while avoiding the associated.

There are other related units within the scope of the NVQ and VRQs that are not listed here as they are outside the remit of this publication.

VRQ evidence requirements

Refer to the technical units for full details.

> ### Key terms
>
> **Compound** – when elements combine together they form compounds.
>
> **Element** – the simplest form of a substance that cannot be broken down by a chemical reaction.

Introduction

The use of electricity and light within beauty therapy goes beyond simply lighting a room or running a piece of electrical equipment. In this chapter you will consider the beneficial effects of the application of light and electrical currents to the tissues of the body.

Structure of matter

All living and non-living things are made of tiny particles called atoms. An atom is the smallest particle that can take part in a chemical reaction –a process where atoms of different elements combine with each other to form another substance or compound. Atoms in turn are made of subatomic particles, namely:

- neutrons: have no electrical charge and are found in the nucleus of the atom

- protons: have a positive charge and are also found in the nucleus

- electrons: have a negative charge and are found circling the nucleus, like planets orbiting around the sun.

It is the number of these subatomic particles that determine one element from another and all the atoms of a given element are the same, that is, they have the same number of subatomic particles. For example, all atoms of helium gas have two neutrons, two protons and two electrons and can be represented in a diagram as shown below.

You can see from the diagram that the electrons are arranged within an 'orbit' or energy level and where there are more electrons, they are arranged in another energy level to the same pattern in all atoms. The first energy level can contain up to two electrons, the second

Helium

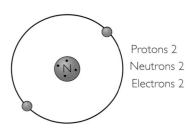

Protons 2
Neutrons 2
Electrons 2

Outer shell containing
2 electrons – full

△ Arrangement of subatomic particles within an atom of helium

energy level can contain up to eight electrons and the third also eight, and further energy levels hold larger numbers of electrons.

It is the outer energy level and the number of electrons contained within it that determines the stability of the atom and its desire to combine with others to form compounds. Stable atoms have 'full' outer energy levels and are resistant to combining with other elements.

Others are known as reactive atoms because they contain less than the maximum number of electrons in their outer energy level and combine readily with other elements to form compounds.

Oxygen only has six electrons in its outer energy level, making it a very reactive element that desires to combine with many other different elements. As a result, there are a large number of compounds that contain oxygen.

Atoms combine because of their need to gain stability by having the maximum number of electrons in their outer energy level. To achieve this, atoms of one element borrow or give up spare electrons to the other element. This giving or borrowing of electrons gives the atoms an electrical charge and the atoms concerned are then called ions. For example, sodium readily combines with chlorine to form sodium chloride or salt. Sodium has 11 electrons – two in the first level and eight in the second level – which means that there is only one electron in the third energy level; chlorine has 17 electrons with seven in the third energy level. To achieve stability, the sodium atom gives its single electron to fill the gap in the outer energy level of the chlorine atom.

The sodium atom becomes a positive ion, or a cation, as it loses a

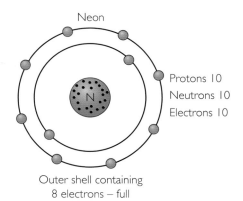

Neon

Protons 10
Neutrons 10
Electrons 10

Outer shell containing
8 electrons – full

△ Arrangement of subatomic particles within an atom of neon

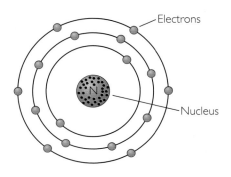

Electrons

Nucleus

△ Arrangement of subatomic particles within an atom of oxygen

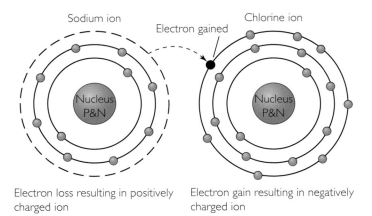

Electron loss resulting in positively charged ion

Electron gain resulting in negatively charged ion

△ Sodium and chlorine atoms combining

negative electron; the chlorine becomes a negative ion or anion because it gains a negative electron.

Ions follow the following laws:

- Ions with the same charge repel or move away from each other.

- Ions with opposite charge attract or move towards each other.

Remember the saying, 'opposites attract, likes repel'.

Key terms

Reactive atom – contains fewer than the maximum number of electrons in its outer energy level.

Stable atom – contains the maximum number of electrons in its outer energy level.

Key terms

Anion – a negatively charged atom.

Cation – a positively charged atom.

Ions – formed when an atom gives or receives an electron.

Types of matter

Atoms and their elements and compounds are arranged into three types or states:

1 Gas: the atoms are widely spaced and expand to fill a container. The atoms can move around freely and at high speed.

2 Liquid: a state where the atoms are more tightly packed than a gas but take up the shape of their container and can still move freely.

3 Solids: have a definite shape as the atoms are tightly packed together in a regular pattern and can move around only slightly.

Solid

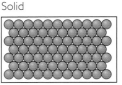

Particles have a regular pattern, are close together, they move slightly and have high density

Liquid

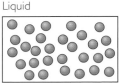

Particles are more widely spaced, move more freely and have a medium density

Gas

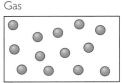

Particles are widely spaced, move randomly at high speed and have a low density

△ Arrangement of atoms in the different states of matter

The state in which the element appears depends on the temperature and pressure that it is exposed to and can change if one or both of these variations are applied. For example, water at room temperature and pressure exists as a liquid but when a low temperature is applied it becomes a solid – ice – and when a high temperature is applied it becomes a gas or vapour – steam.

Electricity and types of current

Electricity is simply an electrical charge as described above, when atoms lose or gain electrons from their outer energy level. There are two basic types of electricity: static electricity and electrical current.

Static electricity

Static electricity is caused by substances rubbing together during which process electrons are transferred from one substance to the other.

In the example in the picture, rubbing a balloon on hair transfers electrons, giving the balloon a negative electrical charge and leaving the hair with a positive charge. The hairs, all having the same charge, repel against each other which sends them apart, but they are attracted to the balloon because it has a negative charge.

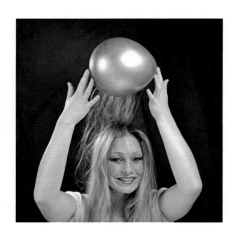

△ Static electricity created with hair and balloon

Electrical current

Electrical current is a flow of electrical charge. In other words, it is the transfer of electrons from one atom to another and then the next atom, from an area where there is an abundance of electrons to an area where there is a lack of them – this is known as a potential difference. The potential difference forces the electrons to make these transfers and is measured in volts.

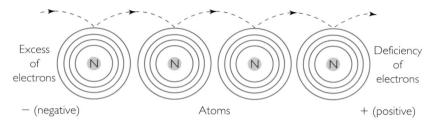

Excess of electrons — (negative)   Atoms   Deficiency of electrons + (positive)

△ Electrons flowing through a length of wire

Conductors and insulators

Materials that are made up of reactive atoms and have free electrons in their outer energy level allow the flow of electrical charge and are known as conductors. Examples of materials that are good conductors are metals, water and the human body.

Material made up of stable atoms and that have no free electrons in their outer energy level (so cannot provide electrons for transfer from one atom to another) are known as insulators. Examples of materials that are good insulators are glass, plastics and air.

Types of current

There are two basic types of electrical current: direct and alternating.

Direct current

Direct current (DC) flows in one direction only and can be obtained from a cell or battery. The pathway taken by the electrical current is called a circuit and the flow of current is from positive to negative. This type of current occurs as a result of a chemical reaction between two elements such as zinc, which has an abundance of free electrons, and carbon which has a deficiency. This sets up a potential difference and the flow of electrons from zinc to carbon, forming an electrical current. In order for the current to flow there must be no break in the circuit.

Alternating current

Alternating current (AC) changes direction as it flows along its circuit and is obtained from the mains supply produced by a generator or dynamo at a power station. With an alternating current the electrons bounce backwards and forwards while still moving forwards in the circuit. The speed at which the electrons bounce backwards and forwards per second is called the 'frequency' and is measured in Hertz (Hz).

Uses of electrical currents in beauty therapy

Galvanic treatments

Galvanic treatments in beauty therapy require the use of a direct current. However, they do not use a direct current from a cell or battery because this cannot produce sufficient voltage to create the required effects and benefits. Instead the equipment is plugged into the mains supply and the alternating current is passed through a rectifier within the equipment, which changes the alternating current to a direct current.

Chemical electrolysis occurs when a direct current is allowed to flow through a solution such as salt water, the molecules within the solution split into ions which have an electrical charge.

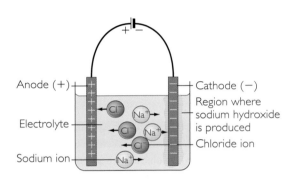

△ Electrolysis of salt water ($NaCl + H_2O$) split into ions

The sodium chloride (NaCl) splits into positively charged sodium ions (Na+), which are attracted to the negative electrode or cathode, and negatively charged chlorine ions (Cl–), which are attracted to the anode or positively charged electrode.

Some water molecules (H_2O) also split into hydrogen cations (H+) and oxygen anions (O–) and are readily used to form new substances at the electrodes.

At the cathode, sodium hydroxide (NaOH) is produced, which is a caustic substance destructive to skin tissue and is sometimes known as caustic soda or lye. This will appear in time as a white substance around the electrode itself.

At the anode, hydrochloric acid (HCl) is produced, which is easily diluted in water to become harmless; there may also be some oxygen and chlorine gas, which will appear as bubbles around the electrode.

There are three uses of direct current in beauty therapy:

1 epilation

2 facial therapy

3 body therapy.

Epilation

Direct current was the original current used in epilation and relies on the chemical electrolysis as described above for its effect. When the current is applied to the growth area of the hair follicle via a probe or electrolysis needle it is very successful at destroying the hair follicle tissue, for the following reasons:

● The tissues of the body contain salt solution so when the current is allowed to flow through the body the salts split into ions.

● These ions are attracted to the active and indifferent electrodes of the epilation equipment according to their polarity and reform to make sodium hydroxide or 'lye'.

- This substance is caustic and can therefore bring about tissue destruction, in this case the destruction of the hair follicle.

- The epilation probe or needle acts as the cathode and has a negative charge.

- The degree of tissue destruction is dependent on the moisture levels in the skin and the intensity of the current.

Advantages

- Effective at tissue destruction, so little regrowth.

- Advantageous on strong, deep-rooted hairs.

Disadvantages

- Difficult to control the degree of destruction, so scarring is more likely.

- Time consuming – current is applied for 10 or more seconds.

'The Blend' is a combination of both high-frequency current (diathermy) and galvanic applied to the hair follicle at the same time via the probe or needle. It is said to have all the benefits of electrolysis but with none of the disadvantages, in other words:

- very effective with little regrowth

- more easily controlled

- as quick as diathermy.

You will find more on the use of these currents and their use in epilation treatment in Chapter 10 Electrical epilation.

Facial treatments

In facial galvanic treatments a direct current is applied so that the current flows from out of the equipment, through the wires to the active electrodes (applicators) into the skin and body tissues to the indifferent electrode (a pad/bar held by the client or placed under their shoulder) and back to the equipment. In the case of facial treatment, the active electrode is the one placed onto the face.

When a direct current is allowed to pass through tissues, the current itself has different effects on the tissue depending on the polarity of the active electrode.

Effects at the cathode (negative electrode):

- creates an alkaline environment

- has a 'slackening' effect on pores, follicles and blood vessels

- increased erythema (as a result of the slackening effect)

- stimulates nerve endings.

> ### Key terms
>
> **Active electrode** – the applicator where the desired effects are taking place.
>
> **Indifferent electrode** – the applicator at which any effects occurring are secondary or not required by the treatment, but which are needed to complete the current circuit.

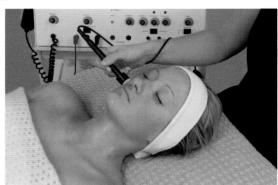

△ Direct current application in facial galvanic treatments

Remember . . .
As stated earlier, 'opposites attract' and 'likes repel'. These simple rules are used to 'force' ionised or charged products into the skin.

⭐ *Hints and tips*
Many of the products used in iontophoresis have positively charged ions in them and so the active electrode is made positive too, but this may not always be the case. It is therefore important to read the product manufacturer's instructions before application.

Remember . . .
Always change the polarity of the active electrode so that it is the *same* charge as the ions in the product.

Effects at the anode (positive electrode):

- creates an acid environment
- tightens and firms tissues
- decreases erythema
- decreased sensitivity
- has an antibacterial effect.

The polarity of the active electrode can be changed so that it can become the cathode (negative) or the anode (positive) by a switch on the equipment.

When you place a product on the skin containing negatively charged ions and the active electrode is also negative, the ions are forced into the skin.

When you place a product on the skin containing positively charged ions and the active electrode is also positive, the ions are forced into the skin.

Direct current in facial therapy can be used for:

- desincrustation
- iontophoresis

Desincrustation

Desincrustation is a facial treatment used as a deep cleanse and so is particularly beneficial for an oily, seborrhoeic or mild acne skin type and conditions but can be used in moderation on any skin that needs deep cleansing.

The product used for desincrustation could be any of the following:

- salt water
- desincrustation gel
- alkaline-based fluids.

Iontophoresis

Iontophoresis is mainly used during a facial treatment to enable the penetration of beneficial products deeper into the skin than can be achieved by normal application on the skin surface.

The products used in iontophoresis could be any of the following:

- iontophoresis gels for specific skin types or problems
- ampoules containing active ingredients such as collagen
- serums.

You will find more on the use of facial galvanic treatments in Chapter 9 Facial electrical treatments.

Body treatments

Body galvanic treatments are mainly aimed at cellulite skin conditions of the body, but can be used to introduce any beneficial product and therefore can be used to treat stretch marks and dilated capillaries or red veins. The firming of the skin tissues at the anode is also beneficial in the treatment of post-natal or pre-mature ageing body conditions.

The action of a direct current alone can, however, be effective on the toxin-based condition of cellulite without a product; this is because of the general action of the current on solutions and its ability to split a compound into smaller ions. These smaller molecules can then be more readily absorbed into the blood stream, removing then from the affected areas to the kidneys where they can be excreted, or to the liver where they can be made harmless.

The products used in body galvanic treatments include:

- gels

- ampoules

- serums or similar products.

All contain beneficial products such as seaweed, caffeine and other natural diuretics.

More on the use and application of body galvanic treatments can be found in Chapter 8 Body electrical treatments.

Electrical muscle stimulation treatments (EMS)

EMS treatments traditionally used a 'faradic current' (named after Michael Faraday who discovered it), which was used to bring about muscle contraction. Modern equipment uses a combination of currents known as 'faradic type currents' rather than just a direct current, so faradic treatments are more accurately known as electrical muscle stimulation (EMS).

The current is allowed to flow in short bursts called a pulse, followed by a rest period and so is described as an interrupted current. This happens very quickly – the time periods are measured in thousandths of a second (ms).

The current causes the muscles to pull tight or contract but there are two additional factors to be taken into account:

- Identical pulses in succession (as shown) will cause the muscle to react less and less, i.e. the muscle will become accustomed to the pulses and will no longer contract.

- Muscles should have a rest from contraction or muscle spasm will result (sometimes referred to as a 'tetanus-type contraction'), where the muscle contracts strongly and for a prolonged period of time.

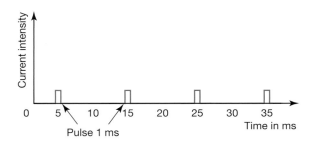

△ Interrupted EMS current

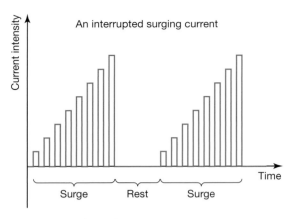

△ Interrupted surging current

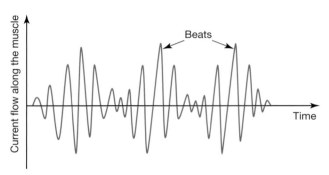

△ Interferential current

To avoid these effects the current is modified to become an interrupted surging current.

Some EMS treatments use an interferential current, which is described as an alternating current with a medium frequency that 'beats' as it flows along the length of a muscle (or muscle fibre).

The general effects of these types of currents are:

- improved tone of specific muscles
- increased metabolism of the specific muscles
- increased elimination of waste products from the area being treated.

Interferential of currents are used in facial treatments to bring about the following effects:

- face lifting
- improved facial contours
- improved skin metabolism
- improved skin texture and colour.

In body treatments, these currents are used to:

- improve posture
- reshape the body in figure correction
- improve body contours
- improve the appearance of cellulite.

Microcurrent

Like many of the advanced facial and body treatments used in beauty therapy, microcurrent was first used in the treatment of medical conditions such as Bell's palsy, sports injuries and as part of a recovery programme after a stroke. During this type of use additional benefits to the skin were noticed and so equipment was developed by the cosmetic industry for use in the treatment of facial and body lifting, stretch marks, scarring and cellulite.

Wave forms

The current used in microcurrent treatments is known as a modified direct current, that is one that is interrupted to form a pulse rather than flowing continuously as in galvanic treatments. The current is also modified to produce different wave forms, which bring about the subtleties in treatment and allow wide use of this type of equipment.

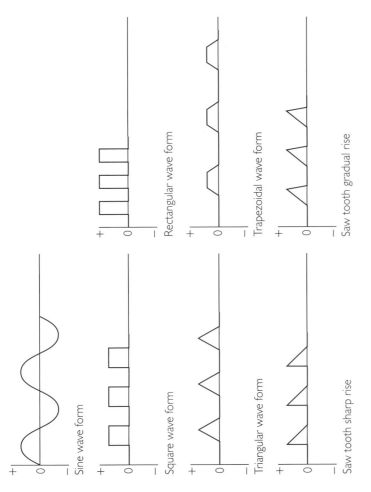

Sine wave form

Square wave form

Triangular wave form

Saw tooth sharp rise

Rectangular wave form

Trapezoidal wave form

Saw tooth gradual rise

△ Different wave forms used in microcurrent treatments

The different wave forms used within a treatment give different beneficial effects, for example:

- the sine wave form brings about effects relating to an increase in the metabolism of the tissues such as improved blood circulation and lymph drainage

- the square wave form brings about the retraining of the muscle tissue and therefore the lifting effect used in non-surgical face-lift and body-lift treatments

- a ramp-shaped wave form brings about a pumping action often used in lymph drainage programmes within a treatment.

Manufacturers of microcurrent equipment have developed variations of these wave forms that are available together in one machine, often with a computer program to change the wave form at different stages of the treatment application.

Other factors that influence the effect on the tissues and therefore the benefits achieved by the treatments are the frequency and the current settings.

Frequency

The frequency of a microcurrent can range between 0.5 Hz to 600 Hz and these different frequencies have different effects.

- A low frequency penetrates the skin and has effect on the deeper tissues such as muscles. A microcurrent with a frequency of 0.5 Hz is therefore used in muscle lifting programmes.

- A high frequency has more superficial effects and brings about an increase in blood circulation in the skin.

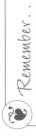

Remember . . .

The frequency or speed of an electrical current is measured in Hertz (Hz).

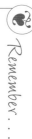

Remember . . .

A galvanic current uses a current measured in milliamps (mA) – 1 thousandth of an amp.

Current setting

A microcurrent is measured in micro amps (μA), that is 1 millionth of an amp, ranging from 10 μA to 650 μA.

The lower the current setting, the deeper the effect. So a current setting of 50 μA is used in treatments of the muscle tissue. The higher the current setting, the more superficial the effect, for example an increase in blood circulation in the skin.

High frequency currents (HFC)

HFC is described as an alternating current with a frequency above 200,000 Hz. High frequency currents are used in electrical epilation and facial and body treatments.

Electrical epilation

HFC is used in epilation to destroy the hair follicle tissue through heat. The alternating current is supplied from the electrical socket via an electrical lead to the epilation machine, in which there is a device called an oscillator which increases the frequency to millions of cycles per second.

▽ Table 5.1 Range of frequencies used in epilation

Class	Abbreviation	Range
Low	LF	30–300 kiloHz
Medium	MF	300–3,000 kiloHz
High	HF	3–30 megaHz
Very high	VHF	30–300 megaHz

When concentrated into the very fine epilation probe or needle these rapid HFCs stimulate the surrounding moisture molecules in the hair follicle to vibrate rapidly causing heat. The heat is greatest in the moist areas and therefore more heat is produced in the lower portions of the follicle. The use of HFC in epilation is also called thermolysis (heat) and short wave diathermy (SWD).

Tissue destruction

The way in which the tissues are destroyed by HFC depends upon the amount of heat generated by the action of the current. VHF and HF currents produce 'electro-desiccation' or drying out of the tissues. MF or LF currents produce 'electro-coagulation' or a cooking/congealing action.

Electro-desiccation:

- deprives the tissue of moisture (as in grilling)
- happens only at high intensity and fast speeds
- area affected around the follicle is small
- used for shallow, straight follicles.

Electro-coagulation:

- converts fluid into a thickened mass (as in boiling an egg)
- provides a wider spread of destruction
- used for deep, strong hairs with a large dermal papilla.

Use of HFC in facial and body treatments

The alternating current from a mains socket passes through the electrical lead to the machine where the voltage is increased by a transformer. The current reaches a 'spark gap' – two pieces of metal with an air gap between them. The now large voltage high-frequency current conducts through the air gap producing the customary sound associated with HF machines. The same occurs when the current passes through the tiny air gaps between the applicator and the skin. In addition, oxygen ions are formed in the air gap and these join up to form ozone gas.

High frequency currents can be applied to the skin directly and indirectly. Table 5.2 describes the effects, benefits and uses of these two methods of HFC.

▽ Table 5.2 Effects, benefits and uses of direct and indirect application of HFC

Method	Effects and benefits	Uses
Direct application of HFC	<ul><li>warming</li><li>increases blood circulation locally</li><li>erythema</li><li>increases skin's metabolism</li><li>stimulates superficial nerve endings</li><li>generates ozone which is germicidal</li></ul>	<ul><li>greasy/oily skin conditions</li><li>mild acne</li><li>to sterilise skin after extraction</li></ul>
Indirect application of HFC	<ul><li>increases activity of sebaceous glands</li><li>increases blood circulation deeper in the tissues</li><li>increases metabolism of skin and muscles</li><li>tightening and toning effect on muscles</li></ul>	<ul><li>dry and dehydrated skins</li><li>improve appearance of fine lines and wrinkles</li><li>improve general appearance of skin</li></ul>

Electrical safety

There is a potential for danger when using electrical currents within beauty therapy treatments but with care and common sense these treatments can be performed to the benefit of the client's condition without causing harm. It is very unlikely that a client or therapist will be placed in a position where they can be fatally harmed by the use of electricity within an electrical treatment, as the currents used are simply too low to have such an effect. However, in the hands of an incompetent or badly trained or thoughtless therapist, beauty therapy electrical treatments can be uncomfortable or at worst cause serious injury resulting in permanent scarring.

In this part of the chapter; electrical safety will be considered at two levels. The first level discusses the safety devices that can be found within the equipment itself and the electrical circuit within the salon building, the maintenance of which the salon owner, together with a professional electrician, is responsible for. The second is at the treatment level, where the therapist is the key person in maintaining the safety of the client.

Electrical safety devices

The salon owner is responsible for the purchase of the correct equipment from a reliable and reputable source and to make sure that all equipment is intended for use within the UK. Equipment displaying the Kitemark means that it has been through rigorous testing and meets the requirements of British Standards for safety. Another symbol you may see is Œ, which indicates the equipment has passed European standards too.

Electrical equipment is also protected by a fuse and/or may be earthed. A fuse is a device that will break the flow of current if it reaches dangerous levels; earthed is where the equipment has a connection to redirect the current flow to a safe area away from the user.

For additional safety, equipment is usually housed within an insulator which, as described earlier is a substance that is poor at conducting electricity. Air, rubber and plastic are efficient insulators and are used to insulate electrical equipment to make them safe. Beauty therapy equipment, for example, often has rubber feet.

A building will also have a fuse box at or near the point where the electricity supply enters and this is fitted near to the circuit board so that the lighting, plug sockets and other circuits intended for individual equipment requiring a high-energy source such as a sauna can be insulated by the use of separate fuses with different ratings.

Other safety devices are a Residual Circuit Device (RCD) and a circuit breaker, both of which are intended to protect the building's electrical circuits. This protects the electrical equipment from being damaged by a surge of electrical current flow or from faulty equipment being used.

Electrical equipment should be checked regularly by a qualified electrician at least every five years but more often if the equipment is in constant use. See the Electricity at Work Regulations 1989 in Chapter 1 Monitoring health and safety.

Therapist's responsibilities for electrical safety

The therapist must always check electrical equipment before use.

- Observe the PAT (Portable Appliance Testing) sticker to see if the machine has recently been checked by an electrician.

- Ensure the mains lead plug is whole and there are no loose parts and the lead itself is whole and there are no breaks in the outer insulating case.

- Check the equipment's applicators or electrodes for breaks and loose connections.

- Test that the equipment is working by switching it on and observing the indicator lamps and/or the meters. Turn the dials back to zero and switch off the machine after these checks.

- If there is anything abnormal, switch off the machine at once and do not use it. Label it as unfit for use and store away from others until it can be checked by a person qualified to do so.

Electrical equipment and water

Because water is an excellent conductor of electricity, care must be taken when the use of water is necessary alongside electrical equipment. Always follow these rules:

- Never place a bowl of water on a trolley shelf above a piece of electrical equipment. Instead place the bowl on a shelf below so that any accidental drips or spillages cannot splash onto the equipment.

- Wipe up any spillages of water immediately with disposable paper.

- Applicators that are required to be damp to allow the passage of electrical current into the body should not be so wet that water is allowed to drip or run.

Contraindications

It is the therapist's responsibility to check the client for contraindications before beginning any form of electrical treatment. The contraindications given below are not exhaustive, but are specific to the use of electrical equipment and explanation of why they are contra-indicated is also given.

- Heart disease, high- and low-blood pressure and circulatory disorders are contraindicated due to the effect electrical currents have in increasing blood circulation and therefore blood pressure, which will place an additional strain on the heart and blood vessels. Electrical treatments may cause the client to feel light headed or faint and additional strain on the heart may make a heart condition worse with potentially serious consequences.

- Diabetes is the inability of the body to control blood sugar levels due to the malfunctioning of the pancreas and reduced levels of the hormone insulin. It can be controlled with diet alone but if severe the client will need to check their blood sugar levels and inject insulin several times a day. A symptom of the condition is problems with blood circulation and the natural healing ability is also impaired, particularly in the extremities of the body such as the hands and feet. Electrical currents that stimulate and require additional energy in the form of sugars can cause the client to feel unwell and may induce hypoglycaemia (where there is too little sugar in the blood), particularly if incorrect levels of insulin have not been injected. Care should also be taken when treating the limbs as even minor damage to the skin of a diabetic can cause serious problems such as ulceration.

- Epilepsy is a neurological disorder that results in seizures. Passing mild electrical currents through the body will stimulate the nervous system, which may induce a seizure.

● Cancer is a serious health condition resulting from the growth of abnormal cells, which may be transported around the body by the lymphatic system. Any treatment that increases lymph flow will aid transportation and therefore spread the disease. When a client is having chemotherapy or radiation treatment the side effects of the treatment cause the client to be quite unwell and electrical treatments will place an additional strain on the body, increasing this effect.

● Dysfunction of the nervous system, including a loss of sensation in an area, is contraindicated due to the therapist often relying on the sensation the client is feeling to determine the treatment intensities. Without the ability to feel the treatment, the intensities can be set too high and damage to the tissues may result. It is important that the therapist performs the relevant skin sensation tests before treatment. See Chapter 7 Skin and body analysis for information on how to perform these tests.

Light and its uses in beauty therapy

Electromagnetic spectrum

Light is made up of alternating electric and magnetic fields and is arranged into bands depending on the wavelength in the electromagnetic spectrum (see Table 5.3). A wavelength is the distance from identical positions on the wave to the next along the direction of travel. This is measured in nanometres (nm), one nanometre being a thousand millionth of a metre. Infra-red is measured in micrometres, with one micrometre being one-millionth of a metre.

The only natural source of light is the sun and the light radiating from the sun is referred to as daylight and is produced by the sun even on a cloudy day. Light from the sun includes both visible light (i.e. visible to the human eye) and non-visible light spectrum; nocturnal animals can see in reduced light when we cannot because this light falls outside of a metre of our visible spectrum.

Visible light has a wavelength within 400 nm (being the blue end of the spectrum) and 700 nm (being the red end). Infra-red light has a wavelength greater than 700 nm, while ultraviolet light has a wavelength shorter than 400 nm. X-rays, gamma rays from radioactive materials, microwaves used for cooking and by physiotherapists for heat treatment and radio waves are all electromagnetic waves. It is the different wavelengths which account for the different effects of the rays.

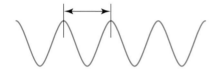

△ Measuring wavelength

▽ Table 5.3 Electromagnetic spectrum

Gamma radiation	X-rays	Ultra violet	Visible light BGYOR	Infra-red	Micro-waves	Radio waves
less than 1 nm	1–160 nm	160–400 nm	400–700 nm	1–1000 μm	1 mm –10 cm	greater than 10 cm

Artificial light sources such as light bulbs also radiate electromagnetic waves. Incandescent light bulbs radiate a yellowish light created by forcing an electrical current to flow through a very fine metal wire; heat is also produced during this process and can be utilised for therapeutic effects. Light can also be formed by passing electrical current through inert gases contained in a glass tube. These are called fluorescent bulbs and can be used to simulate daylight when they are used around a make-up mirror or to create UV light for tanning, depending on the gases contained within the glass tubing.

Ultraviolet light

Ultraviolet rays are electromagnetic waves with lengths of between 400 nm and 100 nm and are absorbed by the skin. It is within the skin that the reactions occur and which cause the beneficial effects. It is usual to refer to three bands of ultraviolet light waves:

UVA has a wavelength of 315–400 nm. The waves produce an 'immediate' tan by darkening pigment already present in the skin which fades within hours. They are thought not to be responsible for skin cancer or to cause sunburn but as they penetrate deep into the dermis they damage the fibres of collagen and elastin resulting in premature ageing.

UVB has a wavelength of 280–315 nm. These waves promote the production of melanin in the melanocytes providing a longer lasting tan. They are also responsible for causing erythema and are a strong factor in causing sunburn and skin cancer. As they do not penetrate the dermis they do not play a part in the ageing process.

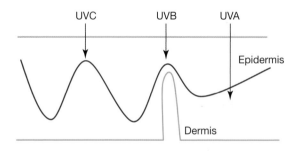

UVC has a wavelength 100–280 nm. These rays are particularly lethal to living cells and are known to cause skin cancer. However, the earth's atmosphere prevents the rays from reaching us (which is why holes in the ozone layer are of much concern). UVC tans in a similar way to UVB. Some lamps that emit small amounts of UVC are of little danger as long as the correct distance of the lamp from the skin is observed.

△ Depth of absorption of UV light

Infra-red and radiant heat

Infra-red is a type of light emitted from a heat source, for example an electric fire or the sun. Like ultra-violet light, infra-red is invisible but we can feel these rays because they produce heat. Like all light rays they are called electromagnetic rays.

A hot object also emits infra-red rays and is called a radiant heat emitter, so there are two types of lamp used in beauty therapy: the radiant heat lamp and the infra-red (IR) lamp.

Both types produce similar effects on the body and have similar physical properties. See Chapter 11 Body massage treatments for more on the beneficial effects of infra-red and its use in treatments.

Inverse square law

When light travels from a source the rays spread out in all directions so that at a greater distance from the lamp, the effect is more widely and thinly spread. So the further away from the lamp the less effect is seen and it will take longer to achieve an effect. In other words, the intensity of radiation varies inversely with the square of the distance from the lamp. Hence the intensity of radiation at 1 ft is four times more than at 2 ft and nine times than at 3 ft. So when a lamp obeys the inverse square law, four minutes at 2 ft and nine minutes at 3 ft are required to produce the same effect as one minute at 1 ft. All lamps, whether infra-red, radiant heat, sun-bed or solarium, obey the inverse square law.

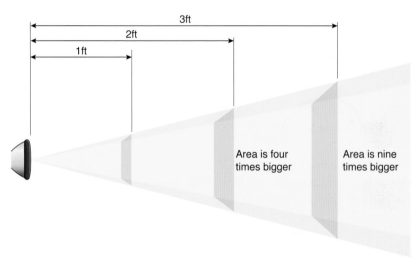

△ Application of the inverse square law

Test yourself

1. What two main types of subatomic particle constitute the nucleus of an atom?
2. In what way does electricity flow through a metal wire?
3. What happens to the molecules of salt when they are dissolved in water?
4. Distinguish between an anion and a cation.
5. Briefly state the chemical reaction that occurs at the cathode when a direct current is passed through a salt solution.
6. Which types of current are used to destroy the tissues of the hair follicle during electrical epilation treatment?
7. What modifications are made to the currents used in electrical muscle stimulating treatments to avoid tetanus-type contraction of the muscles?
8. Why does a loss of skin sensation contraindicate electrical treatment on that area of the body?

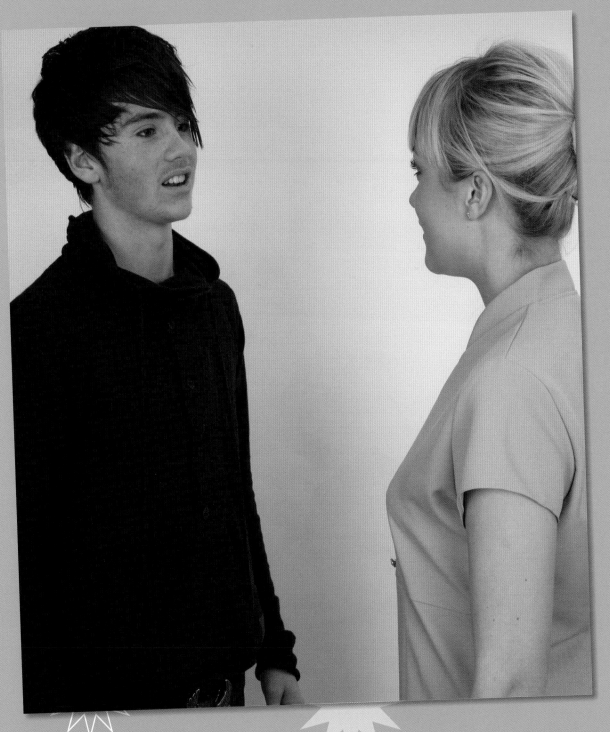

Chapter **6**
PROFESSIONAL PRACTICES

This chapter covers:

VTCT VRQ unit UV20415 Working in beauty-related industries

VTCT VRQ unit UV30468 Client care and communication in beauty-related industries

City & Guilds VRQ unit 301 Working with colleagues within beauty-related industries

City & Guilds VRQ unit 303 Client care and communication in beauty-related industries

LEARNING OBJECTIVES

In this chapter you will learn about the professional expectations and good working practices required to work successfully in beauty-related industries.

The chapter will cover aspects of the NVQ technical units for outcomes 1 'Maintain safe and effective methods of working' and 2 'Consult, plan and prepare for treatment', as well as VRQ units listed above.

In this chapter we will look at:
1. Personal professional standards
2. Working with colleagues
3. Working with clients
4. Working within the law

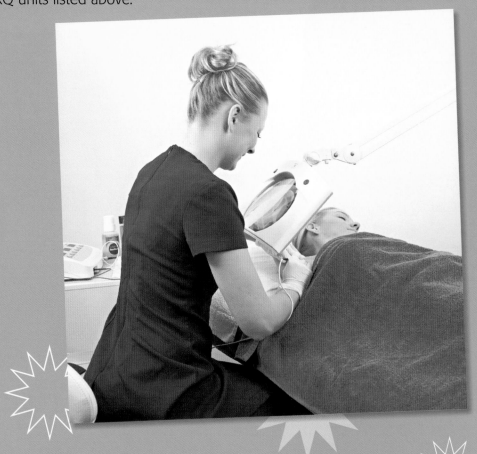

NVQ evidence requirements

You will need to show that you can:

- comply with related legislation in regard to health and safety, consumer protection, discrimination, employment and the treatment of minors
- comply with the rights and restrictions for the service or treatment you are performing
- understand the importance of professional association membership
- comply with beauty-related industry codes of practice and ethics
- provide adequate insurance protection for clients and employees
- show a duty of care towards clients, visitors and colleagues
- behave in a professional manner
- communicate with clients and colleagues in an appropriate manner
- demonstrate appropriate personal appearance, hygiene and protection
- demonstrate client care and professional service procedures
- show punctuality, reliability, integrity, confidentiality, diplomacy and willingness for self-improvement.

VRQ practical evidence requirements

The evidence requirements for the VRQ qualifications for City & Guilds and VTCT are shown below:

City & Guilds VRQ Unit 301 Working with colleagues in the beauty-related industries

Candidates are required to be observed carrying out a consultation, which incorporates client care and communication techniques.

City & Guilds VRQ Unit 303 Client care and communication in the beauty-related industries

Candidates are required to be observed carrying out a consultation, which incorporates client care and communication techniques.

VTCT VRQ Unit UV30468 Client care and communication in the beauty-related industries

You must demonstrate competent performance of all practical criteria on at least three occasions, each for a different client. To include the following range:

Treated the following clients:
- new
- regular

Identified by:
- questioning
- observation

Considered the following factors:
- adverse hair, skin and scalp conditions
- incompatibility of previous services and products used
- lifestyle

Dealt with the following complaints:
- dissatisfied client
- unrealistic client expectations

Sought continuous improvement in:
- client feedback
- client care

Simulation should be avoided.

VRQ knowledge requirements

City & Guilds Unit 301 Working with colleagues within beauty-related industries	Page no.	VTCT Unit 20415 Working in beauty-related industries	Page no.
Learning outcome 1: Be able to work with colleagues within beauty-related industries		**Learning outcome 1: Know the key characteristics of the beauty-related industries**	214
Practical skills/observations		*Underpinning knowledge*	
Communicate effectively with colleagues and clients	183–4	Access sources of information on organisations, services, occupational roles, education and training opportunities within the beauty-related industries	
Behave in a professional manner	184	State the types of organisations within the beauty-related industries	181–91
Assist others to resolve problems	194–6	State the main services offered by the beauty-related industries	181–91
Give clear instruction to colleagues	194	Describe occupational roles within the beauty-related industries	191–2
Provide support and guidance to colleagues	193	State the employment characteristics of working in the beauty-related industries	180
Provide clear and timely feedback to colleagues	184; 194	Describe the education and training opportunities within the beauty-related industries	186
Follow safe and hygienic working practices	196–202	Describe the opportunities to transfer to other sectors or industries	xii
Underpinning knowledge		State the main legislation affecting the beauty-related industries	210–13
Describe roles and responsibilities of team members in a salon	191–2	Describe the basic principles of finance and selling within the beauty-related industries	207–9
Describe the benefits of effective team working and working with colleagues	193–4	Describe the main forms of marketing and publicity used by beauty-related industries	26–7
Describe the different methods of communication	183–4	**Learning outcome 2: Know the working practices associated with the beauty-related industries**	
Describe how to adapt communication techniques for different situations	183–4	*Underpinning knowledge*	
Explain the importance of giving instruction, support and guidance and timely feedback	194	Describe good working practices in the beauty-related industries	Ch6
Describe the processes of giving instruction, support and guidance and timely feedback	194	State the importance of personal presentation in reflecting professional image when working in the beauty-related industries	181
Describe the effects of negative attitude and behaviour on others	183	Describe opportunities for developing and promoting own professional image within the beauty-related industries	186

	Page no.
State when and whom to refer problems to	194
State the basic employment rights and employer responsibilities for working in the beauty-related industries	210–13
Describe the importance of continual professional development for those working in the beauty-related industries	186

City & Guilds Unit 303 Client care and communication in beauty-related industries

VTCT Unit 30468 Client care and communication in beauty-related industries

Learning outcome 1: Be able to communicate and behave in a professional manner when dealing with clients

	Page no.
Practical skills/observations	
Behave in a professional manner within the workplace	184
Use effective communication techniques when dealing with clients	183–4
Adapt methods of communication to suit different situations and client needs	183–4
Use effective consultation techniques to identify treatment objectives	203–4
Provide clear recommendations to the client	203–4
Assess the advantages and disadvantages of different types of communication used with clients	183–4
Underpinning knowledge	
Describe how to adapt methods of communication to suit the client and their needs	183–4
Explain what is meant by the term 'professionalism' within beauty-related industries	180
Explain the importance of respecting a client's 'personal space'	207
Describe how to use suitable consultation techniques to identify treatment objectives	203–4
Explain the importance of providing clear recommendations to the client	203–4

Learning outcome 2: Be able to manage client expectations

	Page no.
Practical skills/observations	
Maintain client confidentiality in line with legislation	188
Use retail sales techniques to meet client requirements	207
Evaluate client feedback	30–1
Underpinning knowledge	
Evaluate measures used to maintain client confidentiality	188; 207
Explain the importance of adapting retail sales techniques to meet client requirements	207–9
Identify methods of improving own working practices	186
Describe how to resolve client complaints	209–10

Introduction

Despite the technical skills that a therapist or nail technician can offer, the most important aspect of working successfully in the beauty industry is to show a high level of professionalism. High standards increase the likelihood of employment and financial reward for the individual and will secure the business' success through improved reputation and return of custom by clients.

Activity

What is meant by the term 'professionalism'? Discuss this with a colleague and together list five words or phrases that express what it means for you.

The client should be central to the business and the experience the client receives during their time in the salon should reflect a high standard of professionalism, from the time of booking their appointment to when they leave after the service. Everyone in the salon plays an important role in the client's experience but it is the therapist or nail technician that will have the greatest opportunity to impress the client.

Personal professional standards

In this section we will be looking at:

- employment characteristics
- personal appearance and hygiene
- personal protection
- communication and behaviour
- membership of a professional body or association
- codes of conduct and ethics
- relevant insurances
- improvement of own professional practices
- continual professional development
- security.

Employment characteristics

An employer will make sure you have a recognised qualification to be employed to perform the services or treatments that the business offers, as failure to do so could invalidate their insurance.

The professional therapist and nail technician must ensure they develop their employability characteristics to enhance their practical and technical skills. These characteristics are sought after by employers and are often used to differentiate between one candidate and another at a job interview. For example, an employer will look for someone with a high standard of personal appearance and hygiene and who has good communication and organisational skills. They require someone who is punctual and reliable as there will be some clients who cancel of their appointments if the therapist is late or takes a lot of sick leave. This will result in a loss of income and will not promote their business.

Personal qualities such as integrity and honesty are important when treating clients as the therapist is placed in a position of trust when giving advice and recommending the purchase of products and services. Diplomacy and confidentiality are other qualities. Often, the therapist is placed in a position during the consultation where they are party to intimate and delicate details of the client's life; they must respect the client's privacy and treat such information as confidential. The client's expectations of the treatment may be unrealistic and diplomacy is needed to inform the client and guide them to the most suitable treatment.

Loyalty is another important quality that is valued by an employer. Remaining loyal to your salon, colleagues and clients involves being tolerant of others' views and behaviour, not judging others or making negative comments about them and not listening to gossip. Challenge sexual, racial and religious discrimination to promote a positive salon atmosphere.

Activity

How would you feel if information you had told someone in confidence was discussed with others? What would be the effect on a salon business if this happened to a client? What action could the salon owner take on the individual who had been responsible for the gossip?

Appearance and hygiene

Image is very important in the beauty-related industry as it promotes client confidence and business reputation. Use this checklist to measure your own personal appearance and hygiene.

Personal appearance and hygiene checklist
Back to basics

1. A high standard of personal hygiene.

2. Fresh breathe free from cigarette or food odours.

3. A clean, pressed overall.

4. Clean, low-heeled shoes.

5. Arms and hands free from jewellery (plain wedding bands are acceptable).

6. Any earrings or necklaces are discreet.

7. Make up is discreet and expertly applied.

8. Long hair is tied neatly away from the face and shoulders.

9. Nails are short, smooth, clean and free of nail enamel.

10. Tights, or socks with trousers, are worn.

11. Any cuts are covered with a clean plaster.

12. Hands are washed immediately before and after physical client contact.

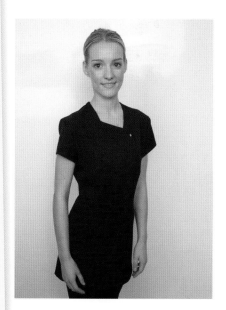

△ A professional-looking therapist

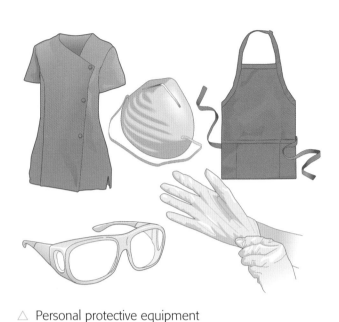

△ Personal protective equipment

Personal protection

As part of the duty of care to clients and colleagues, the therapist must also protect herself from harm and infection when providing services and treatments to clients.

By taking adequate care, the therapist will not contract common work-related health conditions such as dermatitis or musculo-skeletal disorders such as backache, tennis elbow and carpal tunnel syndrome. The therapist and nail technician should ensure that their work area is set up for their comfort as well as that of the client to reduce the risk of the development of such conditions. Ensure that the client is positioned for ease of performing the treatment and that any chair or treatment couch is at the correct working height.

Complying with health and safety legislation is important and in particular the use of recommended personal protective equipment (PPE) following a risk assessment by the employer (see also later in this chapter). Types of PPE include:

- non-latex gloves: worn where there is the risk of contamination from body fluids, such as blood

- dust mask: worn during services where air-borne particles are created, such as during the filing of nail extensions

- eye goggles: worn during the use of light therapy such as Intense Pulse Light (IPL) hair removal or when the risk of a 'flying' object, such as a piece of artificial nail during clipping, can enter the eye.

The therapist should also consider inoculation against the blood-borne virus hepatitis, especially as there is a risk of accidental piercing of the skin with a micro-lance or epilation needle during electrical epilation, facial and advanced electrolysis treatments.

Treating minors

In additional to health and safety requirements, the therapist must be aware of the following points when treating 'minors' (i.e. those under 18 years of age in England and 17 in Scotland).

- The treatment of minors is against the law unless written permission is obtained from the parent or legal guardian.

- When treating clients under the age of 16 years of age the parent or legal guardian should sign the client record *and* be present throughout the treatment.

- Treating minors also requires the therapist to be checked by the Criminal Records Bureau (CRB).

- Never be alone in a treatment room with a minor under the age of 16 years. A parent or guardian should be present throughout the treatment or service.

Dealing with clients of the opposite gender

Another form of personal protection is that of dealing with clients of the opposite gender. To protect yourself from the risk of harm or unfair accusations of improper behaviour it is wise to follow these guidelines:

- Never be alone in the salon when performing treatments or services to clients of the opposite gender. The client should be made aware that a colleague is on the premises.

- Never start a friendship or relationship with a client; always act professionally in this regard.

Dealing with threats

If you are in the unfortunate position to be present during a burglary or similar, do what you are asked and hand over any money that is on the premises. When the burglar has left, phone the police immediately. Do not offer any resistance as this can result in injury.

Communication and behaviour

Communication

Communication at work occurs with different people at different levels in varying circumstances. Choosing the correct method of communication for use with clients, colleagues, those in a more senior position and those with lesser responsibility means that a wide range of communication skills are needed to be successful as well as professional. Remember that the effects of poor communication are:

- ineffective working relationships

- loss of business

- an unpleasant working atmosphere.

Verbal communication

When speaking to clients use appropriate language, avoiding swearing and slang. Make sure you use the correct terminology; using the Latin names for body anatomy with clients is inappropriate but so is the use of common terms such as 'armpit'. 'Underarm' would be more appropriate.

Consider your tone of voice: it may be appropriate to lower your voice when talking to a client about a personal problem, especially when it is not possible to take the client to a private area within the salon. Remember that under no circumstances should you raise your voice in anger when speaking to a client. Dealing with complaints requires you to be calm and to keep your tone of voice even. If you need to reprimand a junior member of staff, do so calmly and in private. Speak clearly when giving instructions or information to a colleague or a client so that they cannot be misheard or misinterpreted. This is especially important when speaking on the telephone.

> ☆ *Hints and tips*
> *Do not accept inappropriate language or behaviour when treating clients of the opposite gender. Stop the treatment or service and explain firmly that you find the language inappropriate and that if it continues you will ask them to leave. If the behaviour continues, carry out your warning, returning payment if necessary.*

> ☆ *Hints and tips*
> *Ensure that a client with hearing difficulties can see your face when you are speaking to them. Gain their attention by gently touching their arm.*

Avoid controversial topics of conversation such as politics, religion and sexuality as your client may have a strong view that is very different to your own. Remember that everyone is entitled to their own opinion and that a different one to yours does not compromise your own.

An important part of good communication is the development of good listening techniques. Asking appropriate open-ended questions requires the client to provide more than a one-word answer and the therapist and nail technician must listen carefully to elicit the relevant useful information. Being able to read the client's body language can also help with determining the client's expectations of the treatment or if he or she is happy with the result.

Making eye contact with a client as they enter the salon or at your first meeting shows a genuine willingness to help and when accompanied with a smile can be friendly and welcoming.

Written communication

Written information is also widely used in the salon to record the client's details during a consultation, writing a stock order, sending emails to clients about a promotion, during the production of marketing materials or during a staff appraisal meeting. The use of appropriate language is very important, as is correct spelling and grammar. Client records should be clear and show step-by-step instruction of procedures so that the treatment can be recreated if desired. Records should be updated at every visit and should be an accurate account of the client's visit and treatment.

Reading written instructions and understanding them is very important as it can lead to serious injury if the instructions are not followed, for example, the safety data sheet for a new chemical treatment or the instructions for a new piece of electrical treatment. If you are in any doubt in such cases you should contact the supplier immediately and not use the product until you are clear.

Visual aids to communication

The use of a visual aid such as a diagram during the client consultation can explain the procedure or treatment more clearly so that it is fully understood by the client.

Behaviour

A professional approach to behaviour involves working cooperatively with others and following the salon requirements. Professional behaviour includes:

- being punctual and reliable
- being polite and courteous
- making decisions within the limits of your responsibility
- referring problems beyond your responsibility to a more senior member of staff
- showing respect for others and their property
- being tolerant of others' views and beliefs
- demonstrating a duty of care towards others.

> ★ *Hints and tips*
>
> *If you know that spelling or English grammar is not your strength, ask someone who has those skills to produce your marketing materials. This can save embarrassment, money and the need to rewrite the materials later.*

Membership of a professional body or association

Some of the many benefits of becoming a member of a professional association include:

- receiving information on new treatments, services, products and developments in the industry
- appearing on the association's register and being recommended to clients
- ability to obtain professional indemnity and other insurances
- access to publications and resources such as aftercare leaflets
- legal advice for the running of a business
- access to continuous professional development (CPD) in the form of education and training.

Codes of conduct and ethics

Many professional bodies and associations produce a code of conduct, which sets the standard for the industry and which their members are expected to abide by. The code may deal with such issues as:

- standards of hygiene
- development of skills and knowledge
- professional practices for service/treatment details
- practising within the law
- standards of behaviour (conduct)
- levels of competence and working within your limitations
- client confidentiality
- ethical selling of products and services.

Relevant insurances

There are three levels of insurance that should be considered when working as a therapist or nail technician:

1 Employers' liability insurance: this provides cover in the event of a member of staff injuring themselves or becoming ill due to their normal duties while at work and is a minimum requirement under the terms of the Employer's Liability (Compulsory Insurance) Act 1969. Note that this insurance is not required if you do not employ anyone.

2 Public liability insurance: this insurance provides cover in the event of a member of the public injuring themselves or becoming ill as a result of being on the business premises, for example slipping on a wet floor. It applies to *anyone* on the premises, whether they are a client, a rep from a company or even the postman. This type of insurance is only necessary if you have

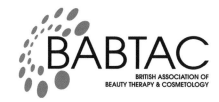

△ The professional association logo of BABTAC. BABTAC are one of the only membership organisations that offer student insurance that covers case studies.

Employer expectations

In order to practice medicine, doctors must be registered and licensed with the General Medical Council and this is known as statutory regulation. There is a move for such a system to be in existence for hairdressers, beauty and complementary therapists and nail technicians but as yet no such law exists. Instead the beauty industry is 'self-regulated'.

Key terms

Statutory regulation – when an industry is controlled by the government by the passing of a law.

Self-regulation – when an industry is controlled by its own members.

Health and safety

Note that employers' liability insurance refers to 'normal duties' while at work; for a therapist or nail technician this largely involves performing services on clients. In the event that a therapist falls and hurts themselves outside of their normal duties, such as falling from a ladder to change a light bulb, the insurance would not apply.

business premises but it also applies if a portion of your home or property is used for business purposes, such as a spare bedroom or a converted outbuilding such as the garage.

3   Professional indemnity insurance: this provides cover in the event that a client suffers financial loss as a direct result of the treatment or service they have received. The client would need to prove that the therapist had been negligent or that an error or omission had occurred that resulted in the financial loss. Professional indemnity insurance will meet the cost of defending any claims and any damages that may be payable as a result. Without insurance the financial security of the business is at risk. In the case of a person operating as a sole trader, this risk extends to their personal financial security. Note however that such insurance will be invalid if the therapist does not comply with industry codes of practice.

Improvement of own professional practices

Professionalism in the beauty-related industries also means improving your own performance. This can be achieved through client feedback, self-evaluation, assessment and reflective practice, accompanied by a positive approach to new developments, treatments and products.

Self-evaluation involves the assessment of personal strengths and weaknesses, implementing a personal development plan and carrying out relevant developmental activities and CPD.

Evaluation of staff performance is a role that is undertaken by a senior member of staff. There should be regular reviews of performance and provision of updates and the senior member of staff will need to be able to analyse feedback and comment on the performance of others. They will also need to develop a plan for improvement and organise development activities. This requires a flexible approach and a willingness to embrace change as well as the ability to share ideas and good practice and set targets that are specific, measurable, agreed, realistic and timed (SMART).

Continual professional development (CPD)

The need for CPD can be as a result of a performance review where development needs have been identified but it is also a requirement because the beauty-related industry is forever changing with the development of new procedures and equipment.

CPD should be a part of every professional therapist and nail technicians' working life because it keeps a therapist up to date with current trends and new technology and ideas, products and skills. It shows good practice and improves performance at work with identified training needs, increases job satisfaction and the prospect of promotion and career progression.

For a business, CPD will increase the number of clients coming into the business and therefore improve its profits. CPD is required by most professional associations and is mandatory in certain professions.

Security

As a therapist, manager or salon owner you have to show a duty of care towards security of the premises in which you work and the property of others, including that of your clients.

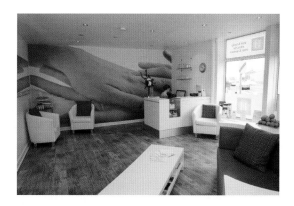

△ A reception area

Handling money

Security at the reception is especially important when receiving payments in the form of cash, cheques, debit and credit card. Looking out for the signs of counterfeit paper money is an important part of a receptionist's job but the therapist may also handle payments and so should also be aware.

When payment is made in cash, accept the money and look carefully at any notes, particularly if they are of a high denomination. Check to see if there is a metallic strip in place and also the quality of the water mark and hologram features. The police and bank will often make known instances of theft of notes of particular serial numbers and when such a list is provided, it is good practice to check each note of the relevant denomination for those serial numbers.

When handling any note it is a good idea to place the note(s) on the till while you count the change into the client's hand. This avoids any disagreement as to the value of the note as you have not yet placed it in the till.

Cheques are becoming an outdated form of payment and will eventually be unavailable. They are unpopular due to the time it takes for a cheque to 'clear' with the result that the payment does not show in the business account for several days.

> ☆ **Hints and tips**
> If you accept a forged or stolen note you must surrender it as evidence to the police and your business is not usually reimbursed the value of the note submitted.

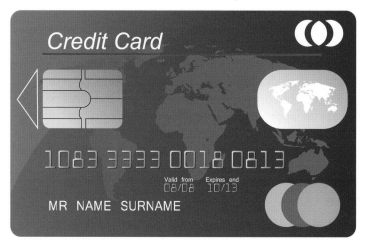

△ Credit card

A financially safer method for both the customer and the business is the use of debit and credit cards. With a debit card the money is instantly taken from the customer's account, although it may still take a few days for the business' account to be credited. It is a safer form of payment because if the customer has insufficient funds in their account the transaction will be refused and they will need to

Key terms

Management hierarchy – the levels of responsibility from director/senior management to middle/junior management and then eventually to supervisory staff and finally service staff.

Span of control – the number of subordinates that a manager is responsible for and has authority over. Organisations with a long chain of control will have narrow spans of control, while those with a short chain of command tend to have wider spans of control.

Line structure – the hierarchical organisation of the members of a team.

Chain of command – the line of command flowing down from the top to the bottom of an organisation.

provide an alternative form of payment. A credit card offers the consumer a 'safety net' in that any loss can be reimbursed by the credit card company in the event of fraudulent activity. Whether a debit or credit card is used, the terminal in the salon is linked to a computer in the customer's bank which recognises the customer's card as it is swiped. The use of a PIN (personal identity number) known only to the card owner is another security feature of this method of payment.

Security of clients' belongings

The security of clients' belongings left at the reception is another consideration of a beauty therapy business and it is usual for a disclaimer to be displayed that exonerates the business from any loss or damage to the property while it is left in such an area. The client should be advised not to leave anything valuable such as a purse, wallet or their mobile phone unattended during a treatment. Any jewellery that is removed should be placed in a safe place and returned to the client immediately at the end of the service.

Security of personal information

Security of personal information obtained from a client and recorded on client record cards must be taken seriously by those working in the beauty and related industries. Under the terms of the Data Protection Act 1998 electronic records must be kept securely with the aid of an electronic password and paper-based records must be kept under lock and key.

Working with colleagues

Business structure

All businesses have a basic structure through which the business as a whole and the various parts of its operations can be directed, monitored and managed – this is known as the management hierarchy. Even a sole trader will have an organisational structure although this will not be formal. In small firms it is likely the owner will have a 'hands on' approach, responsible for all decisions relating to recruitment, marketing and finances. As the business grows the structure will become more important and those in senior positions will need to put more formal arrangements in place.

Line structure

In any profession it is usual to have a variety of staff with different personalities, all of which can contribute to the success of a business. To ensure effective running of the business, staff are usually given different roles and responsibilities. A business is usually organised into functional departments, each headed by a senior manager and below whom there is a chain of command – this is known as the span of control. Each person in the line has authority over those below, while also being responsible for ensuring work handed down to them from their immediate manager is completed. The diagram below shows a typical line structure found in a beauty therapy salon. Of course, the appearance of such a diagram will depend on how many people are employed within the business.

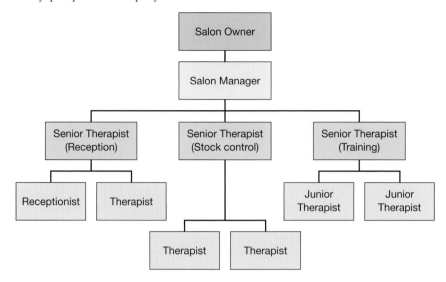

△ A basic line structure showing job roles within a beauty-related business

Advantages

- A line structure is simple to understand, staff know precisely where they are in the structure, who can allocate work to them and to whom they are responsible.

- Managers have a clear understanding of people's roles when allocating work.

- A well-established line authority makes it possible for work to be delegated further down the line; this can widen the experience of subordinates and develop management or supervisory skills.

Disadvantages

- It can involve a very long chain of command, instructions may take a long time to filter from the top and make an impact on the business.

- The flow of information back up the long chain may be a lengthy process, causing considerable delay before problems are identified.

- Individuals may only respond to requests from their superior, creating inflexibility.

Matrix structure

In a matrix structure a senior manager heads a team of specialists drawn from different departments. These specialists are located in departments where they are part of a line authority, thereby being subject to two sources of authority. It is in fact possible for a specialist to be part of several teams or divisions. In a matrix structure, individuals report to managers in more than one department, creating a large number of reporting relationships. It is often used to organise and manage project teams, where people with specialist skills, possibly from different levels, come together to solve complex problems.

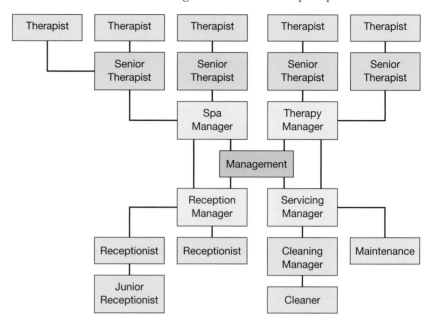

△ A matrix structure

Advantages

- It promotes coordination between departments because it cuts across departmental boundaries. It encourages greater flexibility and creativity by cross-fertilisation of knowledge and skills.

- It allows for the involvement of relatively junior staff, giving them wider experience.

- Staff lower down the structure can gain valuable managerial experience.

- The involvement of specialists from different areas reduces the risk of resources being wasted on projects with no future.

Disadvantages

- Confusion can result because individuals are involved in a large number of different relationships, creating a complex pattern of authority and responsibility.

- Questions may arise as to who has priority over a subordinate's time and what should be reported through the line authority. This can then become a source of conflict and strained relationships as the subordinate may suffer from divided loyalty.

Common elements to both structures

- Major roles and job titles show who is in control and who manages the major business functions within departments.

- Level of seniority of those holding different positions and their respective position in relation to the overall hierarchy is clear.

- The working relationship between individuals is shown, identifying their responsibilities, who has the authority to take decisions and who carries out the work arising from these decisions.

- The extent to which decision making is concentrated in the hands of people at or near the top of an organisation or handed down to lower levels of management.

- The broad channels through which information is communicated throughout organisations, indicating the route by which instructions flow up and down the hierarchy.

Roles and responsibilities

The different roles in the salon are denoted by job title. A person's job title will indicate their authority within the organisation, level of responsibility and their financial reward in the form of salary and benefits.

Table 6.1 shows the different responsibilities for those job roles listed in the line structure.

The role of the manager

There are several important roles that a successful manager will fulfil:

- management of relationships: as a figurehead, leader and coordinator

- information provider: by monitoring and disseminating information

- decision maker: by addressing the needs of the business, problem solving and planning human resources

- trainer: by interviewing potential staff and inducting and training new recruits

- worker: by setting an example to others as an experienced practitioner.

Role of employees

Whatever their job, employees undertake both a functional role (i.e. their job role) and a team role (the way in which they relate to other members of staff).

▽ Table 6.1 Job responsibilities

Salon owner	Salon manager	Senior therapists	Therapists/nail technician/masseuse	Receptionist	Junior therapist
• Customer care	• Treatments/services	• Treatments/services	• Treatments/services	• Reception	• Treatments/
• Pricing of services and retail	• Customer care	• Reception	• Customer care	customer care	services
• Financial records	• Retailing	• Customer care	• Retailing	• Retailing	• Customer care
• Staff discipline	• Selling	• Retailing	• Selling	• Making appointments	• Health and safety
• Health and safety	• Staff discipline	• Selling	• Health and safety	• Selling	• Customer experience
• Customer experience	• Health and safety	• Health and safety	• Customer experience	• Dealing with enquiries	• Setting up for treatments
• Client and staff safety	• Customer experience	• Staff training	• Client record cards	• Health and safety	• Salon cleanliness
• Personal hygiene	• Client record cards	• Customer experience	• Security of the client belongings	• Customer experience	• Client safety
• Marketing	• Security of client belongings	• Client record cards	• Client safety	• Client record cards	• Personal hygiene
• Staff motivation	• Client safety	• Security of client belongings	• Personal hygiene	• Security of client belongings	• Sterilising equipment
• Recruiting staff	• Personal hygiene	• Dealing with suppliers	• Salon atmosphere	• Client safety	• Restocking salon products
• Contracts and wages	• Staff motivation	• Client safety		• Personal hygiene	• Salon atmosphere
• Salon atmosphere	• Recruiting staff	• Personal hygiene		• Stock	
	• Salon atmosphere	• Stock		• Taking payments	
		• Staff motivation		• Salon atmosphere	
		• Maintenance of equipment			
		• Salon atmosphere			

Working as a team

The role a person plays in the team is important as it will have an impact that may or may not be conducive to the atmosphere of the business environment. It is likely that the role a person plays in the team will be moulded by their personality and learned behaviour, rather than by their technical skills and knowledge, but it is possible to provide appropriate training for an individual to develop any required traits.

In order for a team to perform well it is important that there is a good mixture of different types of role to balance and enhance each individual's performance. Most people fit into one of the team roles outlined in the table below.

▽ Table 6.2 Different team roles

The completer	Conscientious worker who searches out any errors and omissions and always meets deadlines. May set standards too high to be practical or may be seen as too fussy, a 'stick in the mud' and slow to make decisions
The coordinator	Mature, trusting and confident. The spokesperson that promotes decision-making and outlines goals. However, could be seen as overbearing and bossy, without always consulting others
The evaluator	Discerning, strategic and level headed, looks at all angles and options before assessing situations, diagnosing problems and choosing the best option
The implementer	Well-disciplined, reliable, efficient and conservative in their approach. They will turn ideas into actual actions or solutions
The investigator	Extrovert, very communicative and enthusiastic. They will explore all the possibilities and develop lots of contacts, but they need stimulus from others to help build and develop their ideas
The plant	Fairly unorthodox, imaginative and creative when left alone, but in need of an appreciative and sympathetic manager
The shaper	Very outgoing, dynamic and usually highly-strung, challenging things and seeking their way around obstacles
The specialist	Dedicated and single-minded
The team worker	Perceptive and accommodating, able to listen and work on ideas. They are sociable and will try to avoid friction

Benefits of working in a team

Teamwork is working together to a common aim or goal. Team work not only benefits the beauty therapy business but can benefit team members too. The benefits of team work are described below.

- More work can be done in less time.

- Team members' strengths can be utilised, increasing their self-esteem.

- Develops trust between individuals and promotes unity within the team.

- Promotes personal responsibility and good working relationships.

Activity

List the human characteristics needed to develop a happy working team and environment.
Working in pairs, decide which team role you think you play and which role your colleague plays. Discuss your observations of each other. Do you agree with your colleague's assessment of you?

- Members strive to do their best so as not to let the team down.

- There is an increase in the abilities of the members as they learn from each other.

- Members share accomplishments when things go well but also the negative aspects, which helps them to strive towards improvements.

Giving and receiving instructions

Whatever role you play in the beauty therapy business, the ability to give and receive instructions is vital to the success of that business. At each position within a hierarchy it is possible that you may have to instruct someone in their role. To do this you should consider the following points.

- Think about where and how you speak to those in a junior position. Be polite and professional, especially in front of clients, and most importantly be clear as to what you would like them to do. Ambiguity leads to confusion and the instruction not being carried out as you wish. The person receiving the instruction may also feel unconfident in their job role and may feel intimidated or defensive when placed in a position where need to receive instructions again.

- If you are reprimanding a colleague remember to do so in a private place away from other colleagues. Be clear, calm and objective; do not let your emotions rule the meeting.

Referring to more senior staff

Sometimes it is necessary to refer work-related to issues to another member of the team. A firm knowledge of personal responsibilities is required to accurately refer an issue that is best dealt with by someone in a more senior position. Issues regarding deviation from salon policy such as inappropriately offering a refund to a client, employment opportunities within the company or disciplinary procedures should be referred to a senior member of the team such as the salon owner, manager or senior therapist, nail technician or spa therapist.

Resolving problems

Dealing with problem clients

Most clients are pleasant and accommodating but there will be those that, for whatever reason, can be problematic to deal with. Situations can occur where differences in culture, language or personality can result in a misunderstanding but it is the duty of the therapist or nail technician to accept and embrace others' differences and try to work within any limitations that might be imposed. A client may act aggressively due to embarrassment, a lack of confidence or as part of a defensive nature. You should keep calm and try to diffuse the situation whenever possible.

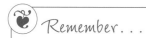 Remember...

It is illegal to refuse to treat a client on grounds of their race, religion, gender, age, disability or sexual orientation.

It is possible to refuse to treat a client if there is a risk of harm to themselves or the client or if the treatment will result in breaking the law, for example dealing with an aggressive drunk or a minor requesting an ear-piercing treatment. The therapist or nail technician should always work within the salon's policy when dealing with problematic clients and the industry's codes of practice for treatments and services.

Dealing with problem colleagues

Staff disagreements

Disagreements among staff can result in a tense atmosphere, which may be detected by clients and result in them taking their custom elsewhere. It is important, therefore, to provide the means by which grievances can be aired and resolved, whether this be in a formal meeting or an informal setting.

Formal grievance procedures provide the means by which employees can sit down to discuss problems at work and are used to solve problems between employees and those between employees and management. Both parties should be allowed to air their views. The desired result is that all parties leave feeling that the problem has been resolved in a constructive and satisfactory way.

Poor performance

It is usual that an employee that is underperforming will be placed on a personal improvement plan. This will involve identifying areas for improvement and providing training and support for those areas. Often, refusal to take part in the plan can result in disciplinary action.

Formal disciplinary procedures are used when there is a serious breach of salon policy or continued unacceptable behaviour such as:

- poor punctuality
- persistent undisclosed absence
- poor performance
- misconduct or bad behaviour
- unsafe conduct
- theft
- inappropriate relationships with clients
- causing physical harm to another.

Disciplinary procedures can ultimately result in dismissal from employment and a manager must be clear when beginning such procedures that there is just cause to do so and record each stage of the procedure accurately. The four stages of disciplinary procedures are:

1 Verbal warning

2 Written warning

3 Final warning

4 Dismissal.

> **Key term**
>
> **Grievance procedures** – formal procedures by which an employee can air a problem so that it can be dealt with to the satisfaction of all parties.

> ☆ *Hints and tips*
>
> *Accepting criticism is not easy! When discussing a problem issue with someone try not to make your comments personal. For example, instead of saying 'You are bad tempered', try saying 'When you speak you sound bad tempered.' This gives the person the opportunity to consider their behaviour as viewed by others.*

It is wise to ensure that at the start of employment all employees are given a written salon policy which gives clear details of the conduct expected and the possible disciplinary procedures that will be invoked if these rules are not adhered to. In this way there can be no possibility of doubt when an employee breaks one of the rules. An employer can dismiss someone instantly if there is unequivocal proof of a serious breach of conduct such as theft.

Working with clients

Service standards

It is important to maintain a high level of customer care and quality of service or treatment to clients as this will ensure their return and increase the profits of the business. The quality of the service provided will largely be down to the training and professionalism of the therapist and their willingness to undertake CPD.

Salon environment

Lighting

Salon lighting should be bright enough for everyone to see clearly what they are doing and to move around safely. However, light that is too bright will cause a glare which may cause discomfort for the client or therapist.

Natural daylight is the best lighting and has the advantage of showing true colour, whereas artificial light can distort colours. When deciding on lighting the following points should be considered:

- Ensure there is enough light to work accurately and safely. Use special lamps for detailed treatments such as nail extensions or epilation.

- Ensure that neither you nor your client is dazzled by bright artificial light.

- Report flickering lights or missing light bulbs so that they can be checked or replaced.

- Consider the type and brightness of the lighting needed for the treatment being performed. A gentle light will encourage a feeling of relaxation and a sense of calm and wellbeing, which is very important for treatments such as massage and aromatherapy.

Heating

The correct temperature for the working environment is 16°C (60–80°F) but this may need to vary considerably when there are clients in a state of partial or complete undress. Certainly in a spa the temperature can be a lot warmer to facilitate the comfort of the clients and bring about some of the beneficial effects.

Within a normal treatment area thermostatically controlled central heating will maintain a comfortable temperature. This is a device which switches off the heating when the required temperature has been reached and turns it back on as the temperature begins to fall.

Whatever type of heating appliance is used, it is vital that it is serviced on a regular basis to ensure it does not emit dangerous fumes.

Ventilation

There should be enough ventilation to keep the air fresh and to prevent a build-up of fumes. Extractor fans and open windows will help to remove the strong odours produced by solvent-based products such as those used in nail technology. Additional specific ventilation requirements may also be required in these treatment areas as prolonged exposure to these fumes can cause nausea and headaches.

Full air conditioning is ideal for keeping a salon fresh and comfortable. Air conditioning works by drawing out stale air and replacing it with fresh air at the correct temperature.

Stale air makes people feel tired and drowsy because of the build-up of carbon dioxide. If air is not circulating, sweat does not evaporate fully from the surface of the skin and therefore the body is unable to cool correctly. This leaves both staff and clients feeling sticky and uncomfortable and will lead to tiredness and fatigue.

Sterilisation and hygiene

The importance of stringent sterilisation and hygiene procedures cannot be stressed enough if cross-contamination of disease from one client to another is to be avoided. The transfer of micro-organisms, bacteria, fungi and viruses and the infestation of parasites can occur through a variety of transmission methods. However, an understanding of the appropriate interventions will reduce the risk of disease and infection spreading.

Bacteria

Bacteria that can cause disease are known as pathogenic or harmful; those that do not are known as non-pathogenic or harmless. We naturally have non-pathogenic bacteria on both the surface of the skin and inside the body in the gut. These harmless bacteria assist the body to function effectively and actually inhibit the growth of pathogenic micro-organisms that cause disease. Bacteria are categorised by their shape.

Bacterial infections of the skin and other external structures such as the conjunctiva of the eye result in the common symptoms or signs of redness, swelling, pain and pus. Internal bacterial infections manifest as different symptoms depending on the structures affected, but can usually be successfully treated with antibiotics. Examples of bacterial infections of the skin and other systems of the body are:

- conjunctivitis
- impetigo
- carbuncles and furuncles
- paronychia or whitlow
- cystitis
- bronchitis.

> ### Key terms
>
> **Sterilisation** – the total destruction of all micro-organisms, including spores, using chemicals or high temperatures.
>
> **Pathogenic bacteria** – micro-organisms that cause disease and are considered harmful to the body.
>
> **Non-pathogenic bacteria** – micro-organisms that do not cause disease; they are harmless and can in fact assist in the effective functioning of the body.

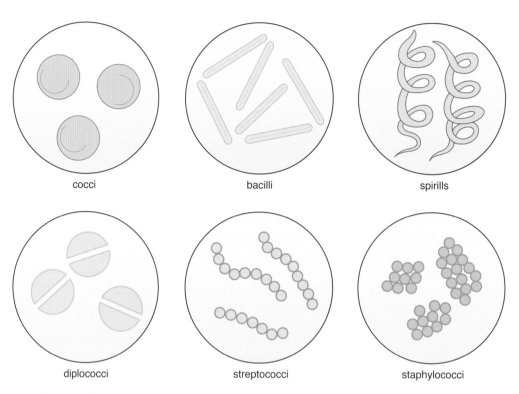

cocci

bacilli

spirills

diplococci

streptococci

staphylococci

△ Pathogenic bacteria

Fungi

Fungi are micro-organisms that rely on a 'host' for their successful existence. Those fungi that feed on dead or decaying matter are known as saprophytic, while those that feed on living matter are known as parasitic. Both types of fungi can cause disease within the human body. The most common fungus that infects the skin is called 'Tinea' and some examples are shown below (note: the second part of the name refers to the part of the body that is affected).

- Tinea capitis: ringworm of the scalp

- Tinea pedis: ringworm of the feet (commonly called Athlete's foot)

- Tinea ungium: ringworm of the nail (also called Onychomycosis).

> ### Key terms
>
> **Parasitic** – micro-organisms that live on living tissue or matter.
>
> **Saprophytic** – micro-organisms that live on dead or decaying tissue.

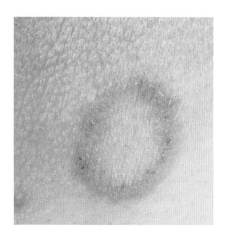

△ Ringworm of the scalp

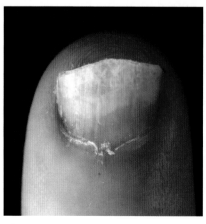

△ Ringworm of the nail

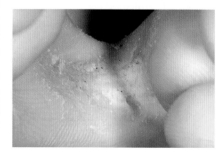

△ Athlete's foot

Viruses

When viewed outside of the body, viruses are merely strands of protein protected by an outer casing. However, when viruses enter the body the casing breaks away, allowing the protein to invade the body's cells where they take over the cell's organelles as their own. This makes them very difficult to destroy and control and they are unaffected by antibiotics. Viral diseases are divided into two main groups – infectious and highly infectious – and include such diseases as:

- hepatitis
- AIDS
- measles
- colds and flu
- warts
- Herpes simplex (cold sores)
- Herpes zoster (shingles).

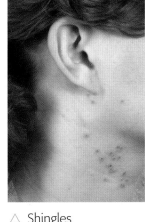

△ Shingles

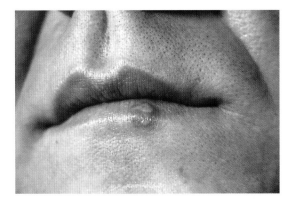

△ A cold sore

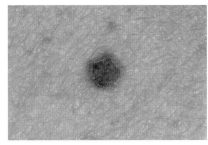

△ Warts

Infestations

Infestation is a term used to describe the transmission of diseases caused by small parasites which live within hairy areas of the body such as the scalp or pubic regions and/or within the epidermis. The parasites 'bite' the skin to obtain food from the nutrients within the blood. As they bite they inject an anticoagulant into the area to prevent the blood from clotting so that they can easily feed. It is this that causes the associated symptoms of itching and redness. A severe allergy to the bite can occur in some individuals, resulting in a much more severe reaction including swelling and/or restriction of movement within the area.

Common examples of infestation include:

- Pediculosis capitis: head lice
- Pediculosis pubis: pubic lice also known as 'crabs'
- Scabies or 'itch mite'.

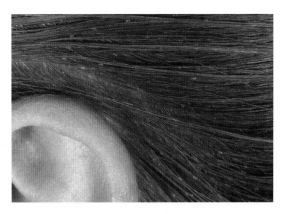

△ Head lice

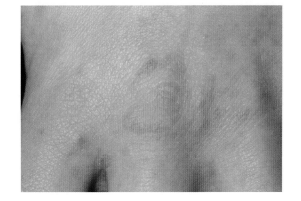

△ Scabies

Transmission methods of disease

Disease can be spread in a number of ways and knowledge of these transmission methods will enable you to provide effective hygiene methods that prevent the spread of disease.

Contact

Contact is the most common method of transfer of micro-organisms from one person to another but this can easily be remedied by the use of simple hygiene precautions. Infections can be transferred in two ways:

1 By direct contact: where an infected area is touched without protection.

2 By indirect contact: where an item such as a towel that has been in contact with an infection is reused on another client.

The following precautions can prevent the transfer of micro-organisms:

- Clean equipment, work surfaces and implements as part of your working routine.

- Fresh laundered towels and bed linen must be available at all times.

- Washing hands is one of the simplest and most effective hygiene procedures. It should become second nature to you in order to protect yourself from infection and also your clients and all those within the salon environment. Use bactericidal hand wash from a dispenser and have the water as hot as possible. Follow this with a thorough drying with a disposable hand towel.

- Cover cuts or abrasions on your hands or the area to be treated on the client with a waterproof plaster.

- Wear disposable gloves for treatments where there is any possibility of coming into contact with blood or body fluids (e.g. depilatory waxing, epilation). There is some concern about the possibility of passing on the HIV virus or hepatitis through some treatments such as electrical epilation, ear-piercing or where the skin is broken. Studies have given contradicting information as to the risks, but procedures must minimise risk of cross infection from any source.

- Sterilise small implements using an autoclave or sterilising fluid.

- Use disposable items such as paper towels, spatulas, tissues and cotton wool where possible and dispose of them immediately after use in a covered waste bin.

Inhalation

Air-borne viruses in the form of droplets suspended in the air can enter the body via the mouth and nose and into the respiratory system as a result of inhalation. Examples include the common cold and the flu virus.

Key terms

Antiseptic – a substance that prevents infection. It inhibits the growth of micro-organisms without destroying them.

Disinfectant – a substance that removes most micro-organisms, therefore preventing information. It will destroy most micro-organisms that are present, but not the means by which they reproduce, thereby allowing the disease to reappear. Disinfectant will not destroy viruses.

Hygiene – the principles and practice of health and cleanliness.

Sterile – the complete absence of micro-organisms and their means of reproduction.

The necessary hygiene precautions to avoid the transmission of such conditions are impractical to administer. It is therefore the therapist's personal responsibility to take care of their own health and avoid activities that can lower the effectiveness of the immune system and make the likelihood of infection more likely.

Ingestion

Micro-organisms and toxins can contaminate food and drink if left uncovered and exposed to the air. When this is ingested the micro-organisms enter the body, causing disease. For this reason there should be NO eating or drinking in the salon environment, except in designated areas. It is also wise to wash your hands before retiring to the staff room to eat your lunch.

Blood

Strict guidelines must be followed where there is a chance that blood or serum may be drawn during a treatment such as epilation or intimate waxing.

Sterilisation methods

The three methods by which micro-organisms can be eradicated from equipment and surfaces are:

1 Heat: both dry and moist heat is used in a salon.

2 Chemicals: used extensively in the industry to clean surfaces and equipment and also as part of some treatments used on the client.

3 Light: irradiation is used to sterilise pre-packed items such as epilation probes and lances. UV light cabinets were popular but have many disadvantages and have become less popular in recent years.

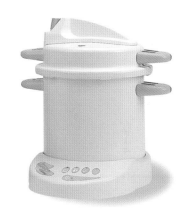

Autoclave

An autoclave is a metal container that is designed to create and withstand heat and pressure. It uses high pressure steam at a temperature of 126°C to sterilise small tools. (Large versions of the autoclave are used to sterilise surgical equipment in hospitals.)

△ Autoclave

● Suitable for tools made of metal or hardened plastic.

● Unsuitable for: tools made of plastic, rubber, glass or those with electrical connectors.

Glass bead steriliser

This is a small, electrically operated metal container about the size of a tumbler which contains thousands of tiny beads. The steriliser heats the beads to a temperature in excess of 300°C and can sterilise items within one minute.

● Suitable for: small metal tools such as manicure and pedicure tools, tweezers and scissors.

● Unsuitable for: large items or those made of plastic, rubber or glass.

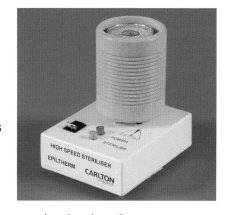

△ Glass bead steriliser

201

UV light cabinet

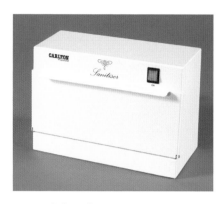

△ UV light cabinet

UV light cabinets use a quartz mercury vapour lamp as a source for ultra violet light; it is the light which destroys the micro-organisms. It is only the surfaces on which the light shines that become sterile.

- Suitable for flat, simple-shaped items made of most materials, with the exception of rubber. It is useful, however, for maintaining the sterile state of equipment after another sterilisation method has been used.

- Unsuitable for: large items or those with a varied and complicated shape where the light cannot reach.

Laser light irradiation

Laser radiation is not a sterilisation method used in salons and clinics but is used by specialised companies to sterilise pre-packed items that are used in salons (and hospitals), such as lances and epilation probes (needles). The items remain sterile until the individual package is opened and the equipment is exposed to the air. However, it remains completely hygienic and is safe to use for treatments/services. This type of item can only be used once and requires specialist disposal.

Chemical

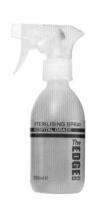

△ Chemical steriliser

Disinfectant is the most common chemical used in a salon. It is used in many locations including hospitals, dentists and laboratories for disinfecting surfaces and soaking equipment. Examples of disinfectants used in the salon environment include Virkon, Barbicide and Cidex.

Client care

The client should be central to the beauty therapy business and as such needs to be considered at every stage of their experience in the salon:

- At reception the client expects a warm, friendly and helpful service. They expect to have their needs met quickly and efficiently and for the atmosphere to be welcoming and free from clutter.

- In the treatment room the client expects the therapist or nail technician to be qualified in the services they are providing and to be offered the most suitable treatment or products to gain the maximum benefit. They also expect to be given advice on homecare and product use and a high level of professionalism to be maintained throughout the treatment.

There are, however, small details that a receptionist and therapist can provide that will ensure the client's return. The following list includes some suggestions that you may already do but others may be new to you and therefore suitable for consideration.

- Providing refreshments and reading materials in salon waiting areas.

- Safe storage of clients' belongings during the treatment or service.

- A well-stocked retail area so that all products are readily available.

- Provision of pillows, props or supports to ensure client comfort during the treatment.

- Provision of blankets or duvets and electric blankets.

- Low, electric couches that allow for the transfer of disabled clients from wheelchairs.

- Variable light, temperature and ventilation of the room to suit both individual client needs and the chosen treatment.

- Performing a hand or head massage during a facial after the face mask application.

Whenever you deal with a client it is vital that you maintain their privacy, modesty and confidentiality. By doing so you will:

- maintain the client's confidence

- increase your professional reputation

- increase the number of clientele

- increase the salon's profit margin

- comply with the requirements of the Data Protection Act 1998.

Consultation techniques

The consultation should be performed in a quiet place such as the treatment room itself. The therapist or nail technician should always be polite and friendly and show sensitivity to the client's condition and/or situation, especially with regard to the client's age and gender and if they have a different cultural or religious background or a disability.

The list below gives some reasons why the consultation is the most important part of a treatment or service for a client.

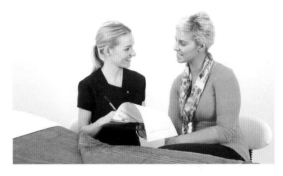

△ Client consultation

- It is the beginning of the relationship between client and therapist or technician, where professional boundaries are set and trust is developed.

- Information is elicited from the client regarding their expectations from the treatment/service. Hopefully the therapist can fulfil these needs if they are realistic but if they are unrealistic other recommendations for treatment can be made.

- The therapist can check the client for medical conditions that may be worsened by the treatment or service and can take steps to protect others from the harmful effects of any disease that is present.

- The therapist can also elicit information surrounding previous similar treatments the client has received, whether at home or in another salon, as well as the problems they have encountered and the success achieved.

- Any limitations to the treatment or service can be established and adaptations can be devised.

- A suitable treatment plan based on the information provided can be devised, with the therapist using her knowledge of products and equipment to maximise the results.

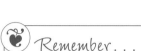

Remember...

Always speak clearly to avoid confusion and use appropriate language and tone of voice when speaking to a client.

★ *Hints and tips*

If you still have doubts about the answers provided by the client, ask another question that is carefully formulated to elicit the information you require.

Activity

Working in pairs, role-play the scenario of a therapist performing a consultation with a client. Take turns to play the client, with the following characteristics:

a) confident
b) angry
c) disappointed
d) nervous
e) lying.

After the consultation role play, the therapist should list the body language displayed by the client.

- The treatment can be explained to the client, including the possible contra-actions, so the client is fully aware of what to expect.

- Once the treatment has been explained to the client, their written consent to begin the treatment can be obtained. This forms a legal agreement that can be referred to in the event of a court case following a disagreement.

Questioning techniques

Using effective questioning techniques is an important part of verbal communication. The use of either open or closed questions will depend on the kind of information the therapist wishes to obtain. A closed question can normally be answered by giving a simple response such as 'yes' or 'no' and is used when a specific piece of information is to be elicited, such as the name of the client's doctor. Closed questions can be used to clarify facts and verify information already given. An open question cannot be answered with a simple 'yes' or 'no' and instead requires the client to give a detailed response. The answers given may be more subjective and include the client's feelings and emotions. Open questions give the client the opportunity to provide what they feel is appropriate information, although this may not be precisely what is required by the therapist who may need to ask further more probing questions.

When questioning a client think carefully about the language and tone of voice that you use, so that your client is not made to feel embarrassed or belittled. Do not be condescending, especially if the client has an obvious learning or physical disability or is of a different race. Do not use terms that may be very familiar to you and other therapists, especially with regard to anatomical structure; try instead to use suitable more common terms but avoid slang terms.

Asking appropriate questions is just one part of the questioning technique. It is also important to listen very carefully to the answers provided by the client and to record them accurately so that they cannot be misinterpreted, as this could result in the wrong service being provided for the client's needs.

Non-verbal communication is also known as body language and includes facial expressions and eye contact. It provides extra information beyond spoken words that you can use to recognise people's emotions, and discover their real intentions.

Contraindications

A contraindication is the presence of a disease or condition that means that the treatment either cannot go ahead or must be restricted or adapted in some way. The contraindications for each treatment are listed in the relevant chapters but can be grouped into those that *prevent* treatment and those that *restrict* treatment.

The disclosure of a contraindication will prompt the therapist or nail technician to undertake certain professional procedures. The presence of medical conditions such as diabetes or epilepsy would need a doctor's permission before treatment can go ahead and the treatment would need to be postponed or another treatment offered that will not affect the medical condition. The therapist/technician should:

- inform the client privately that they cannot have the treatment and rebook the treatment for another time, if appropriate

- seek medical advice or permission from a medical professional, giving as much information about the treatment and any concerns that you have in order for the medical practitioner to be able to make a judgement.

In the event that the therapist/technician suspects that a client has a medical condition they should refer the client to a medical practitioner:

- without causing alarm

- without diagnosing the condition.

The presence of an infectious disease or condition will mean the client cannot have the treatment until the disease has gone and you should recommend that they visit a medical practitioner.

Contraindications that restrict treatment are usually localised to a specific area, for example a cut or abrasion, and mean that the treatment will need to be adapted. When adapting a treatment you should consider:

- the preparation procedures for the treatment, such as the treatment position

- the treatment procedures, for example adaptations to the timings or the applicators used

- avoiding the area affected, for example massaging around bruising.

Contra-actions

At the time of the consultation the client should be made aware of the possible contra-actions to the treatment. The client will then be aware of all the facts in order to make a decision whether or not to continue with the treatment or service. Examples of contra-actions are:

- tiredness

- headache

- nausea

- muscular ache

- increased urination

- increased bowel movement

- heightened emotional state

- change in sleep patterns

- increase in skin blemishes

- change in body temperature – hot or cold.

Contra-actions are symptoms your clients may experience and should be considered as completely normal; not all clients will experience all symptoms. Any contra-action should dissipate (fade) within 12 hours.

Occasionally a client may experience an abnormal contra-action such as an allergic reaction to a product. If the contra-action remains after the period of 12 hours or if the client has any other concerns, they should be encouraged to contact the therapist.

On being contacted by a client with a concern, the therapist should:

- listen to the client's explanation carefully and consider whether aftercare advice has been followed accurately

- if necessary, ask the client to return to the salon

- if the reaction to the treatment is severe, advise the client to seek medical advice

- if swelling of the lips, tongue or soft tissue of the mouth (anaphylactic shock) is evident, encourage the client to urgently seek medical attention

- note any contra-action on the client's record card.

Visual assessment techniques

The visual assessment of a client should be performed after questioning so that trust has been developed and the client/therapist relationship established.

First, the therapist or nail technician should examine the area being treated for signs of infection or any abnormalities. While the diagnosis of any condition should not be made it is important to establish that it is not a contraindication or that the treatment will not aggravate it in any way.

The visual assessment is also used to ascertain the following:

- body and skin type

- body and skin condition

- figure and posture faults

- factors affecting the treatment/service, such as the type and texture of hair.

The individual requirements for the visual assessment for specific treatments or services are discussed within the relevant chapters.

Visual aids

Visual aids are particularly useful when a clear explanation is difficult and can assist in the consultation process as they illustrate to the client what the therapist is trying to convey. Simple diagrams of the skin or the hair in its follicle can be used when explaining the effects of a treatment or product, for example, when explaining the effects of electrical epilation on the hair root.

Manual assessment techniques

Manual assessment techniques include:

- touching the skin to detect its texture and warmth
- palpating an area to feel muscle tone or assess skin elasticity
- weighing and measuring
- assisting the client in the performance of exercise to assess muscle strength or flexibility
- skin sensitivity testing.

The therapist must be confident when touching the client and always have freshly washed hands. Be definite with your touch and do not invade personal space. Keep the hand flat with finger tips together when palpating.

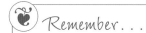

Remember...

Always maintain the client's privacy by keeping the results of your findings confidential. Do not discuss a client's details with anyone without their permission.

Referral to client records

When a client has previously visited the beauty therapy salon, the availability of full accurate client records is an invaluable tool to assist in the consultation process. The records provide information already elicited and can save time set aside for the treatment or service. It is, however, wise to quickly check the client and treatment information to make sure you have the correct record for the client.

Always enquire how the client found the treatment last time and whether there was anything they did not enjoy or found ineffective. This avoids the same treatment being performed when perhaps the client was less than satisfied.

Records should be updated regularly, accurate and confidential. They can be paper-based or stored electronically but must be kept in accordance with the requirements of the Data Protection Act 1998. The Act states that electronic records should be password-protected and that paper-based records must be stored under lock and key. The clients' details should not be passed to a third party without their consent and not used for any illegal activity.

Key terms

Retailing – the exchange of money for goods.

Selling – the process by which a consumer is persuaded to exchange money for goods.

Selling techniques

Why do salons retail?

There are a number of reasons why salons undertake retail selling of products:

- to increase profits: service prices are set for each treatment to be performed in a set time, so a facial that takes one hour may earn the salon £35 but the same client may spend £100 on treatment retail products
- to reinforce treatment benefits: if the client is not offered the opportunity to buy the products used, they will choose their own skincare products without the benefit of the therapist's professional advice

- to create trust and confidence: the client will save money by only buying products that she needs, that will suit her and that are more likely to result in a benefit to her.

Good selling techniques should meet the client's requirements and involves the following stages:

- registering interest
- identifying need
- discussing the features and benefits of the product or service
- closing the sale.

Choosing a retail line

There are a number of factors involved in the choice of a retail line.

- Capital: a large retail line ties up a lot of a salon's capital (money). It is better to start small then invest the profits you make into more and varied retail lines. The lines you choose should fulfil the needs of your clients and the image of your salon.
- Image: the lines you choose should reflect the image that your business portrays. The retail products should be packaged and priced to attract your target market.
- Target market: only buy products for retail that match your target market to prevent unsuitable stock remaining on the shelf.
- Product lines: the number of lines you stock will depend on your available capital, space and the likelihood of them selling. Consider products that enhance treatments such as skincare products, provide appropriate aftercare (such as aftercare lotions) and which complement and relate to the services offered (such as scented products or accessories).

Choosing a supplier

When choosing a supplier, consider the following:

- Price: choose a supplier that offers competitive cost prices and yet is flexible with the retail price to account for special offers or discounts.
- Service: you will need a wholesaler or distributor that is reliable and quick so there is little delay between ordering and delivery, and who offers a personal service so that you can develop a good working relationship.

Wholesaler or distributor?

- Wholesalers give a faster and more personal service. You have control over purchases and they usually offer a wide choice of products from different manufacturers.
- With a distributor, goods may not arrive quickly if the manufacturer is located abroad. If there are production problems with a manufacturing company there may be an inconsistent supply of products and goods.

Whichever you choose, try to develop a good working relationship to ensure continuity of supply as failure to do so may affect your business.

The retail area

The retail area needs to be visible if it is to be successful. Make sure you change product positions to ensure each has an equal chance of selling and to coincide with promotional events.

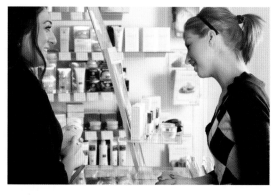
△ The retail area

- Encourage multiple purchasing as it is beneficial to those clients that know what they want. They are able to test and handle the products while the therapist spends more time with those who need advice and assistance. Use 'shelf talkers' – small cards attached to the shelf that offer descriptions to help the client choose. However, there are disadvantages to this approach because high stock levels are needed, which ties up capital and products are handled, leading to damage to packaging and possible theft.

- Use attractive window displays to encourage passing trade to enter the salon. It is said that your salon window is a window to your business, so make it work in a positive way by using it as free advertising for promotional events and special offers.

- Create desire by using posters, props, show cards, display cubes, stands, materials and products to promote the image of your salon.

- Create interest by using a flat-screen TV in your reception area to promote products and services. Place smaller displays of relevant products in treatment rooms and create a 'what's new' area in the reception with products to smell and touch. Mount and frame press cuttings and high profile news items that link to promotional events or the latest trends.

Dealing with complaints

Dealing with complaints will often be a good test of your professionalism. The most common kinds of complaint are:

- being kept waiting without explanation
- dissatisfaction with a treatment or product
- incorrect appointment
- damage to clients' property
- the onset of an injury or disease.

Complaints may be made as they happen, verbally to the therapist or the client may request to see the manager. Alternatively, clients may complain in writing after the incident. At all times the salon's complaint procedure should be followed.

> **Remember...**
>
> Retailing is beneficial to a salon so always bear the following in mind:
>
> - If the client does not buy from you, she will buy from somewhere else without the benefit of your expertise.
> - Choose your retail lines carefully: remember your target market and the image you want to portray.
> - Choose a supplier that can provide you with what you want, when you want it and at a good price.
> - Use your product displays to help you sell.
> - Be honest with your clients and sell them only what is appropriate, effective and good value for money.

- If the complaint is made in person, take the client to a private quiet area and if they are angry or upset, acknowledge this and remain calm.

- Listen attentively to what the client has to say and check facts by asking relevant questions. Repeat the information back to the client to make sure you have understood. Making notes at such an interview is also useful. At this stage, however, do not admit fault.

- Decide whether it is within the limits of your authority to deal with the complaint, following the salon policy, or whether you should pass it on to a more senior member of staff.

- In line with the salon policy agree a way forward so that all parties feel the problem has been resolved in a constructive and satisfactory way, for example, by offering a future free treatment or by refunding the cost of the treatment.

A serious complaint carries a threat of litigation and must be referred to the manager, who will make decisions on appropriate compensation. If the client wishes to take legal action there will need to be a formal record of events with witness statements and physical evidence of the complaint.

Working within the law

Health and safety legislation

The details of the relevant health and safety legislation and how it applies to working in the beauty-related industries can be found in Chapter 1 Monitoring health and safety.

Employment legislation

The employment of individuals within a salon requires compliance with the following legislation (some, but not all, apply to the self-employed too).

Employers' Liability (Compulsory Insurance) Act 1998

This Act states that an employer must have as a minimum insurance to protect an employee in the event that they injure themselves during the course of their normal duties while at work. This also covers the contraction of work-related disease or conditions such as dermatitis and repetitive strain injury (RSI) which are common in beauty-related industries.

Employment Act 2002

This Act governs a parent's rights when expecting a child, including time off to attend antenatal appointments and the right to return after maternity leave. The same rights apply to those adopting a child. Under the terms of the Act, employees can ask for flexible hours if the child is under the age of six or if the child is disabled and under 18. New fathers are entitled to two weeks' paid leave (leave has to finish within 56 days of the birth).

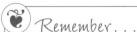

Remember...

When dealing with a complaint remember to use positive body language, maintain eye contact and nod your head occasionally to show that you are listening. Do not cross your arms, frown or show any other negative body language when listening to the client's complaint.

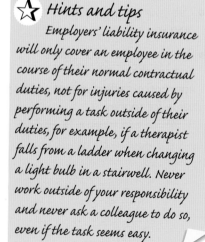

Hints and tips

Employers' liability insurance will only cover an employee in the course of their normal contractual duties, not for injuries caused by performing a task outside of their duties, for example, if a therapist falls from a ladder when changing a light bulb in a stairwell. Never work outside of your responsibility and never ask a colleague to do so, even if the task seems easy.

Working Time Regulations 1998

These Regulations protect workers from developing detrimental effects to their health caused by working long hours and having too few rest periods or breaks or disrupted work patterns. The Regulations state:

- a minimum of 48 hours represents a 'working week'; this includes any overtime and can be averaged over a specific period

- a minimum daily rest period of 11 consecutive hours per day

- a break when the working day is longer than six hours

- minimum rest period of one day per week

- four weeks' annual paid holiday

- night working cannot be over eight hours a night on average

- those aged between 16 and 17 years old have a working week of a maximum of 40 hours.

Payment of Wages Act 1960

This Act covers the right to equal pay for a job, whether the terms of payment are weekly, fortnightly or monthly. An employer should state clearly the terms within which wages or salary are paid when writing the contract of employment.

Employment Rights Act 1996

This Act provides the employee with additional safeguards to their employment such as the right to payslips, statutory sick pay, maternity leave, reasons for dismissal and a statement of particulars and employer's responsibilities; all of these should be stated in the contract of employment. The employer is responsible for paying their employees as long as they are available to work and to ensure that employees are safe while doing their jobs. They should also refund employees' expenses incurred at or during work and act in a reasonable manner towards employees.

The employee's responsibilities are to devote her time during working hours to her employer's business, to not reveal confidential information relating to her employer's business to others and to do her job to the best of her ability.

Employment Protection Act 1978

This Act gives employees the right to receive written particulars of their terms of employment. Most employees are entitled to receive a written statement of the main terms and conditions of their employment within 13 weeks of starting work. An employer with more than 20 employees is also obliged to ensure that every employee has a copy of (or access to) the disciplinary and grievance procedure. An employee is expected to perform their duties and obey their employer. If any order given by a supervisor is within their contract, the employee has an obligation to obey or risk losing his or her job.

> ⭐ **Hints and tips**
> As most beauty therapy businesses are micro businesses, most therapists/employees are paid weekly. Commission on services and/or products can be paid in addition to a 'flat rate'; and weekly payment makes it easier for this commission to be added to an employee's wages.

> **Key term**
>
> **Micro business** – a business with five or fewer employees.

> ⭐ **Hints and tips**
> In a beauty or related industry the employee's responsibility is to wear the correct uniform, use PPE provided, arrive on time and be prepared to work, keep client records confidential and maintain salon hygiene.

Equal Pay Act 1983

This Act is about everyone in the same job being paid the same and on the same terms. The legislation relates to the Sexual Discrimination Act and the Race Relations Act (see 'Discrimination legislation' below).

Consumer legislation

Consumer Protection Act 1987

This is the main piece of consumer protection legislation and protects the client in the case of injury or damage caused by the selling or use of defective products. The Act also relates to the consumer being misled with regard to products, services and facilities.

Cosmetic Products (Safety) Regulations 2008

This is an extension of the Consumer Protection Act within the European Union (EU) and is concerned with a product's presentation, labelling, instructions for use, disposal and any other information or indications provided by the manufacturer. It states that such information should not be misleading or lead to injury or damage to a person or property.

Trade Description Act 1968

This Act protects the consumer from false trade descriptions, whether they are made by a manufacturer, retailer or the service industry. A product or service must be fit for purpose, so it must fulfil the advertised claims, be as described and be of satisfactory quality, including having a reasonable shelf life.

Sale and Supply of Goods Act 1994

This prohibits the use of false trade descriptions. It is important to realise that to repeat a manufacturer's false claim makes a business equally liable. This could be verbally, in words or pictures, on packaging, a sign or in an advert. Goods must be:

- of satisfactory quality (free from fault and defect)
- of reasonable appearance and finish
- safe and durable
- fit for purpose.

The Consumer Safety Act 1978

This Act states the legal safety standards to minimise the risk to consumers from harmful or dangerous products. It prohibits the sale and supply of goods that do not meet with safety requirements or those that are unsafe.

Supply of Goods and Services Act 1982

This Act is also concerned with the quality of products and services, which must be of a satisfactory quality.

Prices Act 1974

This states that advertised and paid prices must be transparent, in other words, prices should be clearly marked so as not to give a false impression. The customer must be clear about the price before buying so they can see they are not being overcharged.

Resale Prices Act 1976

This states that manufacturers are allowed to suggest a retail price but cannot enforce a price at which their goods must be sold. The 'recommended retail price' is only a suggestion of the price a retailer can use.

Discrimination law

New legislation has been passed in relation to the following 'protected characteristics', making it an offence to discriminate on the grounds of a person's:

- race and ethnicity
- religion and beliefs
- disability and/or learning difficulty
- age
- gender
- sexual orientation
- gender reassignment
- marital status, including civil partnerships
- pregnancy and maternity/paternity leave.

The Equality Act 2010 supersedes previous discrimination law and has made the implementation of discrimination law easier to understand. There are seven types of discrimination highlighted, designed to protect those whose status falls into one of the categories listed above. These are:

1   Direct discrimination

2   Associative discrimination: discriminating against someone who is directly involved with someone with a protected characteristic

3   Indirect discrimination: when someone with a protected characteristic is disadvantaged in some way

4   Harassment: when someone is offended by another's behaviour

5   Harassment by a third party: offensive behaviour by someone not in direct contact with the person

6   Victimisation

7   Discrimination by perception.

Want to know more?

For up-to-date information on beauty-related industries, health and safety, codes of practice and career opportunities, visit the Habia website: www.habia.org

For information on professional associations offering insurance and other benefits to their members please visit one of these websites:

www.babtac.com

www.itecworld.co.uk

www.fht.org.uk

www.beautyguild.com

For more information regarding health and safety legislation and to monitor the latest information visit the Health and Safety Executive website: www.hse.gov.uk

For the latest on employment legislation visit: www.direct.gov.uk/en/Employment

Test yourself

1. Give five desirable employment characteristics.

2. Name three ways in which the therapist can protect themselves from harm when providing treatments and services to clients.

3. What are the benefits of becoming a member of a professional body or association?

4. Name the types of insurance needed when working in the beauty therapy industry.

5. What is the importance of continued professional development?

6. What security procedures should a therapist consider when working in the beauty therapy industry?

7. Name four benefits of working in a team.

8. What are the four stages of a formal disciplinary procedure?

9. Name three methods of sterilisation.

10. When would you use closed questioning techniques during a consultation?

Chapter 7
SKIN AND BODY ANALYSIS

It will cover aspects of the following NVQ technical units:

B13 Provide body electrical treatments

B14 Provide facial electrical treatments

B20 Provide body massage treatments

B21 Provide UV tanning services

B23 Provide Indian head massage

B24 Carry out massage using pre-blended aromatherapy oils

B28 Provide stone therapy treatments

B29 Provide electrical epilation treatments

LEARNING OBJECTIVES

In this chapter you will learn about the skin and body analysis procedures that are important to the success of every beauty therapy treatment.

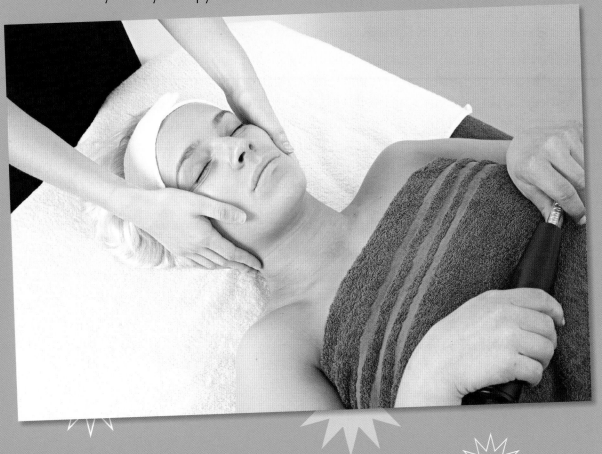

This chapter will also cover aspects of the following VRQ units at Level 3:

City & Guilds

- Unit 305 Provide body massage
- Unit 306 Provide facial electrotherapy treatments
- Unit 307 Provide body electrotherapy treatments
- Unit 308 Provide electrical epilation
- Unit 309 Provide massage using pre-blended aromatherapy oils
- Unit 311 Provide Indian head massage
- Unit 312 Provide UV tanning
- Unit 313 Provide self tanning
- Unit 314 Apply and maintain nail enhancements
- Unit 319 Intimate waxing for female clients
- Unit 321 Apply microdermabrasion
- Unit 322 Apply stone therapy massage
- Unit 328 Airbrush design for nails
- Unit 329 Design and apply nail art

VTCT

- Unit UV30403 Provide facial electrotherapy treatments
- Unit UV30404 Provide body electrotherapy treatments
- Unit UV30405 Apply & maintain nail enhancements
- Unit UV40407 Airbrush design for nails
- Unit UV40424 Provide body massage
- Unit UV30425 Provide massage using pre-blended aromatherapy oils
- Unit UV30430 Apply microdermabrasion
- Unit UV30450 Provide UV tanning
- Unit UV30451 Provide self tanning
- Unit UV30474 Provide electrical epilation
- Unit UV30475 Apply stone therapy massage
- Unit UV30476 Design & apply nail art

Introduction

Skin and body analysis facilitates the customisation of treatments to the face and body. From this analysis the therapist should be able to identify:

- the client's skin type and condition, including any differences due to age, race and gender and the care/treatment it has received
- the client's body type and condition
- any lifestyle factors such as postural faults.

The collation of this information can inform decisions made by the therapist in terms of the most beneficial treatment and products to use and can also suggest appropriate aftercare and homecare advice, including recommendations for changes in lifestyle. This enables the client to receive the best possible treatment for the condition presented, which in turn promotes trust and confidence in the therapist. It helps to promote return of custom, the professionalism of the therapist and salon and ensures the success of the business.

Both skin and body analysis relies on the effective use of questioning techniques and visual and manual assessments.

Skin analysis

A thorough analysis of the skin is imperative for any facial treatment to be successful, but should not be overlooked during nail and body work too, including the different forms of massage. This analysis should include the appendages of the skin such as the nail and hair where appropriate.

A thorough skin analysis includes a visual and manual assessment to determine:

- skin type: dry, oily, combination or normal

- skin condition: dehydrated, moist, sensitive, mature, congested, oedematous

- skin tone and texture

- differences relating to age, race and gender

- nail and hair condition

- presence of non-infectious treatable skin, nail and hair conditions.

Skin type

Skin type is defined by the activity of the sebaceous glands in the skin and is described as normal, dry, oily, combination. When the sebaceous glands produce sufficient sebum the skin appears normal and is smooth and flexible to the touch, with no apparent shine and is blemish free.

Oily skin

Oily skin has over-active sebaceous glands and subsequent production of sebum, resulting in a shiny and oily appearance. There is likely to be the presence of comedones, papules and pustules as the pores and hair follicles become blocked with the excess sebum. The excess sebum on the skin surface also inhibits the skin's natural desquamation process, leading to a thickening of the epidermis and a dull, lifeless appearance.

Dry skin

This is the result of under-active sebaceous glands. Without adequate sebum to trap in moisture the skin can become dehydrated, making it rough to touch and there may be dry flaky patches of skin.

Combination skin

This skin type has areas where the sebaceous glands are over-active and areas where the activity of the sebaceous glands is normal. The shininess associated with this skin type is due to the presence of more sebaceous glands in a particular area, rather than increased activity, for example, the centre of the face, the chest and upper back/shoulder area.

> **Key term**
>
> **Desquamation** – the natural loss of dead epidermal skin cells at the skin's surface.

> ☆ *Hints and tips*
> *Sebaceous gland activity is largely under the control of testosterone, the male sex hormone, which in women is more apparent during and as a result of puberty and occasionally after menopause, as the influence of the female sex hormone, oestrogen, diminishes.*

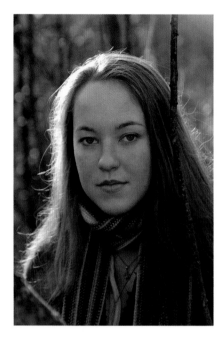

△ Sensitive skin

Key term

Anaphylactic shock – a severe allergic reaction where there is swelling of the tissues, including the lips, tongue and throat, which could lead to asphyxiation.

Skin condition

Skin condition is the result of a number of internal and external factors, including:

- climate and sun exposure
- air conditioning and central heating
- diet and health
- stress and sleep
- alcohol and smoking
- hormones – male and female
- drugs and medication.

These factors can result in sensitive, dehydrated, moist, mature, congested or oedematous skin conditions.

Sensitivity

Sensitivity is the result of an over-zealous immune system that reacts to the presence of an allergen. Usually a sensitive skin is only one aspect of the a hypersensitive immune system and the client may also suffer from (or have a family history of) asthma, hay fever and/or eczema.

There are different types of skin sensitivity and a client may suffer from any of the following:

- heat sensitivity: the client reddens easily when the body temperature rises, for example during exercise
- sun sensitivity: the client always burns when exposed to sunlight or UV light on a sunbed, even if this is then followed by the tanning process
- touch sensitivity: the skin reddens easily even with the most gentle of physical contact, such as during cleansing
- product sensitivity: the client reddens following contact with a product; in some cases they may experience irritation in the form of itching and/or soreness and a rise in the local skin temperature.

A client who experiences all of these types of sensitivity is known as 'hypersensitive' and when combined with a history of asthma, hay fever or eczema, can be very difficult to treat without causing an allergic reaction. In this case a series of thermal, tactile and sensitivity tests with the relevant products is advisable.

A simple thermal test is as follows:

- Prepare a small bowl of very cold water and one of very hot water and in each place a small metal tool such as a cuticle knife or a comedone extractor.
- After a few minutes take out each tool and wipe with a tissue. Test on your wrist that it is a safe but discernable temperature.
- With the client looking away, gently place each tool alternately onto the area to be treated and ask the client to determine whether it is hot or cold.

A tactile sensation test can be carried out in a similar way:

- Prepare an orange stick with cotton wool around the 'hoof end' but leave the pointed end free.

- With the client looking away, gently place each end alternately onto the area to be treated and ask the client to determine whether it is sharp or blunt.

These tests are performed at the time of the treatment and are used to determine the skin's sensation levels, indicating whether an adaptation to the treatment will be necessary. Such adaptations may include the omission of the affected area of the body, a reduction in treatment intensity and/or limiting the choice of equipment used to treat the client's condition.

A sensitivity test involves placing a little of the intended product for use 24–48 hours before the treatment and should be used where there is a history of allergic reactions or product sensitivity.

To perform a sensitivity test:

- Cleanse the area with warm water or an alcohol wipe.

- Place a small amount of the product to be used in the treatment onto the skin.

- Inform the client that a positive reaction can be redness, swelling, irritation and/or itching. If this occurs they need to remove the product immediately and soothe the area with cold water and inform the salon, as the treatment cannot go ahead. If the irritation persists they should consult their GP.

- If no reaction occurs within 24 hours they can remove the product with cool water and the treatment can go ahead.

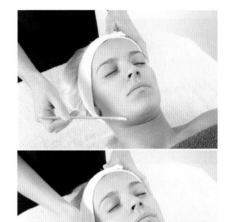
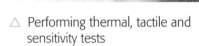

△ Performing thermal, tactile and sensitivity tests

Dehydration

Dehydration is a lack of water in the skin rather than a lack of oil as a result of under-active sebaceous glands. The appearance of the skin includes:

- fine superficial lines (like a 'dried up river bed')

- superficial flaking

- broken capillaries.

Any skin type can become dehydrated as a result of:

- the client's general health as a result of illness, especially fever (due to fluid loss caused by sweating)

- medication

- drastic dieting

- environment, especially low humidity or air conditioning

- exposure to harsh products

- weather conditions such as wind, cold and the sun.

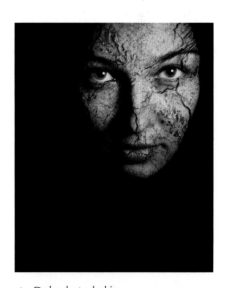

△ Dehydrated skin

Moist skin

This type of skin will appear smooth and soft to touch and when stretched will return quickly to its position, indicating flexibility. It will adhere for a moment when the fingertips are pressed gently against it and then slowly pull away.

Oedematous skin

This condition is caused by fluid retention within the skin tissues and is recognised by slight puffing or swelling in the area, but with no other visual signs such as erythema, irritation or pain being apparent. When gently pressed, the skin will remain depressed for a while after the pressure is released. It may have a tight and shiny appearance.

Oedematous skin can be caused by a variety of factors, such as high salt intake, injury, being immobile or simply from standing on the feet for long periods. Lymph drainage techniques around the affected area can encourage the draining of fluid.

Oedematous skin is often a symptom of an underlying condition such as a systemic illness, for example, heart or kidney disorders. If systemic, the client may also be experiencing aching or tender limbs, stiff joints, weight gain or weight loss and raised blood pressure and pulse rate. If these other symptoms exist the client should be advised to see a medical practitioner.

△ Oedematous skin

> ☆ *Hints and tips*
> *Knowledge of the lymphatic system and how the system drains fluid from the different areas of the body is essential to be able to perform lymph drainage techniques effectively and safely.*

> ☆ *Hints and tips*
> *Puffiness around the eyes is often a sign of blocked or inflamed sinuses, after a cold for example. A facial treatment that soothes inflammation and decongests the sinuses involving the use of products containing aromatherapy oils such as camomile or lavender will be of benefit to the client.*

Mature skin

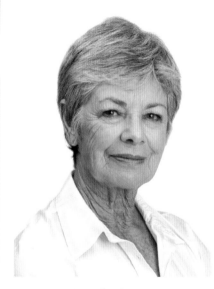

△ Mature female skin

Mature skin conditions are associated with age but can be present in younger clients as a result of poor skin care involving the use of harsh products, inadequate sun protection and harsh environments such as central heating. In such cases the condition is referred to as premature ageing.

The appearance of mature skin is one that lacks sebum and moisture, leading to dry skin and dehydration skin conditions. Lines and wrinkles will be present, formed by the repetitive action of the muscles of facial expression, which cause lines in the skin of the forehead, around the eyes and mouth. There is some loss of skin tone and underlying muscle tone and under the influence of gravity, the tissues begin to drop into folds. This is exacerbated by the loss of the subcutaneous (fatty) layer, especially in women as the result of reduced levels of oestrogen during and after menopause.

> **Key term**
>
> **Exacerbate** – to make something worse.

Congested skin

Under close examination this skin type appears uneven in texture, with the presence of blocked pores, comedones, milia and small lumps under the epidermis, and is associated with an oily skin type. The condition is caused by the accumulation of sebum and waste products that are usually secreted or excreted by the skin becoming trapped under a fine textured or thick epidermis. Congested skin is commonly found on the face, shoulders and chest areas of the body.

Skin tone and texture

Skin texture can be described as fine or coarse and is determined primarily through observing the skin, although touching the skin can confirm the visual assessment. A fine textured skin appears smooth, with no open pores or unevenness such as that found with a congested skin condition. However, on close inspection there may be the presence of fine lines, particularly if the skin is also dehydrated. A coarse skin has open pores and appears uneven and is often associated with an oily skin type, although it can also appear as part of the mature skin type.

Accurate diagnosis of skin tone relies more on the sensitive touch of the therapist rather than observation. Good skin tone relies on the elastic nature of the collagen and elastin fibres in the reticular layer of the dermis. If these are plentiful and in good condition the skin will feel firm to the touch and resilient to gentle pressure – the skin will 'bounce back' against the gentle placing of the fingertips. Skin tone is greatly influenced by factors such as dehydration and is an indication of age and therefore a mature skin condition. A simple test is to take a 'pinch' of skin and gentle pull it away from the underlying fatty and muscular tissue, then release and watch the rate at which the skin returns to a normal state. Poor skin tone will be slow in its return and may remain in a 'peak' for some moments.

Differences in skin relating to age, race and gender

Age

The differences in the skin relating to age can be described as follows:

- Activity of the sebaceous glands slows and the rate at which sebum is produced is reduced, leading to a drier skin condition and then to dehydration as moisture loss increases. This results in the appearance of fine lines within the epidermis.

- There is less resilience in the collagen and elastin fibres leading to a loss in skin tone.

- Muscle tone decreases and underlying adipose tissue diminishes.

- The loss of muscle and skin tone results in the formation of deep wrinkles, based around the character lines formed by facial expression.

- Areas of the body and face with poor muscle tone begin to hang down as a result of the effect of gravity, for example the eyelids, neck and jawline and the breasts, abdomen and buttocks.

- The skin of elderly people is often thinner due to the reduction in collagen and elastin fibres and the reduction in adipose tissue.

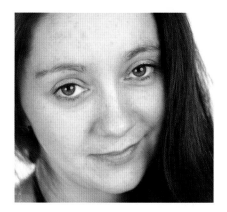

△ Congested skin

Activity

Compare the skin tone of your forearm, the back of your hand and at the knuckle of one of your fingers by performing the 'pinch' test. Is there a difference between the rate at which the skin returns to normal? What could be the explanation for a difference in the rate between the skin of the forearm and that of the back of the hand or knuckle?

Hints and tips

Often, a comparison between different areas of the client's skin is more useful in determining whether to provide corrective treatment for this condition rather than a comparison between the skin of different clients or even yourself.

Race

Differences in the skin relating to race are described below.

White skin

Those people described as having white skin include white American, white British, white African and white Australian ethnic groups.

White skin can vary in shade from very pale to the mid brown of Mediterranean skin with pink, cream and olive as the underlying tone. White skin is usually accompanied by red, fair or mid brown hair and blue, hazel, green or grey eye colour. It is recognised by the reduced levels of the pigment melanin which give the skin its pale colour and this means that it is greatly affected by ultra-violet light and usually burns easily when exposed to the sun. As a result, white skin is prone to premature ageing, with the signs showing in a person in their early thirties, especially if the skin-care routine is poor, without the use of products containing sun protection factors.

Other problems of white skin include an inclination to blemishes due to the activity of the hormones on the sebaceous glands and areas of pigmentation due to sun exposure and the effects of medication. Generally the skin is able to heal itself quite well but with the formation of scarring that appears pink initially and then white as the scar ages. The delicate nature of the collagen and elastin fibres can lead to the formation of striations or stretch marks.

Asian skin

Those described as having Asian skin include Asian British and people from India, Pakistan and Bangladesh and also China, Japan and Nepal. The skin can vary in shade from light to dark brown with a yellow or olive underlying tone. Asian skin is usually accompanied by mid to very dark brown hair and brown or black eye colour.

The presence of melanin in the skin and the mild over-activity of the sebaceous glands give rise to an oily skin type. The melanin offers reasonable protection from the harmful effects of the sun and the onset of ageing is often delayed until the forties or fifties.

Relatively minor skin damage can result in hyper-pigmentation as the skin heals, resulting in an uneven skin colour and Asian skins that originate from the Indian subcontinent are often affected by superfluous hair growth.

Black skin

People who are described as having black skin originate from America, Africa, the Caribbean and Australia and can exhibit a wide variation in skin colour, from the darkest brown/black to mid brown. The skin shows underlying tones of yellow, red and orange and is accompanied by dark brown or black hair and eyes.

This skin type offers a high degree of protection from the harmful effects of the sun and therefore the signs of ageing only appear late in life.

> **Key term**
>
> **Superfluous** – unwanted but not necessarily excessive hair growth. For example, the presence of hair in the underarm is normal but is often removed as it is unwanted.

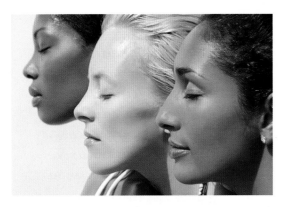

△ Differences in skin related to race

The sheen on a black skin is often mistaken as oily skin type but in fact is a result of the light being reflected from the skin. There is however increased sweat-gland activity.

Black skins are prone to hyper-pigmentation scarring and also keloid scarring if the skin is damaged.

Gender

The differences in skin relating to gender are primarily related to the presence of the male sex hormone testosterone. Testosterone affects the skin as follows:

- A thicker epidermis, making the skin more resilient to infections and less sensitive than female skins.

- More active sebaceous glands, leading to an oily skin type and the presence of congestion, coarse skin texture and blemishes.

- Male pattern hair growth, including facial and body hair which is coarse in texture and sometimes dense. The removal of facial hair, however, can result in the skin becoming sensitised due to the regular exposure to the harsh products involved in soaps and the alcohol found in aftershave lotions.

- The resilience of the collagen and elastin fibres combined with the thicker epidermis and oilier skin often means that men do not show the signs of ageing as quickly as women.

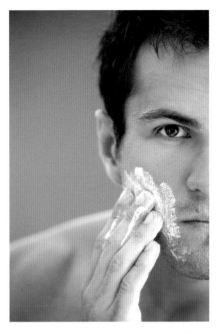

△ Male skin

Hair condition

For some therapeutic treatments it is essential to also consider the presence of hair, including its type, quantity and texture, as this may influence not only the choice of treatment and/or any adaptations. However, the presence of hair in a male hair-growth pattern in women may indicate a systemic disorder that the client is unaware of. Such disorders may require medical treatment before a beauty therapy treatment can go ahead and consequently it is important to consider this as part of the skin and body analysis.

Hair condition should be described as and considered in regard to:

- type: terminal or vellus, curly, wavy or straight

- texture: fine, medium or coarse

- density: sparse, normal or dense; single or compound

- colour: light, dark, red or non-pigmented.

Presence of non-infectious treatable skin, nail and hair conditions

The presence of skin, nail and hair conditions which are not infectious, such as eczema and psoriasis, will inform the decisions made by the therapist. The following points should be considered:

- Severity of the condition: the therapist must consider the safety of the client at all times and if continuing with a treatment is detrimental to the condition, the therapist must make the decision to postpone the treatment until the condition has improved.

☆ *Hints and tips*
When considering the density of hair growth, remember the hair growth cycle. For any hair growth present on the skin, approximately 10 per cent of the hair follicles will be lying dormant in the telogen phase – the resting stage – and may or may not have a hair contained within them. This means that there will be a number of active follicles under the skin surface that will produce a hair later in the cycle.

Key terms

Hypertrichosis – a term used to describe excessive hair for the age, gender or race of the individual.

Hirsutism – a term used to describe a hair growth in a male-growth pattern in females.

223

- Choice of treatment and product: some treatments can actively improve some non-infectious conditions and although this may not be the client's main concern, any improvement will increase client confidence, trust and satisfaction.

- Adaptation of the treatment: such adaptations can include choice of product, intensity levels, variation in pressure and/or technique, treatment timings and aftercare advice.

Nail condition

Nail condition can be an indicator of the general health of the client and the work undertaken as well as the attention the nails receive. The nail technician will consider the nail condition under the following categories:

- nail condition: bitten, damaged, oily, dry, extensions (from another salon or technician)

- cuticle condition: dry, normal, overgrown, split, hangnail

- nail shape: round, square, pointed, fan, oval, trapezoid, narrow, ski-jump, hook

- nail length: short, medium, long.

The information can be used by the nail technician in order to make accurate recommendations for treatment or referral to a medical practitioner as appropriate. The nail technician should ensure that cross infection is avoided and avoid making a nail or skin condition worse.

Body analysis

Body analysis means 'the analysis of the figure and related information to determine figure faults and their causes, and to decide the appropriate treatment plan for their correction'.

Body type or somatype

The shape of a person's body can be divided into three distinct types:

1 Ectomorphs are long and lean with narrow shoulders and hips. They have very little fat or muscle bulk. They are generally good at endurance type sports and activities such as long distance running. The characteristics of ectomorphs are:

- long, thin limbs

- long, thin trunk

- lack of curves

- possibility of problems associated with being underweight.

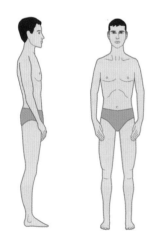

△ A typical ectomorph

2 Mesomorphs have broad shoulders and are narrow waisted and powerfully hipped – the classic triangular shape. Sprinters and gymnasts are often of this type. The characteristics of mesomorphs are:

- defined muscular build

- developed shoulders

- slim hips

- no problems with weight gain when active.

3 Endomorphs are short, wide hipped and have large proportions. They gain weight easily and even when they are not overweight tend to be rounded. The characteristics of endomorphs are:

- round, plump, heavy body

- short neck

- fat deposits

- hands and feet may be small

- short limbs

- prone to weight gain.

Each category is an extreme and few people fit neatly into one of these groups. It is also possible to be more than one type (except endomorph/ectomorph as this is an impossible combination). A person who is overweight may also inhibit the typical appearance of their particular body type, for example, a well-fed mesomorph may look more like an endomorph.

> ☆ *Hints and tips*
> *There is little you can do to change someone's body type. Exercise and eating sensibly will improve their shape but there is a limit to the extent of this improvement and this has to be recognised by those seeking improvements to their figure.*

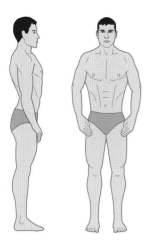

△ A typical mesomorph

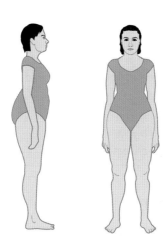

△ A typical endomorph

Read each question then choose your answer from a), b) or c). Some questions may difficult to answer for yourself, so try the quiz with a friend and ask their opinion.

1 Which of the following best describes your body?
   a round
   b square
   c long

2 How would you describe your contours?
   a soft
   b rugged
   c delicate

3 How would you compare the relative size of your trunk with the rest of your body?
   a trunk seems large in relation to rest of body
   b both seem well proportioned
   c trunk seems small in relation to rest of body

4 Are your bones evident?
   a no
   b yes and they appear large
   c yes and they appear small

5 How would you describe your thighs and upper arms?
   a rounded
   b muscular
   c thin

6 How would you describe your neck?
   a short
   b long and wide
   c long and slender

Now look at how you answered each question to determine your overall body shape.

Mostly **a** = endomorph
Mostly **b** = mesomorph
Mostly **c** = ectomorph

Posture

The correct posture is very important in maintaining a good figure and to reduce fatigue in everyday life. Postural faults can lead to back and neck pain, fatigue, figure problems and reduced movement in old age. Correct posture is determined by viewing the client in minimal clothing. Encourage the client to stand easily, with feet together and arms held loosely at the sides. The therapist should view the client from the side and from the front using a plumb line – an imaginary line of gravity that should pass just in front of the ear, through the shoulder joint, through the hip joint, through the front of the knee joint and in front of the ankle when the client is viewed laterally. From the anterior view the line of gravity should run through the tip of the nose, the sternum, pass through the naval, through the pubic symphasis and between the knee and ankle joint.

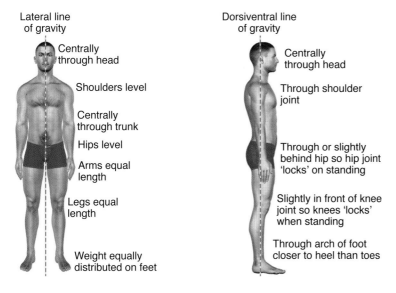

△ How to determine correct posture

When viewed from the front, the spine appears in a straight line but laterally there are four natural curves in the spine:

1 cervical curve

2 thoracic curve

3 lumbar curve

4 sacral curve.

These curves give the body a sound foundation from which movement and everyday activities can be performed without causing injury or discomfort. The curves in the spine are held in place or maintained by the anti-gravity muscles.

Correct posture is maintained by three factors:

1 Anti-gravity muscles: these are groups of muscles that maintain tone (contract) without any movement taking place. They hold the body and therefore the spine in an upright position.

2 Central nervous system control: the posture is maintained by neuro-muscular coordination, the centre for which is situated in the cerebellum of the brain.

3 Postural reflex: this is the body's response to gravity; by coordinating information received from the eyes, ears and skin sensations, the brain sends the correct impulses to the anti-gravity muscles.

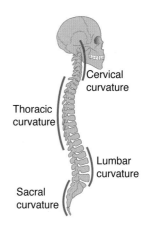

△ The natural curves of the spine

Key term

Anti-gravity muscles – these are found in the anterior and posterior aspects of the body and include the following muscles:

- extensors and flexors of the neck
- pectorals and spinal muscles
- abdominal muscles
- extensors and flexors of the hip and knee.

Postural faults

If a group of anti-gravity muscles are developed to a greater extent or become weaker than that of their antagonist a postural fault will result.

Kyphosis

Kyphosis is an exaggerated curve of the thoracic spine. This condition can sometimes be found in an ectomorph body type and is the result of shortened pectoral muscles and lengthening of the muscles in the upper back between the shoulder blades. Kyphosis is often associated with round shoulders and a forward head tilt.

Lordosis

Lordosis is an exaggerated curve of the lumbar spine. It gives the effect of having a hollow back and is often seen in conjunction with a forward pelvic tilt.

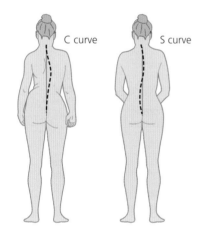
C curve   S curve

△ Kyphosis

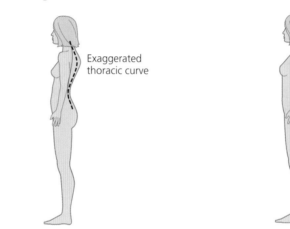
Exaggerated thoracic curve

Exaggerated lumbar curve

△ Lordosis   △ Scoliosis

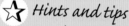

Hints and tips

How the client stands, sits and performs their everyday activities will influence the condition of their muscles and affect the bony structures to which the muscles are attached. For example, a client whose occupation involves holding their arms out in front of them unsupported, such as a hairdresser, may suffer from tension between the scapulae. If this goes untreated it can result in round shoulders and a forward head posture or tilt.

Scoliosis

Scoliosis is a lateral curve of the spine and may be indicated in the thoracic or lumbar regions and to either the right or the left-hand side. Occasionally a client with scoliosis will appear to have an uneven shoulder or hip position.

Any strong deviation from the correct spinal curvature should be considered a medical condition and therefore not treated by the therapist. Instead the client should be referred to a specialist via their GP. It is important however that the therapist should note any such deviation as it will limit or contraindicate treatment and/or exercise.

It is possible that minor deviations from the correct spinal curvature may present themselves during the plumb line diagnosis part of the visual assessment and which are caused by repetitive everyday activity such as carrying bags on the same shoulder. These common conditions can be corrected with stretching and toning exercises aimed at the correct muscle groups.

Here are some other common conditions to look out for during postural analysis:

Forward head posture (tilt)

This is caused by the shortening of the neck flexors and lengthening of the neck extensors (trapezius). A condition known as 'Dowager's hump', where fatty deposits accumulate at the base of the neck around the seventh cervical vertebra can develop if allowed to go uncorrected.

Long-term effects of a forward head posture include:

- rounding of the shoulders

- inward rotation of the arms

- compressed thoracic cavity

- likelihood on an increased lumbar lordosis

- reduced range of motion

- increased wear on articular components of affected joints

- increased muscle tension in some areas causing 'short weakness'

- decreased muscle tension in some areas causing 'stretch weakness'.

Correction: this includes lengthening of shortened muscles and shortening of lengthened muscles through an exercise such as 'chin tucks'.

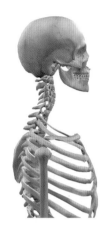

△ Forward head tilt

Round shoulders

This is caused by the shortening of the pectoral muscles and the lengthening of the trapezius and rhomboids and is sometimes associated with having large breasts.

Correction: lengthening of the pectorals and shortening of the trapezius.

1 To lengthen the pectorals: place hands flat on bottom and slowly bring shoulder blades together. Hold in position for a slow count of five and then release. Repeat five times.

2 To shorten the trapezius: lie on your front, hands by the sides, forehead resting on the floor. Inhale as you lift the shoulders up off the floor and exhale as you release. Repeat five times. To progress the exercise as the muscles strengthen, place hands on bottom and eventually use the length of the arms as additional weight.

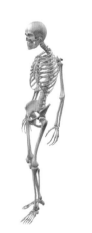

△ Round shoulders

Forward pelvic tilt

This condition is caused by the shortening of the muscles of the lumbar spine and hip flexor muscles and lengthened abdominals and hip extensor muscles. Anterior pelvic tilt involves the pelvic girdle tipping forward, giving the impression of a hollow back. It is often seen in women after pregnancy as a result of poor posture while carrying the weight of the child.

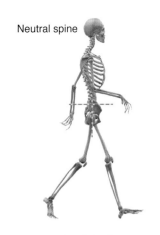
Neutral spine

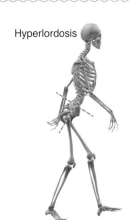
Hyperlordosis

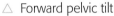

△ Forward pelvic tilt

Correction: lengthening of the lumbar and hip flexors and shortening of the abdominals and hip extensors.

1 Stand with hands on hips, thumbs in back.

2 Roll hips under so that thumbs and the back of the hips come downward (not forward).

3 Use the neutral spine position for normal posture.

4 Alternative: lying on your back (supine) with knees bent and feet flat on floor, pull in stomach muscles to push small of back into floor. Repeat five times. To progress the exercise: lift head and shoulders off the floor, slide hands up front of thighs, progress with arms across chest. Repeat five times.

Other conditions

Winged scapula: a condition where the scapula protrude from the back at the shoulder area.

Knock knees: where the femur is incorrectly set into the hip joint, causing the upper leg to rotate medially, bringing the knees together.

Bow legs: caused by a bending of the long bones of the leg, due to the softening of the bone tissue and the effect of the body weight against gravity.

Flat feet: a condition where the four natural arches of the feet are not supported because of weakened ligaments. This causes the feet to collapse under the weight of the body.

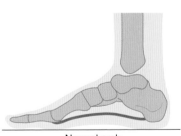

△ Winged scapula

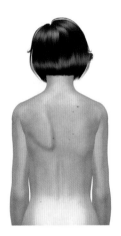

Normal arch

Flat arch

△ Flat feet

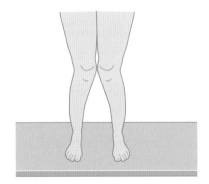

△ Knock knees

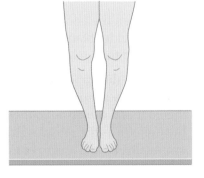

△ Bow legs

Pigeon chest: a condition often associated with severe asthma. It appears as a protrusion outwards of the sternum from high on the chest wall, similar to when a pigeon puffs up his chest feathers.

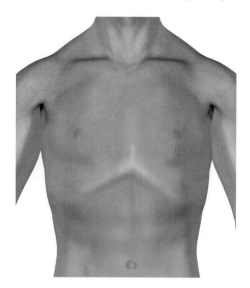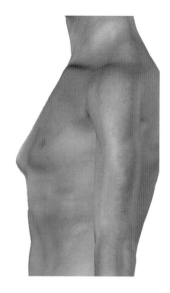

△ Pigeon chest

Correct/healthy weight

In a weight-obsessed society it is hard to break away from the idea that if we are unhappy with the way we look we must lose weight. As a body therapist you must understand the three mechanisms by which a client's 'correct weight' is judged in order to provide a realistic and accurate diagnosis. These three mechanisms are:

1 Weight/height ratio

2 Percentage body fat

3 Body mass index (BMI).

Weight/height ratio

Weight/height ratio is based on whether someone is over- or underweight. It uses charts issued by the government that indicate a weight range according to height, gender and frame size.

The given weight ranges are based on what is considered healthy and are used by doctors in hospitals, surgeries and clinics. However, because body weight can consist of muscle, bone and water as well as fat, the charts alone can prove inadequate in helping a client to improve their figure. It is the proportion of these elements that are important in figure analysis.

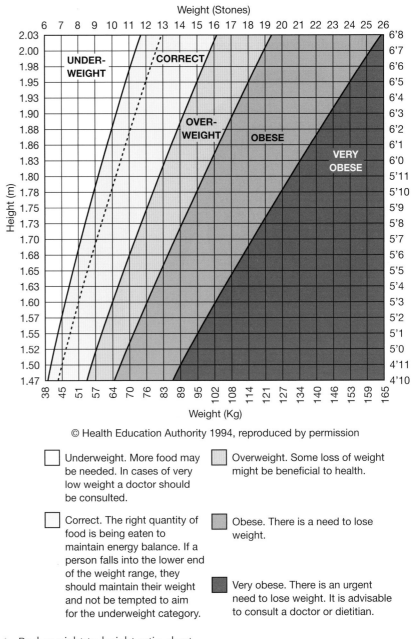

Weight (Stones)

© Health Education Authority 1994, reproduced by permission

Underweight. More food may be needed. In cases of very low weight a doctor should be consulted.

Overweight. Some loss of weight might be beneficial to health.

Correct. The right quantity of food is being eaten to maintain energy balance. If a person falls into the lower end of the weight range, they should maintain their weight and not be tempted to aim for the underweight category.

Obese. There is a need to lose weight.

Very obese. There is an urgent need to lose weight. It is advisable to consult a doctor or dietitian.

△ Body weight to height ratio chart

Percentage body fat

Weight is only one indicator of shape and size. Percentage body fat together with the weight chart is a more accurate way to determine whether someone is underweight, overweight or obese.

It is possible to be the correct weight yet be unhappy with the way you look in the mirror. It could be that improved muscle tone in an area is required in the form of exercise or it could be that the weight of the body is proportionally made up from body fat instead of lean tissue (muscle). It is important therefore to assess the percentage of body fat to achieve an accurate decision as to whether the client is overweight. To do this we use skin fold callipers or specialised scales that measure percentage body fat electronically.

A skin fold calliper is a device which measures the thickness of a fold of skin with its underlying layer of fat. By doing this at key locations, shown by research to be representative of the total amount of fat on the body, it is possible to estimate the total percentage body fat of a person. Skin fold callipers have springs which exert a certain pressure on the skin fold, generally 10 gm/sq mm, and an accurate scale, which measures the thickness in millimetres.

Body mass index

Body mass index is a calculation that is used to assess the degree to which someone is overweight. The formula is:

Weight in kilograms ÷ height squared in metres (m²)

The resulting figure is then compared with the following table:

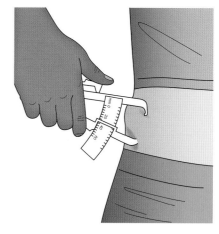

△ Using a skin fold calliper

BMI	Considered to be:
Below 20	Underweight
20–24	Desirable
25–30	Overweight
30	Obese

For example:

Mrs A weighs 70 kg and has a height of 1.68 m.

70 kg ÷ 1.68m x 1.68 m

70 ÷ 2.82 = 24.8

Mrs A is considered to be a correct and healthy weight.

Types of fat

This heading is a little misleading as it suggests that different types of adipose tissue exist, when in fact adipose tissue is structurally the same all over the body. Instead it is the way in which it behaves that leads us to give different names to fat.

Soft fat

This is laid down very easily and is therefore the most easy to rid the body of. In a weight reduction programme, this fat is lost first. It is soft to the touch and it is possible to lift the fat from the underlying muscle tissue (to 'pinch an inch'). Soft fat is common on the stomach, inner thigh, face, backs of arms and the breast area of both men and women.

Hard fat

Hard fat is thought to develop from soft fat when laid down over a period of years. It is difficult to lift away from the underlying muscle tissue and springs out of the fingers. It is thought to have a strong fibrous medium in which the fat cells sit. In a weight-reduction programme, it will be more difficult to remove than soft fat. It is commonly found on the thighs, hips and buttocks of women; in men, the stomach, waist and back can accumulate hard fat deposits.

 Health and safety

Weight gain in the area of and above the waist (apple type) is more dangerous than weight gained around the hips and flank area (pear type). Fat cells in the upper body have different qualities than those found in the hips and thighs and have been proved to lead to the onset of heart disease which can lead to a heart attack.

233

Cellulite

This is not really a type of fat but a condition that affects areas of fatty deposits. It is more common in women due to the effects of the female hormones, but men can also have cellulite.

Cellulite is a condition where toxins accumulate in the tissue fluid and it is made worse when the blood circulation and lymphatic drainage is poor in the area and/or the diet is full of toxins. The condition can be improved by reducing the toxins in the diet, improving general blood circulation in the area to encourage lymph drainage (which is the body's natural waste disposal system) and by undertaking salon and home treatments. Cellulite appears as dimpling in the skin which may be visible without any test, but if unsure, to test for cellulite simply push the skin together in the area being tested and look for the characteristic 'orange peel' dimpling. The most severe forms have a high degree of fluid content where the skin remains indented after compression with the finger tip. In this case the need for natural diuretics in the diet is indicated and should be included within the salon treatment.

Body fat differences due to age and gender

There are variations in men and women regarding the distribution of body fat, as indicated in the diagram below. Men generally have more muscle bulk and therefore can appear in better shape than a woman of the same weight and height.

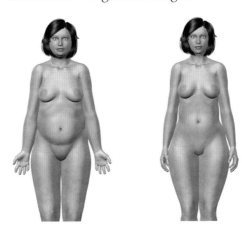

△ Body fat distribution in 'apple' and 'pear' shapes

 Health and safety

Low-impact exercise such as walking helps to maintain the calcium levels in the bones after menopause.

With age, a general reduction in muscle bulk occurs and poor muscle tone is common in both men and women who do not exercise frequently. A condition called osteoporosis (brittle bones)is also common with age and more so in women than in men. This is due to the reduction of oestrogen in the bloodstream after menopause which, when present, maintains the calcium levels in the bones. A reduction in oestrogen leads to the bones becoming brittle and prone to breakage, even with little force.

Want to know more?

Further information can be found at www.nhsdirect.nhs.uk.

Test yourself

1. What are two signs of dry skin?

2. What is another word for comedones?

3. What are the signs of ageing or premature ageing?

4. What are the four main skin types?

5. The activity of which gland in the skin is responsible for skin type?

6. Name five factors that influence the condition of the skin.

7. What factors can lead to the development of oedematous skin condition?

8. Name four distinguishing features of black skin.

9. Name and describe the three main body types.

10. Name three factors that maintain correct body posture.

11. Name the three mechanisms by which a therapist must judge a client's correct body weight.

12. Briefly describe the condition 'cellulite'.

13. What effect can age have on body condition?

14. What is the main difference between males and females of the same weight and height?

Chapter 8
BODY ELECTRICAL TREATMENTS

This chapter covers:

NVQ unit B13 Provide body electrical treatments

City & Guilds VRQ unit 307 Provide body electrotherapy treatments

VTCT VRQ unit UV30404 Provide body electrotherapy treatments

LEARNING OBJECTIVES

This chapter is about improving the body and skin.

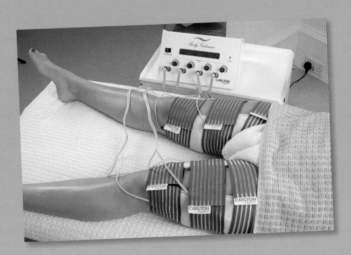

The learning outcomes for NVQ unit B13 are:

1 Be able to maintain effective and safe methods of working when providing body electrical treatments
2 Be able to consult, plan and prepare for treatments with clients
3 Be able to carry out body electrical treatments
4 Understand organisational and legal requirements
5 Understand how to work safely and effectively when providing body electrical treatments
6 Understand how to perform client consultation, planning and preparation
7 Understand the anatomy and physiology for body electrical treatments
8 Understand contraindications that affect or restrict body electrical treatments
9 Understand equipment, materials, products and treatment specific knowledge
10 Be able to provide aftercare advice

You will need to be competent in all of these outcomes to be competent in body electrical treatment, qualify for insurance and perform the treatments on members of the public.

NVQ evidence requirements

For the NVQ your assessor will need to observe you perform these treatments successfully on at least five separate occasions involving at least three different clients.

1 Demonstrate the use of all the following equipment:
- galvanic unit
- electro muscle stimulator (EMS)
- micro-current unit
- lymphatic drainage equipment
- microdermabrasion unit.

2 Demonstrate the use of all these consultation techniques:
- questioning
- visual
- manual
- reference to client records.

3 Treated all the following body types:
- endomorph
- mesomorph
- ectomorph.

4 Treated all the following body conditions:
- cellulite
- poor muscle tone
- sluggish circulation
- uneven skin texture.

5 Take one of the following necessary actions:
- encourage the client to seek medical advice
- explain why the treatment cannot be carried out
- modify the treatment.

6 Meet all these treatment objectives:
- improvement of skin and body condition
- improvement of contour and muscle condition.

7 Provide all these types of advice:
- avoidance of activities which may cause contra-actions
- future treatment needs
- modifications to lifestyle patterns
- healthy eating and exercise advice
- suitable homecare products and their use.

VRQ practical evidence requirements

There are different evidence requirements for the VRQ qualifications, depending on the awarding body.

City & Guilds unit 307 Provide body electrotherapy treatments

- A minimum of four body electrotherapy treatments should be carried out combining the following electrotherapies together:
  – high frequency
  – mechanical massagers
  – galvanic
  – EMS
  – micro-current
  – vacuum suction

- before four final observations in front of an assessor combining:
  – high frequency
  – galvanic
  – micro-current/EMS
  – vacuum suction

- Each of these occasions should be accompanied with a treatment plan

(Please note that information on 'mechanical massagers' is found in Chapter 11 Body massage treatments)

VTCT unit UV30404 Provide body electrotherapy treatments

- Five occasions covering the following range:

Types of equipment:
- galvanic unit
- electro muscle stimulator (EMS)
- micro-current unit
- lymphatic drainage equipment

Consultation techniques:
- questioning
- visual
- manual
- reference to client records

Body types:
- endomorph
- mesomorph
- ectomorph

Body conditions:
- cellulite
- poor muscle tone
- sluggish circulation
- uneven skin texture

All the necessary actions to:
- encourage the client to seek medical advice
- explain why the treatment cannot be carried out
- modify the treatment

Treatment objectives:
- improvement of skin and body condition
- improvement of contour and muscle condition

Types of advice:
- avoidance of activities which may cause contra-actions
- future treatment needs
- modifications to lifestyle patterns
- healthy eating and exercise advice
- suitable homecare products and their use

Note that in all cases, simulation is NOT allowed.

VRQ knowledge requirements

City & Guilds unit 307 Provide body electrotherapy treatments	VTCT unit UV30404 Provide body electrotherapy treatments	Page no.
Learning outcome 1: Be able to prepare for body treatments using electrotherapy		
Practical skills/observations		
Prepare themselves, client and work area for body electrotherapy treatments		241–5
Use suitable consultation techniques to identify treatment objectives		245
Carry out body analysis and relevant tests		224–5, 248
Provide clear recommendations to the client		249–50
Select products, tools and equipment to suit client treatment needs, body types and conditions		252–3
Underpinning knowledge		
Describe salon requirements for preparing themselves, the client and work area		241–5
Describe the environmental conditions suitable for body electrotherapy treatments		244
Describe the different consultation techniques used to identify treatment objectives		245
Explain the importance of carrying out a detailed body analysis and relevant tests		248–9
Describe how to select products, tools and equipment to suit client treatment needs, body types and conditions		252–3
Describe the different body types, conditions and characteristics		217–235
Explain the contraindications that prevent or restrict body electrotherapy treatments		246–7
Learning outcome 2: Be able to provide body treatments using electrotherapy		
Practical skills/observations		
Communicate and behave in a professional manner		248

Follow health and safety working practices	241–3
Position themselves and client correctly throughout the treatment	243
Use products, tools, equipment and techniques to suit clients treatment needs, body type and conditions	252–8
Complete the treatment to the satisfaction of the client	274
Evaluate the results of the treatment	274
Provide suitable aftercare advice	273–4
Underpinning knowledge	
Explain how to communicate and behave in a professional manner	183–4
Describe health and safety working practices	241–3
Explain the importance of positioning themselves and the client correctly throughout the treatment	243
Describe different body types and conditions	217–35
Explain the importance of using products, tools, equipment and techniques to suit clients treatment needs, body type and conditions	252–3
Explain the effects and benefits of electrotherapy equipment and products on the skin and underlying structures	252–4, 257, 263, 265, 269, 271
Explain the principles of electrical currents	158–69
Describe how treatments can be adapted to suit client treatment needs, body types and conditions	256, 261–62, 264, 268, 270, 273
State the contra-actions that may occur during and following treatments and how to respond	251
Explain the importance of completing the treatment to the satisfaction of the client	274
Explain the importance of completing treatment records	249
Describe the methods of evaluating the effectiveness of the treatment	274
Describe the aftercare advice that should be provided	273–4
Describe the structure, growth and repair of the skin	64–70
Describe body types, conditions, diseases and disorders	217–31
Describe the structure, function, position and action of the muscles of the body	100–15
Describe the location, function and structure of the bones of the body	85–97
Describe the structure and function of the circulatory and lymphatic systems for the body	122–36
Outline the structure and function of the digestive system	142–8
Outline the structure and function of endocrine system	136–9
Describe the structure and function of the nervous system for the body	115–22
Explain how the ageing process, lifestyle and environmental factors affect the skin, body conditions and underlying structures	221, 247

Introduction

Body electrical treatments include a wide range of treatments, techniques and equipment that require a high level of expertise and knowledge. New products and equipment come onto the market every year; some have value and are effective in the improvement of skin and body condition, while others are little more than a gimmick. Continued professional development and membership of a professional body will help you keep abreast of the useful developments in this field.

Many of the developments have arisen through use by the medical profession where they are used in the treatment of health-related conditions but have also been found to offer cosmetic benefits too. If your salon has good links to local medical practitioners it is possible to assist in the treatment of clients with particular health conditions.

This unit of your qualification and this chapter will provide the base from which you are able to progress to explore this exciting and rewarding aspect of beauty therapy.

For the principles of electrical current, see Chapter 5 The theory of electrical currents.

 ## Related anatomy and physiology

- Structure and function of the skin
- Structure and location and the body's utilisation of adipose tissue
- Skin characteristics and types, skin characteristics and types relating to ethnic origin.
- The structure and function of the skeleton
- Types of muscle tissue
- Structure and function of muscles
- Position and action of the muscles of the body
- The definition of the terms 'origin' and 'insertion' of a muscle
- The effect of exercise on muscle tone and how it can vary
- The cause of muscle fatigue and how to recognise it
- The function of blood
- Principles of blood circulation, blood pressure and pulse
- Structure and function of the heart, arteries, veins and capillaries
- How to identify erythema and its causes
- Lymph circulation and the interaction of lymph and blood circulation
- Structure and function of the lymphatic system including vessels, nodes and lymph

- Basic principles of the central nervous system, motor points and autonomic nervous system
- The function of the endocrine system and its relationship to weight gain and loss
- The function of the digestive system
- The basic principles of healthy eating
- How ageing affects the body and skin
- How age limits the effectiveness of the treatment.

For the structure and functions and main diseases and disorders of the body systems listed above, refer to Chapter 4 Related anatomy and physiology.

For the effect of the different types of body electrical treatments on the underlying structures of the body, see the individual sections on each type of treatment, later in this chapter.

Maintain safe and effective methods of work (LO1) (LO4) (LO5)

Hygiene procedures

Details on the methods of sterilisation and the disposal of contaminated waste can be found in Chapter 6 Professional practices.

Personal hygiene

High levels of personal hygiene and presentation are expected for the performance of body electrical treatments on clients. Use the following checklist to check the industry's expectations.

Back to basics: Personal appearance and hygiene checklist

1. A high standard of personal hygiene.
2. Fresh breath, free from cigarette or food odours.
3. A clean, pressed overall.
4. Clean, low-heeled shoes.
5. Arms and hands free from jewellery (plain wedding bands are acceptable).
6. Any earrings or necklaces are discreet.
7. Make up is discreet and expertly applied.
8. Long hair is tied neatly away from the face and shoulders.
9. Nails are short, smooth, clean and free of nail enamel.
10. Tights, or socks with trousers, are worn.
11. Any cuts are covered with a clean plaster.
12. Hands are washed immediately before and after physical contact with the client.

Hygiene of the treatment area

To avoid cross-infection from one client to another or to the therapist the following precautions should be taken:

1 Wipe down the couch and trolley with a suitable chemical disinfectant sterilising agent with a low odour so there are no unpleasant aromas lingering throughout the treatment. Spray the surfaces then wipe until dry with disposable paper such as a couch roll.

2 Prepare the trolley with a clean, laundered towel and disposable paper.

3 Prepare the treatment couch using clean, laundered towels. Wash laundry in the hottest water possible using a detergent containing anti-bacterial agents.

4 Use disposable couch roll on all client contact surfaces.

5 Always use a 'cut out' technique when handling products.

6 Dispose of waste material correctly, immediately after treatment.

Hygiene of the client

The following hygiene procedures should be considered for the client:

1 Check for contraindications. Never treat a client who has a contagious condition unless it is very minor, in which case it should be covered with a waterproof dressing while wearing disposable latex-free gloves.

2 The client should shower if facilities are available.

3 Place disposable paper such as couch roll on the floor for the client to stand on when footwear has been removed.

4 Cleanse the client's feet before beginning the treatment using a suitable antiseptic and a clean piece of cotton wool for each foot to avoid the possibility of cross-contamination from one foot to another.

Health and safety practices

Under the terms of the Health & Safety at Work Act 1974 the therapist is responsible for the health and safety of themselves and others while at work including clients and other visitors.

Remember . . .

The main legislation that is relevant to a therapist is presented in the table below. There are others, which are discussed within Chapter 1 Monitoring health and safety.

The treatment room	Health & Safety at Work Act 1974	General safety of staff and visitors to the salon including clients
	Workplace (Health, Safety & Welfare) Regulations 1992	Governs the working environment including ventilation, temperature and lighting, etc.
	Regulatory Reform (Fire Safety) Order 2005	The safe evacuation of the building in an emergency such as a fire
Body electrotherapy equipment	Provision and Use of Work Equipment Regulations 1998	Governs the acquisition of safe and reliable equipment
	Electricity at Work Regulations 1989	Governs the regular maintenance of electrical equipment including the recording of such
Body electrotherapy products	Control of Substances Hazardous to Health 2002 (COSHH)	Governs the exposure of persons to substances likely to cause harm, including flammability and the effect on the tissues
	Cosmetic Products (Safety) Regulations (2008)	Requires cosmetics to comply with correct labelling, to have safe formulation and be fit for the purpose intended
Disposal of waste	The Controlled Waste Regulations 1992	Governs the correct disposal of contaminated waste, i.e. waste contaminated with blood or other bodily fluids

Positioning of client and therapist

The client should be made comfortable on the treatment couch by the use of pillows and bolsters to support the areas being treated and to facilitate the body electrical treatment for the therapist. Work-related health conditions such as repetitive strain injury in the form of carpel tunnel syndrome and back pain are likely from working in the beauty therapy industry. Knowledge of health and safety procedures can help prevent the onset of such conditions.

1　Always use a treatment couch and set work surfaces at the correct height. Adjustable electric couches are available that facilitate this and enable a client to easily and safely get on and off.

2　Never work in an overstretched or bent position. Position the client so that you can perform the treatment easily. If bending is necessary, bend from the knees and not the back.

3　Use your body weight to create more pressure during a treatment rather than strength from the arms.

4　When appropriate, use a larger or stronger part of the body to facilitate the treatment rather than the fingers or thumbs. Alternatively, a piece of equipment could be used instead such as the audio sonic massager.

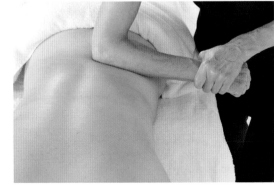

△ Using the forearm in a treatment

243

Plan and prepare for treatment

More detailed information regarding body type analysis can be found in Chapter 7 Skin and body analysis.

Preparation for treatment

In preparation for body electrical treatments consider the treatment area environment and the client.

Preparation of the treatment area environment

- Temperature: the treatment room should be warm and comfortable as the client will be in a state of undress and the body temperature lowers as the body relaxes. The use of a heated under- or over-blanket on the treatment couch is a way of maintaining the client's body temperature and has the additional benefit of warming the tissues before treatment (for more information on the benefits of warming the tissues before treatment see Chapter 11 Body massage treatments).

- Ventilation: there should be a regular exchange of air to maintain air quality in terms of freshness and to remove excess moisture that would otherwise cause condensation. This can be through the use of air extraction.

- Lighting: subdued, dim lighting may be suitable to aid relaxation while brighter lighting is suitable for a more invigorating treatment.

- Privacy: the treatment room should be private in consideration of the client's state of undress. Many clients will feel vulnerable and nervous about revealing their body and having it scrutinised and they must feel confident that there will be no interruptions.

- Volume and type of music/sounds: music and sounds enhance the client's experience of the body electrical treatment and should be suitable and set at a reasonable volume. The sounds of outdoor activities such as rainfall, the sea crashing on a shore or a babbling brook can take the client away from the treatment room and to another place. Choose the music carefully and ask the client what they prefer.

- Pleasant aroma: the use of essential oils in a burner or an aromatic candle can also enhance the client's experience, but again the choice of aroma needs special consideration and the client's preference should be considered.

Preparation of the client

The client should be:

- treated with courtesy and respect throughout the treatment

- addressed by their full name and the therapist should inform them of theirs

- taken to the treatment area and given a brief explanation of the treatment procedure

> ⭐ **Hints and tips**
> When performing body analysis and body electrical treatments on clients, inform the receptionist or other members of staff and emphasise that you should not be disturbed during the treatment.

Equality and diversity

Some clients should not be left alone in the treatment room even when they are undressing due to severe disability or mobility problems. You should not be left alone with either vulnerable adults or minors; they should always be accompanied by a parent or guardian.

- given a thorough consultation and/or a figure analysis if required, including a discussion on the aims of the treatment
- asked to shower if facilities are available
- advised which articles of clothing and jewellery they need to remove and be provided with a gown to wear
- allowed to undress in private
- helped onto the couch and allowed to get comfortable. This should include the placement of bolsters to support key areas of the body.
- Covered with towels and checked that they are warm and comfortable before the treatment begins.

Removal of accessories

The client should be asked to remove all jewellery if possible, including earrings, necklaces, bracelets, anklets and from body piercings. This is because of the use of electrical currents within the treatments. Metal jewellery can attract the current causing heat and minor burns. Removal of accessories avoids any accidental breakage or damage. Where piercings are new or jewellery cannot be removed they should be covered with a suitable dry dressing to insulate them before the treatment begins.

Consult for treatment

Consultation techniques involve the use of:

- questioning techniques including ascertaining contraindications, lifestyle patterns and treatment objectives
- listening techniques (see Chapter 6 Professional practices)
- body language including eye contact and facial expressions (see Chapter 6 Professional practices)
- visual assessment
- manual assessment
- visual aids (see Chapter 6 Professional practices) and referral to client records from previous treatments.

Questioning techniques

Questioning techniques are used to ascertain information regarding:

- the client's personal details such as date of birth or telephone number; it is important to record this information accurately as this can differentiate one client from another with a similar name or initials
- the health of the client including the contraindications to treatment and smoking habits
- the client's diet and exercise habits including fluid intake and alcohol consumption
- the treatment objectives and the client's expectations.

> ★ **Hints and tips**
>
> A client's jewellery should be placed safely in a tissue-lined bowl and returned to the client after the treatment, or placed in a small plastic bag and the client encouraged to place the bag with their belongings to avoid leaving it behind after the treatment.

Contraindications

The contraindications to body electrical treatments are shown in Table 8.1 below. In the event of a contraindication it will be necessary to:

- encourage the client to seek medical advice
- explain why the treatment cannot be carried out
- modify the treatment.

▽ Table 8.1 Contraindications to body electrical treatments

Conditions that prevent treatment	Conditions that restrict treatment
• Fungal infections such as Tinea corporis • Bacterial infections such as impetigo • Viral infections such as herpes zoster • Infestations such as Pediculosis corporis • Eye infections such as conjunctivitis • Severe non-infectious skin conditions such as eczema and psoriasis • Dysfunction of the nervous system • Heart disease/disorder • Current and ongoing medical treatment • Pacemaker • During chemotherapy • During radiotherapy • Recent scar tissue • Undiagnosed lumps, inflammations and swellings • Medication causing thinning or inflammation of the skin, such as steroids, Accutane or retinols • Diagnosed scleroderma • Deep-vein thrombosis	• Diabetes • Epilepsy • High/low blood pressure • History of thrombosis or embolism • Metal plates and pins • Medication • Pregnancy • Body piercings • Anxiety • Varicose veins • Cuts and abrasions • Bruising • Recent dermabrasion or chemical peels • Recent IPL or laser treatment • Recent epilation • Broken bones • Recent fractures and sprains • Skin allergies • Product allergies

Key terms

Steroids – drugs which work mainly by reducing inflammation; they are used to treat a variety of conditions where inflammation occurs.

Accutane – a prescription medicine used to treat severe acne. It is a form of vitamin A and is also known as Isotretinoin.

Retinols – another form of vitamin A; used in anti-ageing products

It is important to remember that some contraindications are infectious and to treat a client suffering from such a condition would pose a risk of cross-infection to the therapist and other clients. This would have a detrimental effect on the reputation of the therapist and the salon, resulting in a loss of client custom and potential new clients and the associated loss of profits for the business.

The other contraindications that prevent treatment are of a medical nature and the client should seek medical advice as outlined in Chapter 6 Professional practices.

Some contraindications that restrict treatment may also require the client to seek medical advice before undertaking a treatment, for example, a client with a history of thrombosis, then adaptation of the treatment can be planned by the therapist. Adaptations may include the following:

- A change in the treatment position, for example, not lying the client flat if they suffer from low blood pressure or raising the limbs if oedema is present.
- Avoiding the area affected by the contraindication by omitting it from the treatment sequence, such as in the case of a broken bone or varicose vein or by avoiding bruising.

- Cuts and abrasions and body piercings may be covered with a dressing and avoided.

- Choosing an alternative treatment that might give a similar effect if the use of body electrical treatment is not advised, for example a body massage.

- The performing of thermal, tactile and sensitivity testing before the treatment if the client is prone to skin and/or product allergies.

- Changing the aftercare advice given, for example, do not give dietary advice to a client with diabetes without consulting with their doctor.

Alternative treatments

Below are some suggested alternative treatments which can be suggested to the client if their contraindications indicate they are unsuitable for body electrical treatment.

- Improve skin conditions: body massage, mechanical massage, aromatherapy, heat therapy.

- Improve underlying muscle tissue: body massage, mechanical massage, exercise.

- Improve body contours: body massage, mechanical massage, diet and exercise, heat therapy.

- Improve blood circulation: body massage, infra-red, aromatherapy, hot stone massage, heat therapy.

- Improve the appearance of cellulite: dry skin-brushing, use of anti-cellulite products, body massage, mechanical massage, aromatherapy, heat therapy.

Lifestyle patterns

The client's lifestyle should be discussed in terms of their:

- occupation

- eating habits

- exercise levels

- fluid intake

- alcohol consumption

- smoking habits.

This information gives a total picture of the client in order for the therapist to understand how the presenting body conditions have developed and it will also inform the aftercare advice needed.

Body electrical treatments are effective but only in partnership with healthy eating and good exercise habits. To gain quick and effective results from these treatments, changes to the client's lifestyle must be considered.

★ **Hints and tips**
It is possible for more than one of the treatment objectives to be applicable to the client but the therapist should try to focus the client's attention to one main objective in order to be successful. Too many objectives can result in limited success in all objectives.

Equality and diversity

Always consider your tone of voice, especially when consulting with minors or vulnerable adults. Ask their parent or guardian for help in explaining the treatment to avoid misunderstanding as they will know how to make things familiar and reassuring.

★ **Hints and tips**
Always be aware of the client's body language which might indicate that you have touched on a sensitive subject or that the client might be lying! You can then adjust your questioning technique appropriately by changing direction or explaining why the piece of information is needed.

Treatment objectives

A discussion should take place surrounding the reason the client has booked the appointment and what they are hoping to achieve from the treatment. This discussion gives rise to the treatment objective, which could be to improve:

- skin conditions
- the appearance of underlying muscle tissue
- body contours
- blood circulation
- the appearance of cellulite.

Communication and behaviour

Good communication is a two-way process and involves the verbal techniques of speaking, asking questions to elicit the required information from the client and using appropriate language and terminology that can aid the client's understanding while avoiding the use of layman's terms.

Visual assessment

During the visual part of the body analysis the therapist will assess the client to determine their body type: ectomorph, endomorph or mesomorph. Body type cannot be changed through the application of body electrical treatments, diet or exercise, and instead is part of the fundamental make-up of a person. Knowledge of this helps the therapist to consider the effectiveness and the limitations of the treatments and the aftercare advice that will be given.

The visual assessment is also used to determine posture and postural and figure faults. The way in which a client stands and sits and their occupation can lead to postural faults that can have an effect on the overall appearance of the body. An improvement in posture can have beneficial effects on body contours, show an improvement in figure faults and improve the client's sense of well-being through the relief of pain and tension. Postural and figure faults are discussed in Chapter 7 Skin and body analysis.

Manual assessment

During the manual assessment the therapists will assess the client for hard fat, soft fat, cellulite and muscle tone. Information on these conditions will inform the therapist's decision as to the type of body electrical treatment that will best improve and benefit the condition.

The therapist should also carry out thermal, tactile and sensitivity tests. Details on how to perform these tests can be found in Chapter 7 Skin and body analysis.

A complete lack of sensation in a wide area can limit the application of body electrical treatments for those clients where their feedback determines intensity levels and treatment times, for example body galvanic. A lack of sensation in a limited area may not affect the treatment if the area can be avoided and the treatment is given adjacent to the area affected.

Referral to client records

Refer to the client's record card for:

- an indication of their health and the presence of contraindications

- the products used previously and potential allergies

- the details of previous treatments, such as the equipment used and in what combination, the intensity levels and treatment times. Ask the client whether these were successful and whether they experienced any long-term effects

- possible contra-actions to previous treatments and/or products.

Treatment planning

Once the therapist has completed their consultation, they can begin to formulate the most appropriate treatment plan for the client. Treatment planning involves collating the information gained from the consultation and using it to decide the:

- proposed treatment including the length and cost

- frequency of treatment – whether weekly, fortnightly, etc.

- body electrical products to use

- body electrical treatments to use and their combination

- adaptations to the routine to suit the client's needs and their treatment objectives.

The proposed treatment plan should be discussed with the client and their approval sought in the form of a signature on the client record. Although this will not protect a therapist from prosecution if the client were to start litigation, it is required as part of the industry's code of practice and membership to a relevant professional body and will influence the outcome of an insurance claim.

Table 8.2 (see overleaf) that can be used for quick reference in order to make effective treatment plans centred on the client and their treatment objectives.

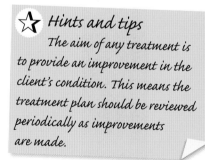

★ *Hints and tips*
The aim of any treatment is to provide an improvement in the client's condition. This means the treatment plan should be reviewed periodically as improvements are made.

▽ Table 8.2 Planning the use of body electrical treatments

Treatment objective or body condition	Galvanic (iontophoresis)	Electro muscle stimulator	Microcurrent	Lymph drainage equipment	Microdermabrasion	Additional requirements for City & Guilds VRQ unit 307 Provide body electrotherapy treatments				
						Galvanic (desincrustation)	Direct High Frequency	Indirect High frequency	Infra-red	Mechanical Massage
Improved skin condition	✓		✓	✓	✓	✓	✓		✓	✓
Improved appearance of muscle tissue		✓	✓					✓		✓
Improved body contours	✓	✓	✓	✓						✓
Improved blood circulation	✓		✓	✓	✓		✓	✓	✓	✓
Improved appearance of cellulite	✓		✓	✓				✓		✓

Treatment times for body electrotherapy treatments

There are no specified treatment times or standard commercial timings for body electrical treatments as the treatment will vary depending on the client's needs and objectives, their reaction to treatment and the combination of equipment and products used. Consequently there are no guidelines that should be used during the practical assessment of this unit.

Contra-actions

The conditions described in Table 8.3 below are brought about by the effects of the treatment but can be avoided if the therapist is careful and works within the manufacturer's guidelines.

▽ Table 8.3 Contra-actions to body electrotherapy treatments

Contra-action	Cause and action to take
Galvanic burn	Insufficient preparation of the skin and/or the equipment; too high intensity; treatment period too long Soothe area with cooling mask or cold water compress
Bruising	Can be caused by too strong suction in lymph drainage treatments or during micro-dermabrasion Apply a witch hazel compress and wait for healing to occur
Irritation	Mild irritation during treatment can indicate beneficial effects, such as increased blood circulation. However, if significant the treatment should be stopped immediately Apply a cold water compress to the affected area
Allergic reaction	Can occur in relation to the products used. These should be avoided in future and an alternative sought Test the alternative product in a sensitivity test before use
Excessive erythema	Can be caused by galvanic, vacuum suction, micro-dermabrasion, infra-red and mechanical massage equipment through prolonged treatment and/or high intensities Treat with soothing cold water compresses or cooling gel masks
Muscle fatigue	Caused by the overworking of muscles during electro muscle stimulation by too prolonged or too frequent treatment. Recognised by the lack of strength, muscle tremors or stiffness and/or cramping Rest the muscles and adjust the treatment times accordingly
Hyper-pigmentation	Caused by aggressive use of the micro-dermabrasion unit or galvanic equipment, particularly on black or Asian skin

The specific dangers associated with body electrical treatments and the safety precautions of each are stated later in this chapter.

Perform body electrical treatments

Types of body electrotherapy equipment

The types of body electrical treatment available are indicated in Table 8.4 below. Note that the additional requirements for City & Guilds unit 307 'Provide body electrotherapy treatments' have also been given. Most are dealt within the context of this chapter but infra-red and mechanical massage can be found in Chapter 11 Body massage.

▽ Table 8.4 Types of body electrical treatment

NVQ & VTCT VRQ unit UV30405 Provide body electrotherapy	Additional for City & Guilds VRQ unit 307 Provide body electrotherapy treatments
• Galvanic (iontophoresis) • Electro muscle stimulator • Microcurrent unit • Lymph drainage equipment • Microdermabrasion unit	• High frequency – direct and indirect • Galvanic desincrustation • Vacuum suction • Infra-red • Mechanical massagers

Effects and benefits of body electrotherapy treatments

The general effects of body electrical treatments are:

- improved skin and body condition
- improved muscle contour and tone
- improved circulation
- induces relaxation.

Types of body electrotherapy products

The products used with body electrical treatments can be divided into three groups:

1 Those used to prepare for the treatment
2 Those used during the treatment
3 Those used post treatment.

Preparation products used before the treatment include cleansing products, which are used to cleanse the treatment area in the absence of shower facilities, and exfoliators, which remove the dead surface skin cells and facilitate the penetration of product and the ease at which the electrical current passes through the epidermis.

Treatment products are used alongside the body electrical equipment, as indicated in the Table 8.5 below.

▽ Table 8.5 Treatment products used alongside body electrical equipment

Body electrical product	Use, effect and benefit
Massage mediums	Oil and cream are used to act as a lubricant to facilitate the applicator's smooth gliding over the skin's surface, such as in vacuum suction Talc is used for the same purpose but is used with mechanical massagers
Galvanic products such as lotions, emulsions and gels	Used to facilitate the flow of current into the tissues by conduction and give additional benefits by providing the vehicle by which electrolytes are taken up by the skin, e.g. collagen ions
Talc	Used to provide 'slip' during direct high-frequency and manual and mechanical massage
Oxygenated creams	Provide additional oxygen molecules which are released as a high frequency current is allowed to pass through. This extra oxygen has a germicidal and antibacterial effect
Conducting gel	Used to hydrate and facilitate the flow of electrical current into the tissues

Post-treatment products are used to enhance the effect of the treatment at home and include products such as anti-cellulite creams, dry bristle brush, moisturising lotions and creams, exfoliators, body washes and buffing cloths.

Benefits of a course of treatment

Most of these body electrical treatments are effective but have an accumulative effect. A course of treatments means that the effects and benefits build on the results of the previous treatment, producing greater effects. For this reason the client should be encouraged to book a course of intensive treatment, with one or two treatments per week to gain maximum effect. Once the desired results are obtained a maintenance approach with fewer, less frequent treatments can be undertaken.

Body electrotherapy techniques

Galvanic

A body galvanic treatment is designed to aid the efficient breaking down and dispersal of cellulite and soft fatty areas of the body. It is based on iontophoresis, which is a process where galvanic current is used to pass active substances through intact skin to the deeper layers, where they remain effective until gradually absorbed by the body. This process is very similar to that of facial therapy; all that differs is the nature of the lotions, emulsions and gels.

The treatment is performed by placing sponge-covered electrode pads onto the problem areas in conjunction with anti-cellulite fluids. These fluids have a diuretic effect and cause the client to pass more fluid as urine and stubborn areas of cellulite to disperse over a period of time. This is especially beneficial to cellulite conditions where a lot of

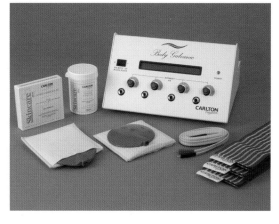

△ Body galvanic unit

253

fluid is present. The client's shape can alter because of the fluid loss although there may be no change in overall weight.

Effects and uses of galvanic

The effects of body galvanic treatment are summarised in Table 8.6.

▽ Table 8.6 Effects of body galvanic treatment

Physiological, psychological and physical effects	Uses/indications
Product penetration under the active pad	Accumulations of soft fat
Interchange of tissue fluids within the cell membrane	Cellulite on thighs, buttocks, abdomen and upper arm
Helps to break down and soften fatty tissues	Accumulations of waste and toxins in a specific area
Increases circulation in the area	Oedema in a specific area
Aids dispersal of fluids and toxins	
Increases tissue and general metabolism	
Relaxation and warming of the tissues	
Skin texture and tone is improved	

Remember...

The 'physiological effects' are those that pertain to and affect a system of the body; a 'psychological effect' is one that affects the mind and a 'physical effect' is one that you or the client can see or feel. They are often inter-related, for example an increase in blood circulation in the skin (physiological) brings about an erythema and increase in skin temperature (physical) which can have a relaxing effect (psychological).

Safety precautions

The following safety precautions should be observed:

1 Remove all jewellery.

2 Observe contraindications such as metal plates and pins.

3 Ensure machine is in good working order, has an up-to-date PAT test sticker, wires and plugs are whole and not broken and that the contacts are firm within the pads.

4 Make sure dials are at zero before contact is made.

5 Never operate the galvanic unit with wet hands.

6 Do not place water or damp electrodes on or above the galvanic unit.

7 Ensure firm contact between electrode and skin.

8 Ensure skin is free from cuts, abrasions and wounds before treatment.

Use of the equipment and products

1 Remove all jewellery.

2 Ensure the skin is clean, as any grease or oil on the skin will prevent the flow of the current and render the treatment ineffective.

3 Saturate sponge covers in warm water, remove excess water and insert electrode pads. Active side of the pad is placed against the sponge of the special cover.

4 Apply the anti-cellulite product either onto the skin with firm massage movements or onto the sponge side of the sponge cover.

5 Place sponge side of the active pad onto the cellulite area and other pad of the pair opposite it or parallel to it depending on area being treated. Secure both in place with elasticated body straps. (Ensure firm strapping and contact with the skin to avoid irritation). *Never overlap pairs of pads*.

6 Ensure that the black lead is inserted into the active (working) pad on the cellulite area and the red lead into the opposite pad. (Pairs of pads should be placed in line or opposite each other.) The non-working pad or indifferent electrode acts as the attracting force for the current.

7 If two regions of the same area need treatment then deal with them on separate occasions. If they are treated within the same session it can alter the interchange of tissue fluid, cause skin irritation and render the treatment ineffective.

8 When all the pads have been correctly placed and secured, ensure that all the polarity switches are on negative (−). This will give a negative charge to all the black leads which will have been placed over the problem areas.

9 Turn current up slowly to a maximum of 2 mA (milliamps). For the first treatment 1 mA for 5 minutes gives an idea of the skin reaction. A treatment set at lower intensity for a longer time is more beneficial to the client. The skin offers resistance to the current and this is measured in milliamps. Initially skin resistance is high and the client *may* experience a prickling sensation. As this resistance lowers it is replaced by a feeling of localised heat. (If this diminishes, the level of current may be raised slightly so that the heat remains constant.) However, if the client complains of burning or pain then STOP.

10 First treatment should be 5 minutes, building to a maximum of 15 minutes. One–two treatments per week with a total of 12 sessions will give maximum results.

11 Treatment begins on the negative pole (active pad) as it is here that penetration of the product occurs to help the tissues to release trapped fluids into the vascular and lymphatic systems. It usually takes about 5–6 minutes for skin resistance to be broken down and for consequent product penetration. To complete the treatment, close pores and cause tissue fluid interchange, switch all the polarity switches to positive (+) and leave for up to 5 minutes, at a low level of skin resistance. (Always switch to zero before reversing polarity.)

12 When the treatment is complete, switch off and turn all dials to zero.

13 Remove straps and pads.

14 Product can be massaged in for full effect.

15 After treatment the skin will have some erythema but should
NOT appear irritated and sore. If it does, then the intensity was
too high or the skin preparation/contact was poor so appropriate
action should be taken. Hydrating the area with steam or using a
spa pool will reduce skin resistance by allowing the current to
pass through to deep areas more easily.

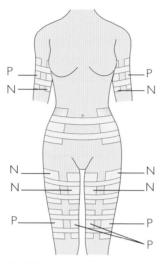

(a) Full body padding – anterior

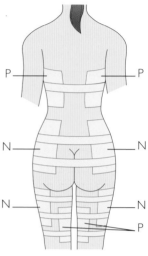

(b) Full body padding – posterior

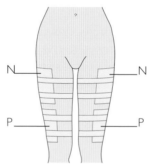

(c) Leg padding – parallel padding

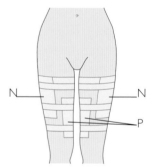

(d) Leg padding – opposite padding

△ Placements of the pads for body galvanic treatment

Adaptation to suit client requirements

It should be remembered that galvanic body treatments will
only help to loosen and relax the various forms of fat and waste
elements which form cellulite. It is therefore essential to perform
other treatments at the same time or immediately after a galvanic
treatment, as this will aid the effective dispersal of the waste products
and toxins from the area.

Treatments that can be performed at the same time as the galvanic
include faradic using specially adapted electrodes. This will half the
treatment time and produce more effective results more quickly.

Treatments to be performed prior to a galvanic treatment include
steam bath, infra red and sauna. All of these aid the softening and
hydrating of the skin and increase circulation.

Treatments to be performed immediately after a galvanic treatment include hydrotherapy baths, G5, faradic, manual massage and exercise.

Results over a few weeks should give a loss of inches and if combined with a diet plan, weight loss should also occur. There may also be a change in shape due to fluid loss locally and/or generally.

Limitations of the equipment and products

Some clients may react to cellulite programmes. The types of reaction may include skin irritation, excessive loss of fluid as urine and discomfort in passing urine. In these cases the treatment should be discontinued and alternative treatments for the treatment objective sought.

Electro muscle stimulation (EMS)

A normal muscle contraction is brought about by an electrical impulse transmitted from the brain along a motor nerve to the muscle. Electrical muscle stimulators replace this natural impulse with one that imitates it and are applied directly to the muscle via the natural motor points. Modern EMS equipment uses a combination of currents known as 'faradic type' which produce a contraction without discomfort. The effect is a natural contraction followed by a period of rest before the contraction period begins again. This brings about an improvement in the tone and to some degree strength of the muscle to which it is applied.

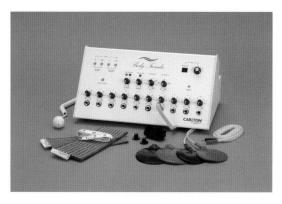

△ A modern EMS unit

Effects and uses of EMS

The effects of EMS treatment are summarised in Table 8.7.

▽ Table 8.7 Effects of EMS treatment

Physiological, psychological and physical effects	Uses/indications
• Strengthens muscles • Tones muscles • Reduces flabbiness • Helps delay ageing process • Increases blood circulation • Produces heat in area • Relaxing • Increases metabolism	• Ageing skin tissue • As a preventative measure to delay effects of ageing • Oedema due to loss of muscle tone • Figure reshaping • Spot reduction • Regain figure after childbirth • Maintain a good figure • Tone and firm during weight loss

Key term

Motor point – the area of the muscle that facilitates contraction. It is where the natural motor nerve comes in contact with the muscle to transmit the impulse to the muscle fibres.

Safety precautions

The following safety precautions should be observed:

1 Remove all jewellery.

2 Ensure skin is free from grease before treatment.

3 Ensure machine is in good working order.

4 Electrolyte must be used on pad, either tap water, saline solution (tsp to 1 pt water) or gel.

5 Make sure dials are at zero before contact is made with the client.

6 Never operate machine with wet hands.

7 Do not place water or damp electrodes on EMS unit.

8 Ensure firm contact between electrode and skin with elasticated straps.

9 Turn current up during exercise time.

10 Turn current up and down slowly.

11 Ensure sufficient rest between surges or muscles will cramp.

12 Avoid excessive number of contractions or muscle fatigue will result.

Use of the equipment and products

Due to the body muscles being large in size and bulk, pads are most commonly used in body EMS treatment. In this way more than one muscle can be treated at a time for more effective use of time. The pads are placed on the motor points of each muscle using one of the following placements or padding techniques.

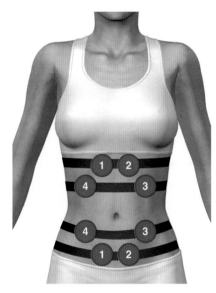

△ Longitudinal padding on the rectus abdominus

1 Longitudinal padding: this is where a pair of pads is placed along the length of a muscle, one at the motor point near the *origin*, the other at the *insertion*. This allows the greatest degree of muscle shortening and full contraction to take place. Useful where a muscle has lengthened in a specific area and needs to be pulled in and shortened, for example the rectus abdominus after childbirth.

2 Duplicate padding: this is when the pads are placed on different muscles in the same area on the same side of the body so that the whole area receives a general tightening and toning effect, for example the thighs.

3 Split padding: this is where the two pads from one outlet are placed on different muscles on different sides of the body. This method is not very successful

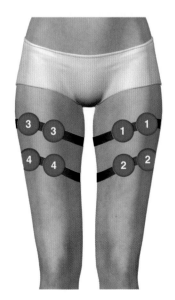

△ Duplicate padding on the thighs

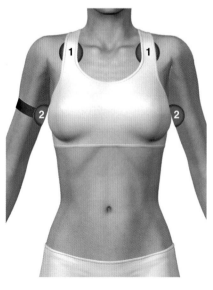

△ Split padding on the pectorals and triceps

as there is only one intensity control. If the muscles vary in strength it can lead to one muscle contracting before the other.

Choosing which method to use will depend on the corrective treatment necessary for the area being worked upon. Care should be taken NOT to pad up pairs of antagonistic muscles.

Procedure

1 Carry out normal safety precautions on the equipment.

2 Prepare the position of the client for body electrical treatment. You will need a bowl of warm water and some cotton wool.

3 The client may keep on her underwear as long as it allows access to the area being treated. Some clients like to wear a bikini. A gown opening at the front may be worn for warmth.

4 Apply the straps in position for the area being treated. They should be firm but not so tight as to restrict blood circulation.

5 When treating the front, the client should lie on her back with the couch slightly inclined; bolsters can be used for comfort.

6 Working systematically, take each pair of pads, dampen the surface with water and place in desired position (see padding layouts), ensuring the pad has good contact with the skin.

7 Check all the pads for accuracy on motor points contact and comfort.

8 Check the equipment is switched off and that all the outlet dials are on zero.

9 Systematically plug in each pair of pads ensuring red with red, black with black. It is useful to have pads from the same area adjacent with each other. The leads will trail over the client but should NOT be allowed to come into contact with water or metal and should not be stretched to the equipment. Position the equipment so that it is close to the working area. Check all dials are on zero or normal settings.

10 Switch on the equipment and check the exercise and resting periods, making sure that the resting period is slightly longer than the exercise period. Do this using the indicator lights or the audio switch.

11 Explain to the client what she should feel and what you are going to do.

12 With your hands on the appropriate muscle turn up the outlet dial until a mild contraction can be felt. Work systematically.

13 Repeat with the other outlets until all are giving a mild contraction. Reposition the pads if necessary, turning the dial to zero before doing so.

14 Pairs of pads can be turned up to give a stronger contraction if desired as the client becomes accustomed to the treatment. Only increase the intensity during the exercise period, NOT the resting period.

15 Duration time of the treatment depends on the physical condition and age of the client (see below).

16 When the treatment is complete, turn the machine off and return all the dials to zero.

17 Remove the pads systematically, unplug and lay them across the machine.

18 Release the straps. The client may now get dressed.

19 Clean the pads with sterilising fluid ready for the next treatment.

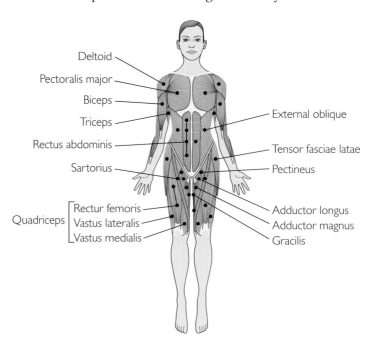

△ Anterior muscles of the body and their motor points

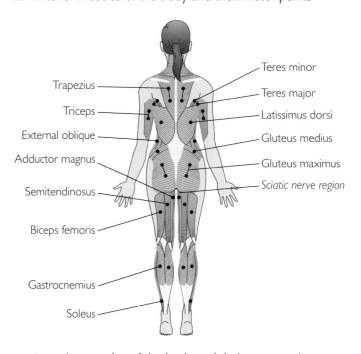

△ Posterior muscles of the body and their motor points

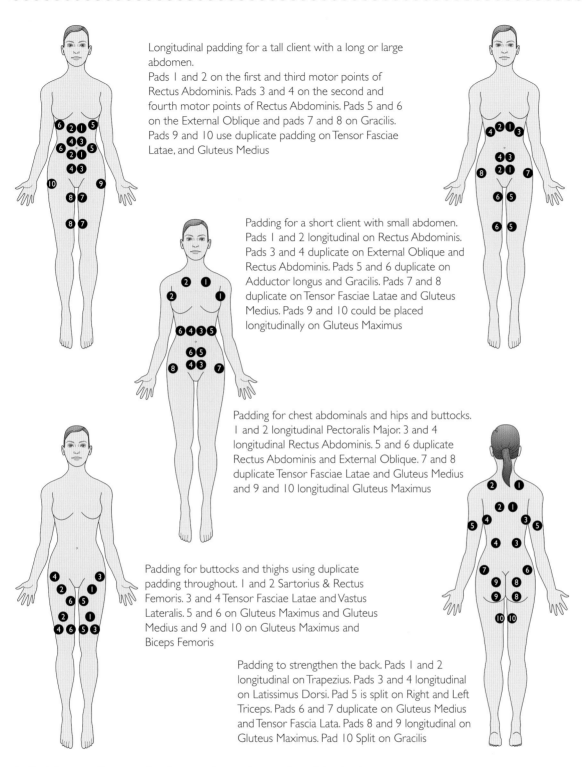

Longitudinal padding for a tall client with a long or large abdomen.
Pads 1 and 2 on the first and third motor points of Rectus Abdominis. Pads 3 and 4 on the second and fourth motor points of Rectus Abdominis. Pads 5 and 6 on the External Oblique and pads 7 and 8 on Gracilis. Pads 9 and 10 use duplicate padding on Tensor Fasciae Latae, and Gluteus Medius

Padding for a short client with small abdomen. Pads 1 and 2 longitudinal on Rectus Abdominis. Pads 3 and 4 duplicate on External Oblique and Rectus Abdominis. Pads 5 and 6 duplicate on Adductor longus and Gracilis. Pads 7 and 8 duplicate on Tensor Fasciae Latae and Gluteus Medius. Pads 9 and 10 could be placed longitudinally on Gluteus Maximus

Padding for chest abdominals and hips and buttocks. 1 and 2 longitudinal Pectoralis Major. 3 and 4 longitudinal Rectus Abdominis. 5 and 6 duplicate Rectus Abdominis and External Oblique. 7 and 8 duplicate Tensor Fasciae Latae and Gluteus Medius and 9 and 10 longitudinal Gluteus Maximus

Padding for buttocks and thighs using duplicate padding throughout. 1 and 2 Sartorius & Rectus Femoris. 3 and 4 Tensor Fasciae Latae and Vastus Lateralis. 5 and 6 on Gluteus Maximus and Gluteus Medius and 9 and 10 on Gluteus Maximus and Biceps Femoris

Padding to strengthen the back. Pads 1 and 2 longitudinal on Trapezius. Pads 3 and 4 longitudinal on Latissimus Dorsi. Pad 5 is split on Right and Left Triceps. Pads 6 and 7 duplicate on Gluteus Medius and Tensor Fascia Lata. Pads 8 and 9 longitudinal on Gluteus Maximus. Pad 10 Split on Gracilis

△ Padding up diagrams for the anterior and posterior of the body

Adaptation to suit client requirements

EMS is a popular treatment with clients as it does not involve a lot of personal effort; it is best offered as part of a combined treatment. Sauna, steam bath and hydrotherapy combined with faradic will help with inch loss on a specific area but must be part of a reducing diet to be successful. The treatment is most effective when used on clients that are 1–2 stone overweight; results on severely overweight clients can be obtained but to a much lesser degree. There may also be a degree of discomfort felt by severely overweight clients as the current may have difficulty passing through excess adipose tissue. Overweight clients should be encouraged to lose weight through dieting, with this treatment as a goal to work towards.

Consider the surge rate and length of time of treatment when deciding on the appropriate treatment time. The surge rate is the rate at which the contractions occur, e.g. 50–60 surges per minute for a healthy client. Therefore, if the treatment lasts 10 minutes, that gives 500–600 contractions during the treatment. A surge rate of 20 for 10 minutes gives 200 contractions. This is suitable where the muscles are weak or have been injured. Subsequent treatment times can be increased gradually by five minutes until a maximum of 30 minutes is reached.

Table 8.8 gives a guide for clients beginning treatment.

▽ Table 8.8 Guide to using EMS treatments with clients

Client type	Surge rate	Treatment time
Weak, traumatised muscles	20	5 minutes
Elderly clients	30–40	10 minutes
Healthy normal muscles	50–60	15 minutes

Limitations of the equipment and products

As it is a passive form of exercise, the benefits of increased circulatory and respiratory systems are not gained so the treatment should not replace active exercise. The therapist should encourage the client to partake in active exercise as she begins to feel the muscles gaining in strength. This should lead to the client becoming aware of her own appearance and physical health and increase the desire to maintain them.

Remember, although this is a passive form of exercise, muscle fatigue may still occur, causing stiffness and discomfort after treatment. This should be avoided by appropriate treatment timings, as shown in Table 8.8.

Poor/uncomfortable muscle contraction may be caused by:

- incorrect placing of pad onto the motor point
- subcutaneous fat overlying the muscle acting as a barrier to the current
- poor skin preparation – oil, talc, etc. present
- electrodes (pads) dry or straps holding pads in place are loose.

There is an initial period before the muscle contracts when the client experiences a 'pins and needles' feeling. The client should be warned of this and that with further intensity of current this feeling should disappear and a contraction felt. If this is not so then the cause is likely to be one of the points listed above.

Microcurrent

Microcurrent treatment has been used for many years for the treatment of sports injury to speed up recovery. It is now one of the most popular treatments used in salons for tightening and firming muscles and skin tissue.

Effects and uses of microcurrent

The effects of microcurrent treatment are summarised in Table 8.9.

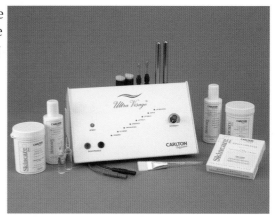

△ Microcurrent body unit

▽ Table 8.9 Effects of microcurrent treatment

Physiological, psychological and physical effects	Uses/indications
Muscles are re-educated, lifted and toned when the microcurrent and particular wave form transmit a series of electrical signals to the area to be treated	Muscle and skin toning after childbirth
Lymphatic drainage is improved. This helps in the treatment of cellulite as lymph fluid is stimulated, toxins are removed and the appearance of 'orange peel' dimpled skin is diminished	Body contouring
Cell permeability is increased, allowing nutrients to pass easily into cells and waste products to pass out	Reduces oedema
Increases energy in the muscles	Improve the appearance of stretchmarks and other scarring
Increases the production of collagen in the skin	Treatment of poor blood circulation
Increases protein synthesis in muscles and skin	Improve the appearance of cellulite
Stimulates healing on a cellular level	Toning of the skin and muscle after weight loss

Safety precautions

The following safety precautions should be observed:

1 Remove all jewellery.

2 Ensure machine is in good working order.

3 Apply plenty of conducting gel to the area to eliminate discomfort.

4 Never operate machine with wet hands.

5 Ensure firm contact between electrode and skin.

6 Ensure skin is free from grease before treatment.

7 Do not place water on or near the microcurrent unit.

Use of the equipment and products

1 Prepare the microcurrent according to the manufacturer's instructions. This could mean preparation of the electrodes with cotton buds or pads with conducting gel.

2 Observe the safety precautions and check the client for contraindications.

3 Remove all jewellery.

4 Explain procedure and experience to the client, e.g. tingling means more gel is needed; pressure is executed during lifts.

5 Cleanse the area with a body wash if shower facilities are not available. It is important to remove grease and dirt from the skin to allow the current to flow into the skin.

6 Exfoliate the area to remove excess epidermal skin cells that could also hinder the passage of the current.

7 Apply conducting gel to the area with a mask brush from a small bowl.

8 Turn on and set the microcurrent unit in accordance with the manufacturer's instructions.

9 Follow the procedure and movements according to the area being treated.

10 Switch the microcurrent unit off.

11 Apply the appropriate moisturising body lotion or cream.

Adaptation to suit client requirements

Table 8.10 gives a guide for clients beginning treatment.

▽ Table 8.10 Guide to using microcurrent treatments with clients

Treatment use	Duration	Frequency
Muscle and skin toning after childbirth and weight loss	20–30 minutes	2–3 times per week
Body contouring	20–30 minutes	2–3 times per week
Improve the appearance of stretch marks and other scarring	15 minutes	Once/twice per week
Treatment of poor blood circulation	15 minutes	Once/twice per week
Improve the appearance of cellulite	20–30 minutes	2–3 times per week

Limitations of the equipment and products

Effects can be slow and require a number of sessions to achieve results but in combination with other treatments such as EMS and galvanic, results can be achieved quickly and are long lasting.

Hydration of the skin before treatment using sauna, steam room or bath or spa pool ensure the comfort of the client by facilitating the flow of current through the skin and tissues, helping to maximise results.

Lymph drainage equipment

Lymph drainage equipment uses the application of reduced pressure within a glass or perspex cup. The cups are applied directly to the area being treated while being attached to the vacuum massage unit via plastic hosing. The unit creates the vacuum by means of a pump and expels the air into the atmosphere. The resulting vacuum causes the tissues to arc up inside the cup with resulting stimulation, vascular interchange and erythema.

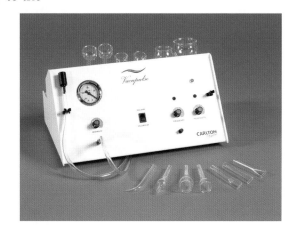

The gliding cup method is applied to the body in patterns of flowing strokes which relate directly to the lymphatic system and move towards the nearest lymph node to speed up the removal of waste products in the area.

The static application can be combined with faradic to produce additional muscle contraction. This is very effective in cases of reshaping the body where the fat accumulations are overlying areas of reduced muscle tone.

△ Vacuum suction unit

Effects and uses of lymph drainage equipment

The effects of lymph draining equipment are summarised in Table 8.11.

▽ Table 8.11 Effects of lymph drainage equipment

Physiological, psychological and physical effects	Uses/indications
● Increases blood circulation ● Increases lymph flow ● Skin texture is improved ● Skin metabolism is improved ● Breaks down and promotes absorption of adipose deposits ● Erythema produced ● Warming of the skin ● Relaxing ● Maintains a client's interest in weight reduction by causing a sense of achievement ● Reduces oedema	● Areas of poor circulation ● Areas of oedema of non-systemic nature ● Cellulite ● Aids slimming by making adipose tissue more available as a source of energy ● Prevents chilblains ● Out-of-proportion figure ● Abdominal weight accumulations ● Heavy upper arms ● Subcutaneous accumulation on the back, i.e. 'dowager's hump'

Safety precautions

The following safety precautions should be observed:

1 Check equipment before placing on client.

2 No more than 20 per cent arcing should be allowed to occur inside the cup.

3 Use fast, rhythmical strokes to avoid too much arcing.

4 Check glass for cracks or chips.

5 Do not pull off cup but release vacuum first.

6 Do not use on loose, crêpey or vascular skins.

7 Avoid breast area as it is too sensitive.

8 Avoid abdomen during menstruation or if the client is prone to hernia.

Use of the equipment and products

1 Prepare and position the client on the couch so they are comfortable; use bolsters and pillows if necessary.

2 Apply oil to the treatment area and then wash or wipe hands to remove the oil. This is important so that the glass cup does not slip in your hands.

3 Switch on the machine and check pressure by blocking the air inlet at the tube and adjust the reading on the equipment. Choose size of cup and attach to the tubing.

4 Keep the client warm throughout treatment by exposing the immediate treatment area only. Work in a similar order as for body massage if treating the whole body. Infrared lamp can be used throughout the treatment to keep treatment area warm.

5 Assess the softness and firmness of the area and adjust the pressure to suit. Start with a low percentage of arc then increase as the client's tolerance increases, but no more than 20 per cent.

6 Place the cup at the start of the stroke and allow the skin to arc, lift the cup and with a sweeping motion, move it smoothly toward the nearest lymph node. Release the cup with a quick flicking action of the wrist, removing finger from air hole orby slipping a finger under the cup to break the suction. Never try to pull off the cup as this may rupture blood vessels, causing bruising.

7 Work in overlapping strokes rhythmically and quickly, adopting a pattern of work as shown in the diagram. Always work towards the lymphatic nodes.

8 When the treatment is complete, the client should be encouraged to be rest for half an hour, wrapped warmly, to achieve maximum effect.

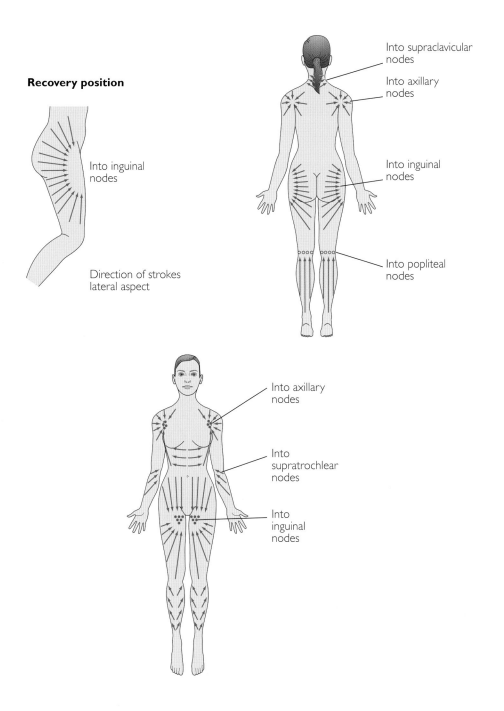

Recovery position

Into inguinal nodes

Direction of strokes lateral aspect

Into supraclavicular nodes

Into axillary nodes

Into inguinal nodes

Into popliteal nodes

Into axillary nodes

Into supratrochlear nodes

Into inguinal nodes

△ Direction of strokes is towards the lymph nodes

Adaptation to suit client requirements

The possible adaptations to suit different clients' requirements are indicated in Table 8.12.

▽ Table 8.12 Guide to using lymph drainage equipment with clients

Treatment use	Duration	Frequency
Out-of-proportion figure	10–30 minutes	Daily or at least twice a week until result achieved
Abdominal weight accumulation	10–30 minutes	Daily or at least twice a week until result achieved
Swelling of ankles/knees	10–20 minutes	As necessary
Heavy arms	5–10 minutes	Daily or at least twice a week until result achieved
Large buttocks	10–30 minutes	Daily or at least twice a week until result achieved
Dowager's hump	45–50 minutes	Daily or at least twice a week
Cellulite	10–15 minutes or until skin reaction is seen	Daily or at least twice a week until result achieved

Limitations of the equipment and products

The treatment is capable of body reshaping, either with or without a diet programme, but the former is more effective. When used statically, with or without pulsation, there is increased stimulation but toxins and fat accumulations remain in the area so it is normal to precede and follow this application technique with the gliding cup method.

Microdermabrasion

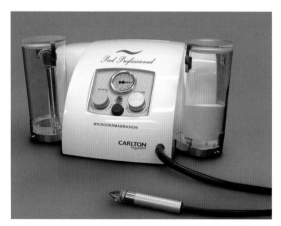

△ Microdermabrasion unit

Microdermabrasion is the mechanical peeling of the upper layers of the epidermis to improve the texture and regenerative qualities of the skin. It is used to treat skin conditions such as scar tissue, stretch marks, pigmentation and the effects of ageing. The treatment involves the use of safe, non-organic crystals of uniform shape and size in conjunction with a vacuum pump that initially blasts the crystals onto the skin and then sucks them up again for disposal.

The treatment was developed by plastic surgeons and dermatologists for the effective treatment of scarring and pigmentation and has been used for about 20 years. It is now available for use by the beauty therapist.

Effects and uses of microdermabrasion

The effects of microdermabrasion are summarised in Table 8.13.

▽ Table 8.13 Effects of microdermabrasion

Physiological, psychological and physical effects	Uses/indications
• The healthy balance of 70 per cent living epidermal cells and 30 per cent dead skin cells is restored • Regeneration of the epidermis gives a healthy and well-functioning protective layer • Congestion and blockages are removed from the pores and neck of the hair follicles • Increase in blood circulation of the skin, giving a brighter and clearer appearance • Nutrients and oxygen are brought to the skin cells, improving their metabolism • Lymph drainage of the skin is improved and therefore the removal of waste products • Localised swelling is reduced	• Stretch marks • Scar tissue • Areas of pigmentation e.g. after UV light exposure • Treatment of ingrown hairs • Areas of skin congestion and blockage, e.g. acne or oily skin • Treatment of lines and wrinkles, e.g. ageing of the hands, age spots • Areas where skin regeneration is required

Safety precautions

The following safety precautions should be observed:

1 Check equipment before using on client.

2 Ensure machine is in good working order.

3 Do not use on loose, crêpey or vascular skins.

4 Do not operate the machine with wet hands.

Use of the equipment and products

1 Prepare and position the client on the couch so they are comfortable; use bolsters and pillows if necessary.

2 Cleanse the area to be treated and dry thoroughly.

3 Use the preparation such as peels that are recommended by the manufacturer for use with microdermabrasion unit.

4 Use the microdermabrasion unit at settings recommended by the manufacturer.

5 Remove excess crystals if necessary.

6 Apply post treatment products as recommended by the manufacturer.

7 Apply moisturising lotion containing SPF if area is exposed to daylight (omit if clothing provides the protection needed).

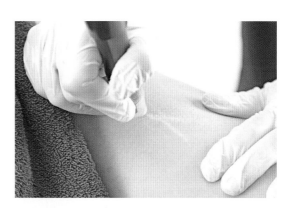

△ Microdermabrasion unit in use on stretch marks

Adaptation to suit client requirements

The possible adaptations to suit different clients' requirements are indicated in Table 8.14.

▽ Table 8.14 Guide to using microdermabrasion equipment with clients

Treatment use	Duration	Frequency
Scarring, including stretch marks	30 minutes	Six treatments with 4–6 days between each session then reassess
Pigmentation	15–30 minutes depending on the surface area affected Treat area once then concentrate on the pigmentation area	Six treatments with 5–7 days between each session
Ingrown hairs	10–20 minutes	As required
Anti-ageing treatment	45–60 minutes	Six treatments with 7 days between treatments

Limitations of the equipment and products

1 Do not use in areas where the client may have received dermal fillers, botox or glycolic peels within the previous 12 weeks.

2 Do not use if the client has been taking medication that thins the skin such as accutane, steroids or retinols.

3 Do not use where there are areas showing signs of psoriasis and eczema.

4 Do not over treat an area or recommend too frequently as *internal puncture bleeding* may result from damage to the dermal blood capillaries present in the basal layer of the epidermis.

> **Key term**
>
> **Dermal fillers** – a material which is injected and used to correct scarring, wrinkles and other depressions in the skin.

High frequency

This section is an addition for those learners studying for a Vocational Related Qualification (VRQ) rather than the NVQ. It is a requirement of the awarding body City & Guilds that you also study high frequency as a body electrical treatment.

High frequency is an alternating current of at least 200,000 Hz that produces low energy. When allowed to pass through the skin and tissues of the body, the water molecules in the tissues are 'excited' by the energy and begin to vibrate, causing heat. This is the main therapeutic action of the current used in body electrical treatments.

The current can be delivered to the skin by two methods:

1 Direct application through a glass electrode containing a partial vacuum; this method has an additional benefit in that ozone gas is produced which is drying and antibacterial to the skin.

2 Indirect application by means of a saturator which the client holds while the therapist performs massage movements.

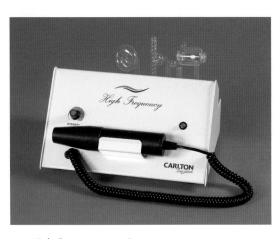
△ High frequency unit

Effects and uses of high frequency

The effects of microdermabrasion are summarised in Table 8.15.

▽ Table 8.15 Effects of high frequency

Physiological, psychological and physical effects	Uses/indications
Direct application	
Warming to the skin	Areas of poor blood circulation
Blood vessels dilate locally and an erythema is produced	Mild acne skin conditions found at the chest and upper back areas
The increased blood supply brings nutrients and oxygen to the tissues, increasing cell metabolism	After extraction of comedones as an anti-bacterial treatment
The blood supply aids in the removal of waste products from the tissues affected	
Drying and antibacterial effect at the skin surface	
Indirect method	
Mild sedative effect on sensory nerve endings	Areas where there is muscular tension and pain
Blood circulation deep in the muscle tissue is stimulated	Areas of poor blood circulation such as the limbs
Deep warmth is created, promoting relaxation of the muscle fibres	Areas of toxin build up such as after exercise or cellulite
Increase in nutrients and oxygen delivered to the muscles which is available for muscle contraction	Useful in the treatment of hard fat
The increase in oxygen locally dispels lactic acid – a waste product of anaerobic muscle contraction during strenuous exercise	Areas of oil dry skin
Glands of the skin are stimulated to produce more of their secretions	

Safety precautions

The following safety precautions should be observed:

1 Remove all jewellery and metal from the area being treated.

2 Do not use the indirect method if a client presents with metal plates and pins.

3 Metal parts of the couch and the trolley should be insulated using dry towels.

4 Ensure machine is in good working order.

5 Never operate machine with wet hands.

6 Ensure firm contact between electrode and skin.

7 Ensure skin is free from grease before treatment.

8 Do not place water on or near the high frequency unit.

Use of the equipment and products

Direct method of application

1 Prepare the client for body electrical treatment and position on the couch, ensuring their comfort by use of bolsters and pillows as necessary. For treatment of the upper back the client should lie on their front with bolsters under the ankles.

2 Warn the client of the noise that the equipment makes.

3 Apply a light application of talc or an oxygenated cream to the area to be treated.

4 Place the electrode onto the skin and then switch on the high frequency unit; for a large area use the roller electrode.

5 Increase the intensity while moving the electrode until a warm sensation can be felt by the client.

6 Move the electrode firmly and rhythmically over the skin to aid relaxation until a mild erythema is apparent or 10 minutes has elapsed. Do not break contact with the skin throughout the procedure; maintain firm even pressure of the electrode on the skin.

7 Before removing the electrode from the skin, reduce the intensity slowly and switch off the high frequency unit.

8 Remove excess talc with damp cotton pads and apply a treatment body mask to the area if desired.

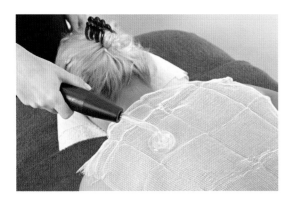

△ Direct application of high frequency to the back

Indirect method of application

1 Prepare the client for body electrical treatment and position on the couch ensuring their comfort by use of bolsters and pillows as necessary.

2 Place the saturator bar into the high frequency unit and give to the client to hold – one hand on the saturator and one on the holder. Support the client's arms as she relaxes with bolsters or pillows if necessary.

3 Apply massage medium to the area; oil, cream or talc can be used as preferred.

4 Place one hand on the client and maintain contact while the high frequency unit is switched on and the intensity increased.

5 Increase the intensity until warmth under the hand can be felt and then begin the massage routine.

6 Do not break contact with the client throughout the massage, so omit tapotement movements.

7 Be aware that the current is attracted to the surface in contact with the client, so use the whole palm of the hand for a general suffusion of warmth to the area or the tips of the fingers for a more concentrated application, over a fibrous adhesion, for example.

8 Massage the area for 15–30 minutes.

9 When completed, one hand should remain in contact with the client while the intensity is reduced and the unit switched off.

10 Remove the massage medium if necessary and continue with the body treatment.

Adaptation to suit client requirements

The possible adaptations to suit different clients' requirements are indicated in Table 8.16.

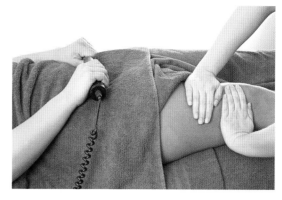

△ Indirect application of high frequency to the legs

▽ Table 8.16 Guide to using high frequency with clients

Treatment use	Duration	Frequency
Mild acne skin conditions found on the chest and upper back areas (direct)	10 minutes	Once per fortnight, reducing to once per month as condition improves
Areas where there is muscular tension and pain	15–20 minutes	As required
Areas of poor blood circulation such as the limbs	20–30 minutes	Once/twice per week
Areas of toxin build up such as after exercise or cellulite	20–30 minutes	Once/twice per week
Useful in the treatment of hard fat	20–30 minutes	Once/twice per week
Areas of oil dry skin	15–20 minutes	Once per week

Galvanic (desincrustation)

Galvanic (desincrustation) is a requirement of the VRQ for City & Guilds but not for the NVQ qualification.

Galvanic (desincrustation) is used in body electrical therapy in the treatment of acne-type conditions found in the chest and upper back/shoulder regions. The procedure is the same as for the face and is covered in detail in Chapter 9 Facial electrical treatments.

Aftercare advice for body electrical treatments

The aftercare advice for body electrical treatments is important as it improves the effectiveness of the treatments and prevents possible contra-actions occurring.

Remember...

Just to remind you, the contra-actions to massage are:

- galvanic burn
- bruising
- irritation
- allergic reaction
- excessive erythema
- muscle fatigue
- hyper-pigmentation.

Avoidance of activities which may cause contra-actions

For 12–24 hours following treatment the client should be advised to:

- Avoid heat treatments such as sauna, steam room or bath, spa pool, infra-red, hot bath or shower.
- Avoid strenuous exercise to give the body time to rest after the treatment.
- Avoid touching the area as this may make the area sore and irritated.
- Avoid tight clothing.
- Avoid bathing or showering immediately after the treatment to allow the treatment to be fully effective on the skin (galvanic).

Future treatment needs

Because results rely on an accumulative effect, further treatment should be booked in order to see the intended results. In most cases a maintenance programme involving fewer treatments and at monthly intervals is advised. Additional treatments such as aromatherapy massage would also be beneficial.

Modifications to lifestyle patterns

- Follow an 'elimination' diet; drink diuretic teas instead of tea or coffee.
- Avoid smoking and drinking alcohol.
- Exercise to increase the body's metabolism.
- Do stretching exercises in areas where there is muscle tension.

Suitable homecare products and their use

- Use an anti-cellulite product at home, 2–3 times per week, massaged into the area after bathing.
- Dry skin brush before a bath.
- Body wash.
- Exfoliators and buffing cloths.

Methods of evaluating

Methods of evaluating a body electrical treatment include:

- visual
- verbal
- written feedback
- repeat business.

Want to know more?

The following professional bodies offer membership, information on changes in practices including health and safety, insurance and continued professional development.

www.babtac.com

www.itecworld.co.uk

www.fht.org.uk

www.beautyguild.com

Habia is the lead body and can provide up-to-date information. They can be found at:

www.habia.org

Specific health and safety information for the Hair and Beauty sector can be found at: www.habia.org/healthandsafety.

NVQ assessment checklist

To complete this unit you must have the following theoretical and practical skills. Check against the list below and refer back to the relevant section for information on anything you are unsure about.

1. **Be able to maintain effective and safe methods of working when providing body electrical treatments**

❏ **1.1** set up work area to meet organisation and manufacturers' instructions

❏ **1.2** use industry hygiene and safety practices throughout the service to minimise the risk of cross-infection

❏ **1.3** position the person and themselves to minimise fatigue and the risk of injury and allow ease of body electrical application, maintenance and removal

❏ **1.4** clean all tools and equipments using the correct methods

❏ **1.5** position equipment, products and materials for ease and safety of use

❏ **1.6** adopt a positive, polite and reassuring manner towards the client throughout the treatment

❏ **1.7** maintain the client's modesty, privacy and comfort at all times

❏ **1.8** check the client's wellbeing at regular intervals according to organisational policy

❏ **1.9** dispose of waste materials safely and correctly

❏ **1.10** complete the treatment within a commercially viable time

❏ **1.11** keep records are up to date, accurate, easy to read and signed by the client and practitioner

❏ **1.12** leave the treatment area and equipment in a suitable condition for future treatments

2. **Be able to consult, plan and prepare for treatments with clients**

❏ **2.1** use effective consultation techniques in a polite and friendly manner to determine the client's treatment needs

❏ **2.2** obtain signed, written and informed consent prior to the treatment from the client or minor for a minor a parent or guardian

❏ **2.3** explain to the client what the treatment entails in a way they can understand

❏ **2.4** ask the client appropriate questions to identify their medical history, body type, body condition and life style pattern

❏ **2.5** identify any contra-indications to body electrical treatments by asking the person questions and recording the responses

❏ **2.6** provide client advice without reference to a specific to a specific medical condition and without causing undue alarm and concern

❏ **2.7** carry out thermal and tactile test to accurately determine the client's skin response to heat and pressure stimuli

❏ **2.8** carry out a test patch, if necessary, to determine skin sensitivity and to avoid adverse reactions

❏ **2.9** recommend alternative treatments which are suitable for the client's condition and needs if contra-indicated for body electrical treatments

❏ **2.10** explain and agree the projected cost, likely duration, frequency and types of treatment needed

❏ **2.11** agree in writing the client's needs, expectations and treatment objective, ensuring they are realistic and achievable

❏ **2.12** check that the client's skin is clean and prepared to suit the type of equipment to be used

❏ **2.13** select suitable equipment and related products to suit the treatment objectives

3. **Be able to carry out body electrical treatments**

❏ **3.1** explain the sensation created by the equipment being used

❏ **3.2** explain the treatment procedure to the client in a clear and simple way at each stage in the process

❏ **3.3** safely use the correct treatment settings, applicator and accessories on the body throughout the treatment in accordance with manufacturers' instructions

❏ **3.4** adjust the intensity and duration of the treatment to suit the client's body type and condition and the areas of the body being treated

❏ **3.5** take prompt remedial action if the client experiences discomfort or contra-actions

❏ **3.6** apply a suitable post-treatment product to the treated area, if required

❏ **3.7** check the finished result is to the client's satisfaction and meets the agreed treatment objectives

❏ **3.8** give client suitable aftercare advice

4. **Understand organisational and legal requirements**

❏ **4.1** explain their responsibilities under relevant health and safety legislation, standards and guidance

❏ **4.2** explain the importance of not discriminating against clients with illnesses and disabilities and why

❏ **4.3** state the age at which an individual is classed as a minor and how this differs nationally

❏ **4.4** explain why it is important, when treating minors under 16 years of age, to have a parent or guardian present

❏ **4.5** explain why minors should not be given treatments without informed and signed parental or guardian present

❏ **4.6** explain the legal significance of gaining signed, informed consent to treatment

❏ **4.7** explain their responsibilities and reasons for maintaining their own personal hygiene, protection and appearance according to accepted industry and organisational requirements

❏ **4.8** explain the manufacturers' and organisational requirements for waste disposal

❏ **4.9** explain the importance of the correct storage of client records in relation to the Data Protection Act

❏ **4.10** explain how to complete the client records used in their organisation and the importance of and reasons for keeping records of treatments and gaining client signatures

❏ **4.11** explain the organisation's requirements for client preparation

❏ **4.12** explain their organisation's service times for body electrical treatments

❏ **4.13** explain their organisation's and manufacturers' requirements for treatment area, equipment maintenance and equipment cleaning regimes

5. **Understand how to work safely and effectively when providing body electrical treatments**

❏ **5.1** explain how to set up the work area for body electrical treatments

❏ **5.2** explain the necessary environmental conditions for body electrical treatments

❏ **5.3** explain the type of personal protective equipment that should be worn for micro-dermabrasion treatments and why

❏ **5.4** explain the importance and reasons for disinfecting hands and how to do this effectively

❏ **5.5** explain how to position themselves and the client for body electrical treatments

❏ **5.6** explain the reasons for maintaining client modesty, privacy and comfort during the treatment

❏ **5.7** explain why it is important to maintain standards of hygiene and the principles of avoiding cross-infection

❏ **5.8** explain why it is important to check the client's wellbeing at regular intervals

6. **Understand how to perform client consultation, planning and preparation**

❏ **6.1** explain how to use effective consultation

❏ **6.2** explain why it is important to encourage and allow time for clients to ask questions

❏ **6.3** explain the importance of questioning clients to establish any contra-indications to body electrical treatments

❏ **6.4** explain possible contra-actions which may occur during the treatment and how to deal with them

❏ **6.5** explain why it is important to record client responses to questioning

❏ **6.6** explain the legal significance of client questioning and the recording of client responses

❏ **6.7** explain how to give effective advice and recommendations to clients

❏ **6.8** explain how to work out body mass index (BMI)

❏ **6.9** explain how to visually assess muscle tone

❏ **6.10** explain how to assess body fat, fluid retention, posture and skin type

❏ **6.11** explain the reasons why it is important to encourage clients with suspected contra-indications to seek medical advice

❏ **6.12** explain the importance of and reasons for not naming specific contra-indications when encouraging clients to seek medical advice

❏ **6.13** explain why it is important to maintain client's modesty and privacy

❏ **6.14** explain the characteristics of different body types and body conditions

❏ **6.15** explain the importance of using electrical treatments in conjunction with other treatments, healthy eating and exercise to maximise results

❏ **6.16** explain the types of treatments that could be given in conjunction with, or after, body electrical treatments

❏ **6.17** explain the types of alternative treatments which could be recommended in the event of contra-indications to electrical treatments

7. **Understand the anatomy and physiology for body electrical treatments**

❏ **7.1** explain the structure and function of the skeleton

❏ **7.2** explain the structure and function of muscles, including the types of muscle

❏ **7.3** explain the effect of exercise on muscle tone and how it can vary

❏ **7.4** explain the positions and actions of the main muscle groups in the part if the body specified in the range

❏ **7.5** state the definition of 'origin' and 'insertion' of a muscle

❏ **7.6** explain the causes of muscle fatigue and how to recognise it

❏ **7.7** describe the basic structure and function of skin .

❏ **7.8** explain the skin characteristics and skin types of different ethnic client groups

❏ **7.9** explain the structure, location and the body's utilisation of adipose tissue

❏ **7.10** explain the function of the endocrine system and its relationship to weight gain and loss

❏ **7.11** explain the function of the digestive system

❏ **7.12** explain the basic principles of healthy eating

❏ **7.13** explain how ageing affects the body and skin

❏ **7.14** explain how age limits the effectiveness of the treatment

❏ **7.15** explain the function of blood and the principles of circulation, blood pressure and pulse

❏ **7.16** explain the structure and function of the heart and arteries, veins and capillaries

❏ **7.17** explain how to identify erythema and its causes

❏ **7.18** explain the structure and function of the lymphatic systems, including lymphatic vessels, nodes and lymph of the body

❏ **7.19** explain the principles of lymph circulation and the interaction of lymph and blood within the circulatory system

❏ **7.20** explain the basic principles of the central nervous system, motor points and autonomic system

❏ **7.21** explain the effect of electrical treatment on the muscles, skin, circulatory, skeletal, lymphatic, endocrine, digestive and nervous systems

8. **Understand contra-indications that affect or restrict body electrical treatments**

❏ **8.1** explain those contra-indications which prevent body electrical treatment and why

❏ **8.2** explain those contra-indications which restrict treatment and why

❏ **8.3** explain the importance of and reasons for not naming specific contra-indication when referring client to a general practitioner

9. **Understand equipment, materials, products and treatment specific knowledge**

❏ **9.1** explain how to prepare and use the equipment and products for body electrical treatments

❏ **9.2** evaluate the use and limitations of products used for body electrical treatments

❏ **9.3** explain methods of disinfecting, sterilising and maintaining equipment

❏ **9.4** explain the benefits and effects of electro-therapy machines which combine different currents and their effects

❏ **9.5** explain the benefits of products available for electrical treatments and their effects

❏ **9.6** explain the type of currents produced by galvanic units, EMS units, micro-current units and lymphatic drainage equipment

❏ **9.7** explain how to select, use and adapt the use of body electrical equipment to suit different body types, body conditions and treatment objectives and why

❏ **9.8** explain the importance of cleansing the skin prior to treatment

❏ **9.9** explain how to carry out and interpret thermal, tactile and skin sensitivity tests

❏ **9.10** explain the dangers associated with body electrical treatments

❏ **9.11** summarise the physical effects created by the use of the equipment

❏ **9.12** explain why some body treatments should be conducted in a certain direction

❏ **9.13** explain the types of post-treatment products available and why they are necessary

❏ **9.14** explain how to evaluate the effectiveness of body treatments

❏ **9.15** explain the benefits of a course of treatment

❏ **9.16** explain why it is important to give aftercare advice

10. **Be able to provide aftercare advice**

❏ **10.1** explain the lifestyle factors and changes that may be required to improve the effectiveness of the treatment

❏ **10.2** explain post-treatment restrictions and future treatment needs

❏ **10.3** explain products for home use that will benefit and protect the client and those to avoid and why

❏ **10.4** explain how current eating and exercise habits can affect the effectiveness of treatment

❏ **10.5** explain how healthy eating and exercise can improve the effectiveness of the treatment

Test yourself

1. Why is it important to discuss the client's lifestyle during a consultation for body electrical treatments?

2. Which best describes the body type known as an ectomorph?

    a) Tall and thin
    b) Short and fat
    c) Tall and muscular
    d) Muscular and short

3. Why is it important to review a client's treatment plan periodically?

4. Name four contra-actions to body electrical treatment.

5. What product can be used to insulate a cut in the area when performing body electrical treatments?

6. Which chemical is produced under the cathode during galvanic treatments?

    a) Sodium chloride
    b) Sodium hydroxide
    c) Hydrogen chloride
    d) Hydrochloric acid

7. Give three uses of galvanic in body electrical treatment.

8. Give three uses of Electrical Muscle Stimulation in body electrical treatment.

9. Define the following terms:

    a) Longitudinal padding
    b) Duplicate padding
    c) Split padding

10. Which of the following is the correct percentage of pressure within a vacuum suction applicator in order to prevent bruising?

    a) 10 per cent
    b) 20 per cent
    c) 30 per cent
    d) 40 per cent

11. Give four uses of vacuum suction in body electrical treatment.

12. Give four uses of microcurrent in body electrical treatment.

Chapter 9

FACIAL ELECTRICAL TREATMENTS

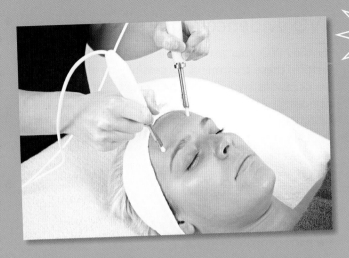

This chapter covers:

NVQ unit B14 Provide facial electrical treatments

City & Guilds VRQ unit 306 Provide facial electrotherapy treatments

City & Guilds VRQ unit 321 Apply microdermabrasion

VTCT VRQ unit UV30403 Provide facial electrotherapy treatments

VTCT VRQ unit UV30430 Apply microdermabrasion

LEARNING OBJECTIVES

This chapter is about improving face and skin condition using electrical equipment. It covers the skills involved to formulate a specific course of treatment which is tailored to meet individual client needs.

The learning outcomes for NVQ unit B14 are:

1 Be able to maintain safe and effective methods of working when providing facial electrical treatments
2 Be able to consult, plan and prepare for treatments with clients
3 Be able to carry out facial electrical treatments
4 Understand organisational and legal requirements for providing facial electrical treatments
5 Understand how to work safely and effectively when providing facial electrical treatments
6 Understand how to perform client consultation, treatment planning and preparation
7 Understand the anatomy and physiology that relates to facial electrical treatments
8 Understand the contraindications and contra-actions that affect or restrict facial electrical treatments
9 Understand how to carry out facial electrical treatments
10 Understand how to provide aftercare advice

You will need to be successful in all of these outcomes to be competent in facial electrical treatments, to qualify for insurance and be able to perform the treatment on members of the public.

NVQ evidence requirements

For the NVQ your assessor will need to observe you perform these treatments successfully on at least five occasions involving three different clients. This includes:

1 Demonstrate use of the following tools and equipment:
- direct high frequency unit
- galvanic unit
- electro muscle stimulator
- micro-current unit
- lymphatic drainage equipment
- microdermabrasion unit
- micro-lance.

2 Use the consultation techniques of:
- questioning
- visual
- manual
- reference to record cards.

3 Treat the skin types of:
- oily
- dry
- combination.

4 Treat skin conditions of:
- sensitive
- mature
- dehydrated
- congested.

5 Be able to take the necessary actions of:
- encouraging the client to seek medical advice
- explaining why the treatment cannot be carried out
- modification of the treatment.

6 Have different treatment objectives that are:
- improved skin condition
- improved contour and muscle condition
- improved skin texture.

7 Provide advice that covers:
- avoidance of activities which may cause contra-actions
- future treatment needs
- modifications to lifestyle patterns
- suitable homecare products and their uses.

VRQ practical evidence requirements

There are different evidence requirements for the VRQ qualifications, depending on the awarding body.

City & Guilds Unit 306 Provide facial electrotherapy

A minimum of four formative facial electrotherapy treatments using a combination of the following:
- direct high frequency
- indirect high frequency
- galvanic iontophoresis
- galvanic desincrustation
- micro-current
- vacuum suction
- EMS

Which must include the following:
- skin analysis, including current use of skin care products, client profile, lifestyle factors and client expectations
- how facial electrotherapy treatments were selected and adapted to suit the treatment needs, skin types and conditions

- contra-actions that may occur during and following treatments and how to respond.

Four final summative observations of facial electrotherapy treatments using a combination of the following electro therapies:
- high frequency
- galvanic
- micro-current
- vacuum suction.

City & Guilds Unit 321 Apply microdermabrasion

A minimum of two formative assessment microdermabrasion treatments, including:
- skin analysis identifying findings, to include current use of skin-care products, client profile, lifestyle factors, client expectations

- how microdermabrasion techniques were selected and adapted to suit the treatment needs, client skin types and conditions
- contra-actions that may occur during and following treatments and how to respond.

One final observation carrying out a microdermabrasion treatment.

VTCT Unit UV30403 Provide facial electrotherapy treatments

Five occasions using all types of equipment:
- galvanic unit
- electro muscle stimulator (EMS)
- micro-current unit
- lymphatic drainage equipment

Consultation techniques:
- questioning
- visual
- manual
- reference to client records

Carried out a minimum of one of the necessary actions:
- encouraging the client to seek medical advice
- explaining why the treatment cannot be carried out
- modification of treatment

Skin types:
- oily
- dry
- combination

Treated all skin conditions:
- mature
- sensitive
- dehydrated
- congested

Met all treatment objectives:
- improved skin condition
- improved contour and muscle condition
- improved skin texture
- congested

Provided all types of advice:
- avoidance of activities which may cause contra-actions
- future treatment needs
- suitable home care products and their use

VTCT Unit UV30430 Apply microdermabrasion

Minimum of three occasions covering the following range:
- Used all consultation techniques:
  - questioning
  - visual
  - manual
  - reference to client records

Met all the treatment objectives:
- improved skin condition
- improved contour appearance
- improved skin texture

Dealt with at least one necessary action:
- encourage the client to seek medical advice
- explain why the treatment cannot be carried out
- modification of treatment

Treated all skin types:
- oily
- dry
- combination.

Treated all skin conditions:
- sensitive
- mature
- dehydrated

Treated all areas:
- face
- body

Treated all body conditions:
- appearance of cellulite
- uneven skin texture

Provided all types of advice:
- avoidance of activities which may cause contra-actions
- future treatment needs
- modifications to lifestyle patterns
- recommended use of home care products

In all cases, simulation is NOT allowed.

VRQ knowledge requirements

City & Guilds unit 306 Provide facial electrotherapy treatments	VTCT unit UV30403 Provide facial electrotherapy treatments	Page no.
Learning outcome 1: Be able to prepare for facial treatments using electrotherapy		
Practical skills/observations		
Prepare themselves, client and work area for facial electrotherapy treatments		291–2
Use suitable consultation techniques to identify treatment objectives		203–6; 288–90
Carry out skin analysis and relevant tests		288
Provide clear recommendations to the client		288–300
Select products, tools and equipment to suit client treatment needs, skin types and conditions		288; 291
Underpinning knowledge		
Describe salon requirements for preparing themselves, the client and work area		291–2
Describe the environmental conditions suitable for facial electrotherapy treatments		291
Describe the different consultation techniques used to identify treatment objectives		203–6; 288–90
Explain the importance of carrying out a detailed skin analysis and relevant tests		288
Describe how to select products, tools and equipment to suit client treatment needs, skin types and conditions		292–305
Describe the different skin types, conditions and characteristics		217–24
Explain the contraindications that prevent or restrict facial electrotherapy treatments		290
Learning outcome 2: Be able to provide facial treatments using electrotherapy		
Practical skills/observations		
Communicate and behave in a professional manner		183–4
Follow health and safety working practices		286–7
Position themselves and client correctly throughout the treatment		291–2
Use products, tools, equipment and techniques to suit clients treatment needs, skin type and conditions		292–305
Complete the treatment to the satisfaction of the client		308

City & Guilds unit 306 Provide facial electrotherapy treatments	VTCT unit UV30403 Provide facial electrotherapy treatments	Page no.
Evaluate the results of the treatment		207
Provide suitable aftercare advice		308
	Underpinning knowledge	
Explain how to communicate and behave in a professional manner		183–4
Describe health and safety working practices		286–7
Explain the importance of positioning themselves and the client correctly throughout the treatment		291–2
Explain the importance of using products, tools, equipment and techniques to suit clients treatment needs, skin type and conditions		292–305
Describe the effects and benefits of electrotherapy equipment and products on the skin and underlying structures		293–4; 297–9; 302–3
Explain the principles of electrical currents		160–9
Describe how treatments can be adapted to suit client treatment needs, skin types and conditions		292–305
State the contra-actions that may occur during and following treatments and how to respond		290
Explain the importance of completing the treatment to the satisfaction of the client		308
Explain the importance of completing treatment records		207
Describe the methods of evaluating the effectiveness of the treatment		308
Describe the aftercare advice that should be provided		308
Describe the structure, growth and repair of the skin		64–70
Describe skin types, conditions, diseases and disorders		70–7
Describe the structure, function, position and action of the head, neck and shoulder muscles		104–7
Describe the location, function and structure of the bones of the head, neck and shoulders		91–5
Describe the structure and function of the nervous, circulatory and lymphatic systems for the head, neck and shoulders		115–35
Explain how the ageing process, lifestyle and environmental factors affect the condition of the skin and underlying structures		289

City & Guilds unit 321 Apply microdermabrasion	VTCT unit UV30430 Apply microdermabrasion	Page no.
Learning outcome 1: Be able to prepare for skin treatment using microdermabrasion		
Practical skills/observations		
Prepare themselves, client and work area for microdermabrasion skin treatment		291–2
Use suitable consultation techniques to identify treatment objectives		288
Advise the client on how to prepare for the treatment		291–2
Carry out a skin analysis		288
Provide clear recommendations to the client		305; 308
Select products and tools to suit client treatment needs, skin types and conditions		291; 306
Underpinning knowledge		
Describe salon requirements for preparing themselves, the client and work area		291–2
Describe the environmental conditions suitable for microdermabrasion skin treatment		291
Describe the different consultation techniques used to identify treatment objectives		203–6; 288–90
Describe how to select products and tools to suit client treatment needs, skin types and conditions		305–7
Describe known contraindications that may restrict or prevent microdermabrasion treatment		306
Describe the importance of carrying out a skin analysis		288
Describe the effects and benefits of a microdermabrasion treatment		305–6
Learning outcome 2: Be able to provide skin treatment using microdermabrasion		
Practical skills/observations		
Communicate and behave in a professional manner		183–4
Follow health and safety working practices		286–7
Position themselves and client correctly throughout the treatment		291–2
Use products, tools and techniques to suit clients treatment needs, skin types and conditions		305–7
Complete the treatment to the satisfaction of the client		308

City & Guilds unit 321 Apply microdermabrasion	VTCT unit UV30430 Apply microdermabrasion	Page no.
Record and evaluate the results of the treatment		207
Provide suitable aftercare advice		308
Underpinning knowledge		
Explain how to communicate and behave in a professional manner		203
Describe health and safety working practices		286–7
Explain the importance of positioning themselves and the client correctly throughout the treatment		291–2
Explain the importance of using products, tools and techniques to suit clients treatment needs, skin types and conditions		305–7
Describe how treatment can be adapted to suit client treatment needs		290
State the contra-actions that may occur during and following treatments and how to respond		290
Explain the importance of completing the treatment to the satisfaction of the client		308
Explain the importance of completing treatment records		207
Describe the methods of evaluating the effectiveness of the treatment		308
Describe the aftercare advice that should be provided		308
Describe the structure and function of the skin		64–70
Describe the main diseases and disorders of the skin		70–7
Describe skin types, conditions and characteristics		217–24
Describe the growth cycle and repair of the skin		64–70
Explain how natural ageing, lifestyle and environmental factors affect the condition of the skin		289

Introduction

Facial therapy has long been one of the most sought after treatments by clients who wish to improve their skin. As a therapist, making accurate recommendations and encouraging clients to have facial electrical treatments can produce significant skin-enhancing results if performed regularly and correctly. These results can be achieved faster and more effectively than those of manual facial treatments.

Clients' objectives can range from improving skin condition, improving contour and muscle condition and improving skin texture; all of these can be enhanced by facial electrical treatment.

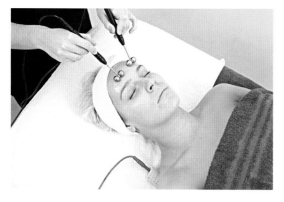
△ Receiving facial electrical treatment

Maintain safe and effective methods of working when providing facial electrical treatments

Safe and effective methods of working are of paramount importance when performing any facial electrical treatment. For general health and safety advice please refer to Chapter 1 Monitoring health and safety. Health and safety requirements relating specifically to performing electrical treatments are given below.

- Never operate machinery with wet hands.
- Keep machinery away from all sources of water to prevent electrical shock.
- Ensure leads, plugs and sockets are in safe working order with no fraying wires.
- Do not overload plug sockets.
- Avoid trailing wires to prevent tripping.
- Place equipment securely on your trolley where intensity dials are easy to see and reach.
- Ensure all dials are set to zero before introducing any electrical machinery to the client's skin.
- Do not come into contact with metal while performing facial electrical treatments; make sure metal sections of your trolley and treatment couch are thoroughly covered.

requirement because metal conducts electricity and burning could occur to an area where jewellery has been left on). Ask the client to lie under the towels in a supine position and wait for your return to the treatment room.

Wash your hands for hygiene, ensure the client is sufficiently covered and place a pillow or bolster support for comfort as required. Verbally check that the client is warm and comfortable and inform them that you are about to begin.

Carry out facial electrical treatments

It is essential that a therapist has a clear understanding of the theory of the skin's structure. Details of relevant anatomy and physiology relating to this chapter can be found in Chapter 4 Anatomy and physiology. For information on how the different electrical currents work for the different pieces of facial electrical machinery covered within this chapter see Chapter 5 Theory of electrical currents.

⭐ **Hints and tips**
Some of the electrical machines used for facial electrical treatment can be noisy. Always inform the client of this before you start your treatment, otherwise the sound will be unexpected and may cause alarm.

High frequency

The high frequency machine uses an alternating current at a high frequency of up to 250,000 hertz (Hz). The current passes easily through the skin producing a warming effect. This alternating current does not stimulate a muscle contraction as the pulses are too short. The effects are local to the point of contact which means the effects are relatively superficial.

There are two different methods of applying high frequency to the client:

1 Direct application

2 Indirect application

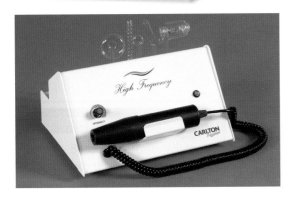

△ High frequency unit

⭐ **Hints and tips**
Use electrical treatments in conjunction with other treatments to maximise results.

Direct high frequency

This method follows its name and involves placing a glass electrode directly onto the client's skin. This treatment is particularly effective on clients who suffer with oily and congested skin, acne and seborrhea, as ozone gas is produced by this method which is of great benefit to these skin conditions.

There are a number of different glass electrodes that can be used for direct high frequency:

- Large bulb or mushroom electrode

- Small bulb or mushroom electrode

- T-shaped electrode used for treatment of the neck

- Roller electrode (which is more commonly used on treatment of the body).

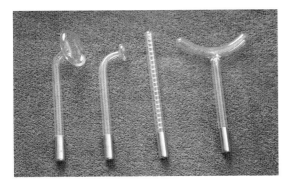

△ Direct high frequency applicators

- Ensure machinery is kept clean at all times and wipe down with a sterilising solution before and after each use.
- Store machinery correctly and in a safe environment.

Health and safety specific to performing electrical treatments

Electricity at Work Regulations (1989)

This piece of legislation requires electrical equipment to be safe to use and checked at regular intervals by a qualified electrician. This means every six months for frequently used machinery and annually for less frequently used machinery. Checks must be performed and recorded. It is the responsibility of the employer or a self-employed person to ensure this regulation is adhered to.

Consumer Protection Act (1987)

If a client is injured or harmed by a piece of faulty or malfunctioning machinery that does not meet safety standards they may have the right to sue for damages.

Personal Protective Equipment (PPE) Regulations (2002)

PPE must be worn when performing micro-lancing and microdermabrasion treatment. Disposable powder-free nitrile or powder-free vinyl gloves should be worn to protect the therapist against the risk of contact with body tissue fluid. Protective eye shields should also be used over the client's eyes when performing microdermabrasion techniques to prevent irritation to the eye area from the crystals used.

Controlled Waste Regulations (1992)

Disposal of contaminated waste should follow the requirements of the Controlled Waste Regulations (1992). If micro-lances have been used for treatment they must be disposed of in a sharps container. Disposable gloves and tissues used to assist with micro-lancing must be disposed of in a yellow clinical waste bin as they will contain residues of blood and tissue fluids.

Sterilisation of machinery and applicators

Facial electrical machinery should always be wiped over with a sterilising solution before and after treatment and prior to being stored correctly. You also need to ensure the machine applicators are thoroughly sterilised too. These applicators come in a variety of materials, from glass and plastic through to conducting metal. After each use, wash the applicators in hot soapy water and, if possible, place in an autoclave or chemical sterilising solution for 20 minutes. A UV cabinet can be used for sterile storage until the applicators are required again. While cleaning, check that each applicator is safe to use and is not broken, cracked or has sections missing.

Health and safety

Never use a piece of unsafe machinery. It should be referred immediately to the appropriate person for checking, maintenance or replacement.

 Remember...

Look out for the Portable Appliance Testing (PAT) sticker on all your electrical machinery to check when the machine was last inspected and when it is due to be checked again.

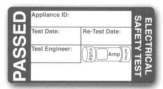

△ PAT testing sticker

★ *Hints and tips*
As long as your client is not allergic, you may need to use a plaster to cover their jewellery if it cannot be removed for treatment.

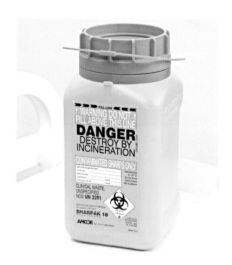

△ Sharps box

Benefits and effects of direct high frequency

- Drying effect
- Germicidal and antibacterial
- Healing of papules and pustules
- Heat producing
- Increase in blood circulation
- Mild soothing effect on nerve endings
- Increases lymphatic circulation
- Astringent effect of tightening pores.

Specific contraindications to direct high frequency

- Sunburn
- Excessive metal filling or metal plates and pins
- Asthma, as the ozone gas can instigate an asthmatic attack
- Acne rosacea
- Hyper sensitive skins.

Sparking

Sparking occurs when the electrode is held just off the skin and there is a gap between the skin and electrode. The current jumps between this gap and an intense amount of ozone is produced at this point. As ozone is germicidal and destroys bacteria this can be of some benefit to the client, however, sparking must be performed with great care. If the gap is too large the spark may destroy tissue and lead to a burn or even scarring.

Treatment procedure for direct high frequency

1. After cleansing and skin analysis, place a thin layer of oxygenating cream over the client's face. This will increase the amount of oxygen present, which, when ionized, will create more ozone for an enhanced affect.

2. Apply a layer of gauze over the oxygenating cream.

3. Warn the client of the noise that the unit will emit, the sensation they may feel (slight warming) and the smell of the ozone gas.

4. Place a medium bulb glass electrode into the saturator and turn the machine on, checking the intensity control is at zero.

5. Apply the electrode to the client's skin and slowly turn up the intensity up to the client's tolerance.

6. The therapist's spare hand should not be placed on the client's skin as it will draw the current away from the electrode.

> **Key term**
>
> **Seborrhea** – a condition where the sebaceous glands produce an excessive secretion of sebum or an alteration in its quality, resulting in an oily coating, crusts or scales on the skin.

> **Health and safety**
>
> A shock can be caused very easily when using high frequency current. To prevent this, ensure that all jewellery is removed, metal sections of couches and trolleys are covered, and you place and remove the electrode to and from the skin correctly.

> **Hints and tips**
>
> Place a layer of gauze over the client's skin when performing direct high frequency. You can then fold the gauze over on itself a couple of times which will form a safe buffer to create more intense ozone without having to spark.

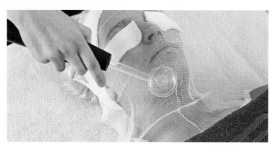

△ Performing a direct high frequency treatment

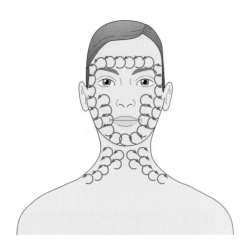

△ Using circular movements for direct high frequency treatment

 Health and safety

During direct high frequency, the glass electrode can be changed during the treatment time if necessary. However, always remember to turn the intensity to zero before removing or applying a different electrode.

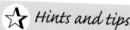 **Hints and tips**
It is a good idea to apply direct high frequency after you have performed extractions due to the germicidal and antibacterial effect of the treatment.

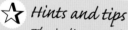 **Hints and tips**
The indirect application of high frequency is not a method that is required to be practically assessed for the NVQ standards. It is, however, important that you learn and understand it as a method of facial electrical treatment.

7 Use small circular movements, slowly covering the whole of the face.

8 After 5–7 minutes turn the intensity down to zero, remove the electrode from the client's face and turn the machine off.

9 Continue with your facial treatment as normal.

10 Provide thorough aftercare advice.

Treatment frequency

Depending on how oily the skin is, the client could receive direct high frequency on either a weekly or fortnightly basis as required, moving on to monthly treatments when appropriate.

Indirect high frequency

This method is also referred to as a Viennese Massage, whereby the client holds the saturator in their hands and the therapist is part of the circuit. The current flows through the saturator and charges the client while the therapist massages their skin. The current is transferred from the client's face to the therapist's hands, creating a warming and deeply relaxing effect. This treatment is indicated to clients with dry, sluggish and dehydrated skin.

Benefits and effects of indirect high frequency

- Warming
- Relaxing and soothing
- Increases lymphatic circulation
- Increases blood circulation
- Increases sebaceous gland activity
- Improves the appearance of fine lines
- Improves the overall appearance of the skin.

Specific contraindications to indirect high frequency

- Pregnancy, of both the client and therapist, as they are both used to transfer the current
- Sunburn
- Hypersensitive skin
- Recent facial injectable treatment

The health and safety and sparking dangers identified for direct high frequency also apply to indirect high frequency.

Treatment procedure for indirect high frequency

1 When you reach the point in facial treatment where you would normally massage, lightly cover the saturator in talc (to avoid slip) and give it to your client to hold. Ensure they hold one hand on the glass electrode and one hand on the saturator.

2 Apply a massage medium onto the client's skin for slip and glide.

3 Ensure all the intensity dials are set at zero and turn the machine on.

4 With one hand on the client's face, turn the machine up slightly and begin to massage in small circular movements.

5 Turn the machine up to your client's tolerance level and place your other hand on the client's skin.

6 Perform a full facial massage for 10–20 minutes, without losing contact on your client's skin at any point, otherwise a shock will be felt by the client.

7 Warmth will begin to be felt by both the therapist and the client; erythema will be present on the client's skin.

8 At the end of the massage, remove one hand from the client, turn the intensity down to zero and switch the machine off. Remove the other hand only when the machine is off.

9 Take the saturator from the client's hands.

10 Remove the excess massage medium.

11 Continue your facial treatment as normal, with mask, toner, moisturiser and SPF.

12 Provide thorough aftercare advice.

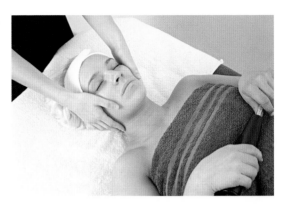

△ Client receiving treatment with indirect high frequency

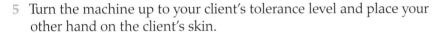

Saturator held in one hand   Holder held in other hand

△ Electrode for client to hold during indirect high frequency

Treatment frequency

For very dry or dehydrated skin a client could receive an intensive course of indirect high frequency twice a week for six weeks. Treatment could also be performed weekly or monthly as required.

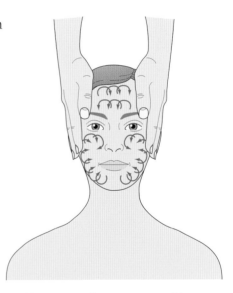

△ Movements for treatment with indirect high frequency

Galvanic

Galvanic treatment works on the scientific principle that similar charges repel and opposites attract. Galvanic current uses a direct current that flows in one direction only and has polarity. Two electrodes are required to complete the circuit; one electrode is negatively charged (−) and called the cathode, while the other is positively charged (+) and is called the anode. The inactive electrode is held by the client and the active electrode is applied to the skin by the therapist. Be careful because the active electrode can be positive or negative (the anode or the cathode). The polarity of the electrodes depends on the setting on

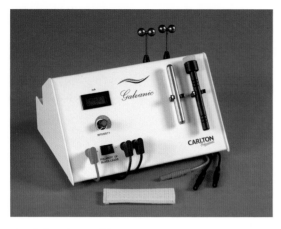

△ Galvanic machine

the galvanic unit; it is the responsibility of the therapist to change this according to the treatment and product requirements.

There are two methods of galvanic application to the face and these have different effects:

1 Desincrustation: this is a deep cleansing treatment to remove the build-up of sebum.

2 Iontophoresis: this is the application of specially manufactured products which are repelled deep into the skin. It is suitable for many skin types.

Dangers of galvanic current

There is a danger of burns if the galvanic current is applied incorrectly. Ensure there is plenty of product on the client's face during treatment, that you set the intensity of the machine correctly in accordance with manufacturer's instructions, and that you keep the active electrode moving on the skin at all times.

There is also a danger of shock with galvanic current. Ensure the intensity is set correctly and not increased beyond a safe level and that the electrodes are not lifted off the skin without the intensity being turned down to zero first.

Specific contraindications to galvanic treatment

- Loss of tactile sensation
- Metal plates, pins or excessive dental work
- Hypersensitive skin
- Highly nervous client
- Acne rosacea
- Pregnancy

Desincrustation

This facial electrical treatment is used on oily, congested and combination skin and has a deep cleansing effect. In desincrustation treatment the negative cathode (–) is the active electrode and placed onto the client's skin while the positive anode (+) is the inactive electrode and is given either to the client to hold or tucked under their shoulder to complete the electrical circuit. An electrolyte solution is placed onto the skin. Under the cathode (–) an alkali, sodium hydroxide, is produced which will soften sebum. Keratinised cells will be broken down, blockages will be released and pores deep cleansed.

Benefits and effects of desincrustation, cathode (−)

- An alkali (sodium hydroxide) is produced which destroys the acid mantle

- Deep cleansing

- Increased cell renewal

- Increases circulation

- Increases waste removal

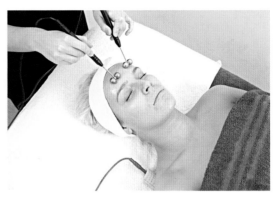

△ Performing galvanic treatment

After desincrustation has been performed for 5–10 minutes the polarity must be reversed to return the skin to an acid pH, in order to restore the acid mantle for protection and improve the skin's resistance to infection.

Benefits and effects of the anode (+) when the polarity is reversed

- Hydrochloric acid is produced, which restores the acid mantle

- Tightening and firming effect on the skin

- Vasodilation and erythema can be seen

Treatment procedure for galvanic desincrustation

1 Cleanse skin so it is free from make-up and grease.

2 Cover the inactive electrode with dampened lint and give to the client to hold or place it touching the skin under their shoulder.

3 Place either a saline solution or negatively charged desincrustation gel on the client's skin.

4 Switch the machine on and check the intensity is at zero. Switch the machine to match the polarity of the product on the client's skin.

5 Place the cathode (active electrode) firmly onto the skin and while keeping it moving, turn up the intensity until the client feels a slight tingle; this is usually between 0.5 and 1.5 milliamps – do not exceed this intensity.

6 Circle over the skin keeping in contact at all times for 4–5 minutes for general cleansing and 8–10 minutes for oily skins.

7 Reduce the intensity over bony areas.

8 When complete, reduce the current to zero, switch off the machine and remove the electrode from the client's skin.

9 Remove all product from the client's skin with plain damp cotton pads.

10 Comedone extraction can now take place if required, as the blocked sebum will have been softened and extraction will be much easier to perform.

11 Re-apply fresh product to the client's skin.

⭐ *Hints and tips*
For an oily, congested skin, before changing over the polarity you could apply oxygenating cream and gauze and use direct high frequency for 5–7 minutes.

12 Switch the polarity of the machine to positive.

13 Repeat the procedure for 2–3 minutes to tighten pores, soothe and restore the skin's acid balance.

14 Complete the rest of the facial treatment.

15 Provide thorough aftercare advice.

Iontophoresis

This treatment is recommended for dry, dehydrated, mature and sensitive skins but can be used for all skin types depending on the product and active ingredients found within it. Iontophoresis means the 'movement of ions'. Products of iontophoresis can be either positive (+) or negatively (–) charged. It is the product that informs us which polarity to set the machine at because the product and the machine match and repel, thus pushing the product deep into the skin.

Benefits and effects of iotophoresis

- Increase in cell metabolism
- Tightening and firming effect on the skin
- Vasodilation, erythema can be seen
- Increase in blood circulation

Treatment procedure for iontophoresis

1 Reach the point of the facial where you are ready to apply the mask.

2 Place the inactive electrode into dampened lint and give to client to hold or place it touching the skin behind the shoulder.

3 Apply the appropriate gel or contents of an ampoule onto face.

4 Turn the machine on and check the machine is on the correct polarity to match the product you are using and the intensity is at zero.

5 Place the active roller electrode onto the client's skin, switch the machine on and slowly turn the dial until a slight tingling sensation is felt. This is usually between 0.5 and 1.5 milliamps – do not exceed this intensity.

6 Commence roller movements for about 5–7 minutes; if the skin is sensitive reduce the intensity and treat for longer.

7 After this time, slowly switch the machine to zero and then to off.

8 It is not always necessary to remove the product from the skin, however, excess sticky gel should be removed.

9 *Do not reverse the polarity for iontophoresis.*

10 Tone the skin if required.

11 Complete your treatment with moisturiser and SPF.

12 Provide thorough aftercare advice.

Treatment frequency

Desincrustation should be performed depending on the skin's requirements, either weekly, fortnightly or monthly. Iontophoresis can be performed once a week and then monthly.

Electro muscle stimulator (faradic)

The electro muscle stimulator or EMS is a treatment which stimulates the superficial facial muscles. It is used on clients who show signs of premature ageing and loss of muscle tone; it can also be used as a preventative to delay the visible signs of ageing. The facial electrode consists of a plastic block, which is placed on the motor point of the facial muscles. It is used to stimulate groups of facial muscles rather than individual ones.

EMS uses a low frequency, interrupted direct current of 10–120 Hz (Hertz) to perform a muscle contraction. The client will feel the muscles contracting and relaxing and this should be explained to them during consultation. There may be some immediate improvement to the contours of the face, but the effects are temporary and the client should be advised that only regular treatments will sustain the desired results.

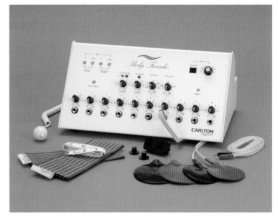

△ Faradic machine

Benefits and effects of EMS

- Increases blood circulation and skin colour
- Improves muscle tone and facial contours
- Increases muscle metabolism
- Can be used as a preventative measure to delay the signs of ageing
- Stimulates sensory nerve endings

Specific contraindications to EMS

- Hypersensitivity
- Sinus congestion
- High blood pressure
- Highly nervous client
- Epilepsy
- Diabetes
- Rosacea
- Migraine sufferers
- Excessive metal plates, pins or dental work

Treatment procedure for EMS

Ensure you follow the specific manufacturer's instructions for treatment procedure as EMS machines can vary.

1   Cleanse the skin.

2   Check all the intensity dials are set to zero and turn the machine on.

3   Cover the applicator block with a damp cotton pad.

4   Set all the dials correctly for the individual client's needs.

5   Test the current on the back of your arm to ensure safety.

6   Change the damp cotton pad over so your client has a new one.

7   Place the block on the client's skin when there is no contraction present. The intensity should be turned up on the surge only so the client can feel the current increasing. Ask them to tell you if the setting becomes uncomfortable.

8   Hold the electrode over each set of muscles for 6–8 contractions; these will be increased each time the client has another treatment.

9   Always turn the intensity down to zero before moving onto a new muscle group.

10 Treat both sides of the face equally; treatment time is 10–15 minutes.

11 After EMS has been performed, manually massage the client's face to break down any lactic acid which may have accumulated in the muscles during treatment.

12 Apply an anti-ageing mask to the client's skin.

13 Remove the mask and apply a moisturiser and SPF.

14 Provide thorough aftercare advice.

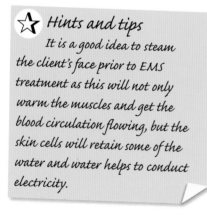

△ Faradic treatment being performed

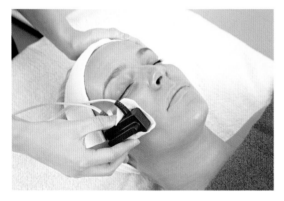

☆ *Hints and tips*
It is a good idea to steam the client's face prior to EMS treatment as this will not only warm the muscles and get the blood circulation flowing, but the skin cells will retain some of the water and water helps to conduct electricity.

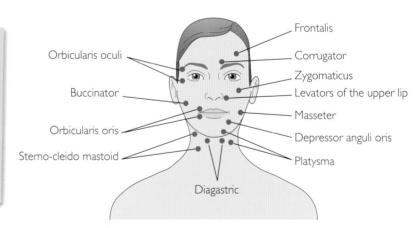

Frontalis
Orbicularis oculi
Corrugator
Zygomaticus
Buccinator
Levators of the upper lip
Masseter
Orbicularis oris
Depressor anguli oris
Sterno-cleido mastoid
Platysma
Diagastric

△ Superficial facial muscles

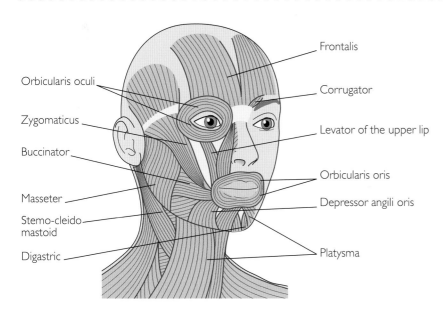

Frontalis

Orbicularis oculi

Corrugator

Zygomaticus

Levator of the upper lip

Buccinator

Orbicularis oris

Masseter

Depressor angili oris

Sterno-cleido mastoid

Digastric

Platysma

△ Motor points of facial muscles

Treatment frequency

It is important to avoid causing muscle fatigue, so care must be taken when recommending frequency of treatment. Do not exceed two treatments a week. A course of 12 treatments is recommended, followed by maintenance to retain the desired results.

Micro-current

Micro-current uses a very low-intensity, interrupted direct current, which is measured in microamps. This unit of electricity it so small it is barely felt by the client. The effects of micro-current are used as an anti-ageing treatment. The effects are seen immediately, making micro-current treatments very popular with clients. However, the effects are temporary and the client should be advised that only regular treatments will sustain the desired results.

Micro-current is modified by waveforms which are interrupted by varying pulses. These pules have different widths ranging from one millionth of a second through to 2 seconds and it is these varying pulse widths that achieve different results. The wave forms are:

- Sine: the most gentle effect; most likely to be the wave form used first as it produces superficial effects such as increased blood circulation and light toning.

- Ramp: produces a 'pumping' action required in lymph drainage. It rises sharply and decreases gradually after it has peaked.

- Square: - this wave form produces the 'lifting effect' and is a deep treatment, although the rise and intensity duration are the same.

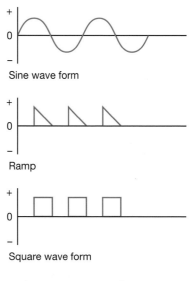

Sine wave form

Ramp

Square wave form

△ Micro-current wave forms

Benefits and effects of micro-current

- Increases blood circulation
- Increases lymphatic circulation and the removal of waste
- Reduces puffiness due to lymphatic drainage
- Stimulates renewal of collagen and elastin fibres
- Stimulates cell renewal
- Temporary removal of fine lines and plumps wrinkles
- Assists the healing process of visible scar tissues
- Refines pores
- Improves appearance and texture

Specific contraindications to micro-current

- Electrical implants such as a pacemaker
- Metal plates and pins and excessive dental work
- Migraine sufferers
- Epilepsy
- Pregnancy

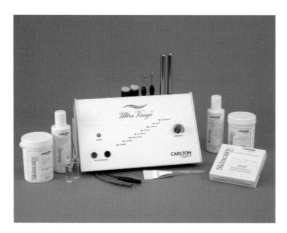

△ Micro-current machine

Treatment procedure for micro-current

Micro-current treatment can be performed in different ways, depending on the type of equipment you have available. Some machines require you to manually select the intensity and duration; other machines have these automatically programmed in. Always follow the manufacturer's instructions, as these will differ from machine to machine.

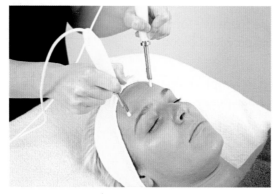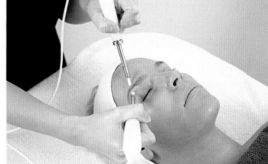

△ Micro-current treatment being performed

Chapter 10
ELECTRICAL EPILATION

This chapter covers:

NVQ unit B29 Provide electrical epilation treatments

City & Guilds VRQ unit 308 Provide electrical epilation

VTCT VRQ unit UV30474 Provide electrical epilation

LEARNING OBJECTIVES

This chapter is about the skills involved in assessing, preparing and conducting electrical epilation to remove unwanted hair using an alternating current and blend techniques.

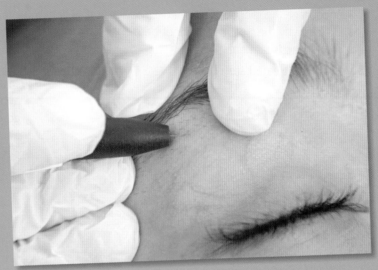

The learning outcomes for NVQ unit B29 are:

1 Be able to maintain safe and effective methods of working when providing electrical epilation treatments
2 Be able to consult, plan and prepare
3 Be able to carry out electrical epilation treatments
4 Understand the organisational and legal requirements of providing electrical epilation
5 Understand how to work safely and effectively when providing electrical epilation treatments
6 Understand the use of client consultation for electrical epilation treatments
7 Understand anatomy and physiology relevant to electrical epilation
8 Understand the contra-indications and contra-actions of electrical epilation
9 Understand the use of equipment and materials in electrical epilation
10 Understand how electrical epilation treatments are used
11 Understand how to provide aftercare advice following electrical epilation

You will need to be competent in all of these outcomes to be competent in electrical epilation treatments, qualify for insurance and perform the treatments on members of the public.

NVQ evidence requirements

For the NVQ your assessor will need to observe you perform these treatments successfully on at least six separate occasions involving four different clients. This includes:

- Two observations each for the upper lip, chin and bikini line

You must practically:

1 Demonstrate the use of all these consultation techniques:
- questioning
- visual
- reference to client records

2 Take one of the following necessary actions:
- encourage the client to seek medical advice
- explain why the treatment cannot be carried out
- modify the treatment

3 Areas to be treated are:
- upper lip
- chin
- bikini line
- eyebrows
- underarms
- neck
- breast

4 Types of needle includes:
- one piece
- two piece
- insulated
- gold

5 Hair types are:
- fine
- coarse
- curly

6 Skin types and conditions are:
- dry
- oily
- sensitive
- dehydrated
- mature

7 Electrical epilation treatments are:
- alternating current
- blend

8 Provide all these types of advice:
- avoidance of activities which may cause contra-actions
- future treatment needs
- dealing with regrowth between treatments

VRQ practical evidence requirements

There are different evidence requirements for the VRQ qualifications, depending on the awarding body. The lists below show the requirements for two major awarding bodies: City & Guilds and VTCT.

City & Guilds unit 308 Provide electrical epilation

The final summative observation should be undertaken when the candidates have completed a minimum of five formative treatments using the following methods of electrical epilation:

- short-wave diathermy
- blend epilation.

Candidates are required to cover all of the following face and body areas in the five treatments:

- lip
- chin
- eyebrows
- underarms
- breast tissue
- bikini
- legs.

The areas of the face and body listed above can be combined during the five treatments. At least three of the five treatments must include the lip and chin.

Each observation should include:

- findings of the skin and hair analysis
- the type and size of needle that was selected to suit the client's hair and skin types
- how electrical epilation techniques were adapted to suit the client's treatment needs, skin and hair.

Types and conditions

- contra-actions that may occur during and following treatment and how to respond.

For the final observation the candidate will be assessed carrying out two electrical epilation treatments on the upper lip and chin using either of the following methods:

- short wave diathermy
- blend epilation.

The method selected must meet the needs of the client's hair and skin.

VTCT unit UV30474 Provide electrical epilation

Six observations are required, covering the following range:

Used all consultation techniques:

- questioning
- visual
- reference to client records.

Dealt with a minimum of one of the necessary actions:

- encouraging the client to seek medical advice
- explaining why the treatment cannot be carried out
- modification of treatment.

Treated all areas:

- upper lip
- chin
- bikini line
- eyebrows
- underarms
- neck.

Used all the types of needle:

- one piece
- two piece
- insulated
- gold.

Dealt with all hair types:

- fine
- coarse
- curly.

Dealt with all skin types and conditions:

- dry
- oily
- sensitive
- dehydrated
- mature.

Carried out all electrical epilation treatments:

- alternating currents
- blend.

Given all the types of advice:

- avoidance of activities which may cause contra-actions
- future treatment needs
- home care
- dealing with regrowth between treatments.

In all cases, simulation is *not* allowed.

VRQ knowledge requirements

City & Guilds unit 308 Provide electrical epilation	VTCT unit UV30474 Provide electrical epilation	Page no.
Learning outcome 1: Be able to prepare for electrical epilation		
Practical skills/observations		
Prepare themselves, client and work area for electrical epilation treatments		322–4
Use suitable consultation techniques to identify treatment objectives		324–6
Carry out skin and hair analysis		217
Select products, tools and equipment to suit client treatment needs, skin types and conditions		334–5; 338–41
Provide clear recommendations to the client		325–7
Underpinning knowledge		
Describe the different consultation techniques used to identify treatment objectives		324–6
Explain the contraindications that prevent or restrict electrical epilation treatment		327–8
Describe health and safety working practices		321–4
Explain the importance of carrying out detailed hair and skin analysis		217
Describe how to select products, tools and equipment to suit client's needs		334–5; 338–41
Describe the environmental conditions suitable for electrical epilation treatments		322
Learning outcome 2: Be able to provide electrical epilation		
Practical skills/observations		
Communicate and behave in a professional manner		325–6
Follow health and safety working practices		321–4
Position themselves and the clients correctly throughout treatment		324
Use products, tools, equipment and techniques to suit client's treatment needs		334–5; 338–41
Insert the needle into the hair follicle with regard to depth and angle		337
Complete the treatment to the satisfaction of the client		338–41
Record and evaluate the results of the treatment		343
Provide suitable aftercare advice		341–3
Underpinning knowledge		
Describe how to select the needle type and size to suit hair and skin types		334–5
Describe how to work on different hair growth patterns and treatment areas		338–41
Explain the consequences of inaccurate probing		337
Explain the principles, uses and benefits of galvanic, short-wave diathermy and blend		319–21

Introduction

Electrical epilation is the process of permanently removing hair by means of an electric current. The primary aim of the therapist is to bring about permanent removal of unwanted hair without skin damage. A therapist's job role in the treatment of electrical epilation can be varied; their work may be within the beauty therapy industry or they could work within a medical clinic.

Epilation is more than a beauty treatment and involves a great deal of client psychology as excessive or unwanted hair growth can be very distressing for a client. The psychological benefits of this treatment are an improvement in confidence and self-esteem, which will impact vastly on the client's quality of life.

As a treatment, epilation requires a lot of patience and skill to perform safely and effectively. However, once mastered it is a highly sought after and rewarding treatment to offer.

The relevant anatomy and physiology relating to this unit can be found in Chapter 4 Anatomy and physiology. The theory of the electrical currents that relate to this unit can be found in Chapter 5 Theory of electrical currents.

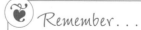 Remember...

Hair growth has three stages: anagen, when the follicle is actively producing a hair, catagen (changing stage) where the follicle has stopped producing hair but is breaking away from the blood supply and finally telogen, where the follicle is at rest.

Hair growth

After epilation the follicle will go through a healing process, repairing itself to the best of its ability. It may eventually begin to produce a new hair which, when it appears at the skin surface, should be epilated again. This will ensure that the follicle is in anagen. With consecutive treatments the new hairs will become finer and take longer to reappear until eventually the dermal papilla is destroyed and no new hair is formed.

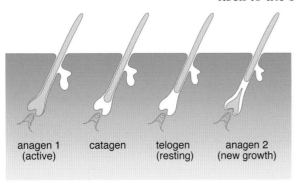

△ Three stages of hair growth

The purpose of electrical epilation is to bring about the permanent removal of the hair by cutting the hair off from its nutrient and oxygen supply: the dermal papilla. This can only be successfully accomplished when the hair is in anagen. At any other stage of growth the shortened follicle hinders the process, making it less successful, if at all. When the electrical epilation is correctly delivered to a hair follicle in anagen by means of a needle, it causes destruction of the hair follicle without damaging the skin. Note that the inner and outer root sheaths are affected as well as the dermal papilla; this loosens the hair, allowing it to be removed from the follicle with tweezers but without tension (plucking).

If a hair is removed by epilation when the follicle is in catagen or telogen this may stimulate the follicle into anagen and the resulting new hair should be treated as soon as it appears. Too long between treatments can result in the hair follicle being in telogen and an unsuccessful treatment given. For effective removal, treatments should be given weekly at first and then the time between treatments extended to suit as the regrowth slows down.

Recognising the hair growth stage

Table 10.1 below shows the different hair growth stages.

▽ Table 10.1 Hair growth stages

Anagen	If a correctly epilated hair (one that comes out without resistance from the follicle after treatment) is removed by tweezers and placed on a cotton wool pad it can be studied closely and it will be seen to have a fully formed bulb with the entire length of tissue sheath intact. This is the best stage to epilate the hairs.
Catagen	In this stage the hair has broken away from the bulb and is therefore club ended. Depending upon the stage of catagen it will have varying amounts of tissue sheath intact.
Telogen	In this stage the hair is ready to fall out of the follicle. It will still appear club ended but with no tissue sheath attached.

Methods of electrical epilation

Permanent hair removal can be achieved using a number of methods of electrical epilation:

- Short-wave diathermy (thermolysis): this works by heat coagulating or cutting off the blood supply to the hair follicle.

- Galvanic electrolysis (electrolysis): this works by bringing about a chemical reaction within the tissues to destroy the hair. Electrical epilation owes its reputation to the thoroughness of this method.

- Blend (combination of electrolysis and thermolysis): this method combines the chemical thoroughness of galvanic with the fast heat from short-wave diathermy to bring about hair destruction.

Short-wave diathermy

Short-wave diathermy uses a high-frequency alternating current to produce heat which destroys the hair root.

Rapid oscillations of the high-frequency current causes fast vibration of water molecules within the tissues, causing friction. This friction causes a temporary release of energy in the form of heat. It is the moisture within the tissues that is heated, not the needle. The heating occurs at the tip of the needle, creating a high-frequency field of current (this refers to the heating pattern radiating from the needle). The high-frequency field is strongest and at its most intense close to the tip of the probe and in practice will concentrate around the tip.

To destroy the hair, the papilla must be coagulated. Coagulating the blood supply in the papilla means that the nourishment to the hair is reduced so it will grow back finer until it is eventually destroyed. The current is able to reach the papilla because water is a good conductor of electricity and the dermis is very moist.

Short-wave diathermy is a fast method; however, the main disadvantage is a higher percentage of regrowth. It is recommended to treat the hairs in an anagen stage of hair growth as the blood supply in the papilla is at its richest and so destruction at this stage provides quicker and more satisfying results.

Galvanic

Galvanic uses a direct current whereby the electrons flow continuously in one direction. The current flows from the epilation unit through the needle holder to the needle, then into the follicle, through the client and via the shortest path back to the indifferent electrode where the current returns to the epilation unit. Direct current always flows from negative to positive; this is from the negative needle (cathode) to the positive indifferent electrode (anode) which is held by the client.

When a direct current is made to come in contact with the moisture in the follicle a chemical reaction takes place. When direct current is passed through a conducting stainless steel needle into the follicle it causes the water and salt in the follicle to break up into their component parts or ions. These ions realign to make new substances

> **Key term**
>
> **Coagulation** – A process by which the blood thickens, preventing the passage of oxygen and nutrients.

> **Key term**
>
> **Thermolysis** – a process which occurs when current is applied to the follicle; the tissues are destroyed by the 'heating effect'.

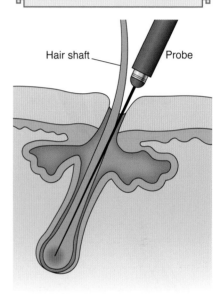

△ Short-wave diathermy in the follicle

Hair shaft — Probe

> **Key terms**
>
> **Electrolysis** – this is the process of the application of a direct current. It is a term often used to describe any form of epilation but actually refers to the galvanic method.
>
> **Lye** – otherwise known as sodium hydroxide, it is produced under a direct current when using galvanic or blend electrical epilation. It has a caustic effect to the papillae and is an alkaline.

319

which are sodium hydroxide (lye) and chlorine and hydrogen gas. Lye is an alkaline and it is this that brings about the destruction of the follicle by its caustic and corrosive nature, not the direct current. The amount of lye produced is small and is soon neutralised by the skin's tissues, which are slightly acidic.

Hydrogen gas can sometimes be seen frothing out of the follicle opening; chlorine gas appears at the positive indifferent electrode (anode) in the form of extremely mild hydrochloric acid.

Units of lye

The term 'units of lye' was devised by the co-inventor of the blend, Arthur Hinkel, as a means of measurement for the minute amounts of lye made in the follicle. Prior to this, industrial measurements in gallons were used.

One unit of lye (UL) is the amount of lye made when 0.1 milliampere of direct current flows for one second.

Formation of lye:

- Salt (NaCl) + Water (H_2O) = Na + H + Cl + OH

Ion realignment means that:

- Chlorine gas (Cl_2) being negative forms at the indifferent/positive electrode (anode).
- Hydrogen gas (H_2) being positive forms at the needle/negative electrode (cathode).
- Sodium Hydroxide or lye (NaOH) forms at the needle/negative electrode (cathode).

Galvanic is a more effective method than short-wave diathermy because:

- lye is attracted to the moisture at the dermal papilla
- lye is fluid and can reach all parts of the follicle
- distorted and curved follicles are more effectively treated
- the moisture gradient of the skin ensures the action is maintained at the dermal papilla where it is required.

The only disadvantage of galvanic current is that it is slow. The formation of lye takes time and the current needs to flow for many seconds for the chemical reaction to take place – 10 seconds on average in each follicle. When treating hairs individually, this means few hairs are removed at each treatment. However, direct current is very effective in destroying the follicle.

Hair shaft — Probe

△ Lye in the hair follicle

△ Blend epilation unit

Blend

The blend technique uses both direct current (galvanic) and an alternating high-frequency current (short wave diathermy) at the same time.

Both currents retain their own characteristics in the treatment of the follicle. The direct current produces lye, the alternating high-frequency current produces heat. The heating effect is kept very low and is merely warmth; this prevents the follicle from becoming dehydrated, which would inhibit or prevent the formulation of lye. The warmth makes the lye more active in the follicle and by warming the lye quickens the process of tissue destruction. With the presence of warmth the lye becomes more turbulent and can therefore fill any shape of distorted or curved follicle. The warmth also increases the porosity of the surrounding follicular tissue, allowing the lye to diffuse into it and making the treatment more thorough.

The follicle is treated very effectively but in less time than by direct current alone. By combining alternating current with direct current it reduces the treatment time per follicle by a half: direct current only =10 seconds on average, blend = 5 seconds on average.

The blend method is more effective, results in less hair regrowth, is more comfortable and gives the therapist and the client far more choices than diathermy or galvanic alone. As a result, client motivation is high and they invariably go on to have other parts of their body treated because it is much more comfortable.

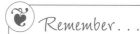

> ★ **Hints and tips**
> It is a scientific fact that a rise in temperature accelerates the rate of chemical reactions.

> **Remember . . .**
> A successful therapist will remove the hair without pulling and without causing skin damage.

Maintain safe and effective methods of work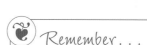

Legislation

Health and Safety legislation is extremely important during the preparation and delivery of epilation treatment. Below are the main pieces of legislation that relate to epilation treatment. For more information on health and safety see Chapter 1 Monitoring health and safety.

Local Government Miscellaneous Provisions Act 1982

The Act requires that any person who is carrying out electrical epilation should be registered with the local authority due to the high risk of cross-infection from blood or body fluids. The environmental health officer (EHO) will visit the premises to ensure that there is adequate provision for hygiene and sterilisation, including appropriate methods for the disposal of contaminated waste and sharps, both of which are generated during electrical epilation treatment.

> **Remember . . .**
> Failure to register with your local authority can result in a fine.

Personal Protective Equipment at Work Regulations (PPE) 2002

PPE in the form of disposable powder-free, nitrile or vinyl gloves must be supplied by the employer and used by the therapists when performing electrical epilation treatment. Disposable masks could also be worn if required.

Controlled Waste Regulations 1992

This Regulation governs the correct disposal of contaminated waste. Electrical epilation waste is contaminated waste and should be placed in yellow bin bags for incineration. Used epilation needles should be disposed of in a sharps box. Arrangements for disposal should be made with your local authority.

Provision and Use of Work Equipment Regulations 1998

This Regulation ensures that the electrical epilation equipment is suitable for its intended use, that it is safe, well maintained and inspected to retain its condition.

Electricity at Work Regulations 1989

This Regulation governs the regular maintenance of electrical equipment by a qualified electrician and the keeping of records.

Preparation of the treatment area

Your treatment room should be clean, tidy and hygienic. Electrical epilation is an invasive treatment in terms of consultation and performance and so hygiene should be of the highest standards.

The client is likely to be embarrassed by their hair growth so they should be made to feel comfortable and relaxed in a calm and quiet atmosphere. Lighting will need to be clear and bright; the use of a magnifying lamp with lighting (mag light) is essential to provide suitable lighting and increased vision of the treatment area. Soft and calming background music will help to create a peaceful ambience for the client.

You should also consider the heating and ventilation of the treatment room because if your client is nervous they may be hot and sticky.

△ Mag light

Personal appearance and hygiene checklist

The treatment room/cubicle should be:

- calm
- private
- well ventilated
- well lit
- suitably relaxing – music playing
- clean and tidy at all times.

The treatment couch should be prepared with:

- freshly laundered towels
- clean couch roll
- bolsters or supports for client comfort
- headband if working on the face.

The trolley should be prepared with:

- epilation unit
- needle holder
- hygienic sterilisation preparations for the skin
- sterilised tweezers
- lined, sealable bin for the disposal of contaminated waste
- disposable gloves
- selection of individually packed needles of different diameters
- sharps box for used probes
- bowl for jewellery
- cotton wool
- facial mirror
- consultation form and client record card.

A foot switch is available with certain machines and is preferable for some methods of epilation. This will need to be tucked neatly under the couch with any trailing wires securely out of the way.

Hygiene procedures

Specific hygiene procedures to following for electrical epilation treatment are as follows.

1 Use individual needles pre-sterilised by gamma radiation and dispose of in a sharps box immediately after use.

2 The therapist's hands should be washed and nails scrubbed with an anti-bacterial hand cleanser immediately before and after treatment.

3 Open cuts/wounds should be covered during treatment.

4 The use of disposable gloves is essential

5 All tweezers, scissors and chuck caps should be sterilised before and after each use.

6 Use disposable cotton wool and tissues, clean towels and couch roll over the treatment couch.

7 Use a skin-sterilising agent to clean the area to be treated. If working on the face all make up should be removed prior to treatment.

For further information on sterilising methods see Chapter 6 Professional practices.

Preparation of the therapist

The therapist needs to have high levels of personal hygiene and look presentable in a clean and smart uniform with their hair securely tied back and nails neat and short. Personal qualities of the therapist are a caring attitude, patience and practice to achieve skills to a professional standard. For electrical epilation the therapist will need to be particularly discreet and understanding of the client's specific requirements.

Preparing the client

- When the client arrives for treatment they should be treated with courtesy and respect.

- Always address the client by their name and inform them of yours.

- Take the client to the treatment area and briefly explain the treatment procedure.

- Carry out a thorough consultation and discuss the aims of the treatment.

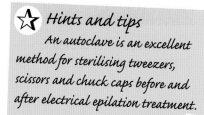

△ Preparation of the treatment trolley

 Remember...

It is essential that the client's details are kept securely and, due to the sometimes intimate nature of this treatment, may also require special considerations to maintain confidentiality.

Hints and tips
An autoclave is an excellent method for sterilising tweezers, scissors and chuck caps before and after electrical epilation treatment.

 Health and safety

Sterilise your probe holder by wiping it over with a disinfectant solution before and after each client.

You must adhere to current guidance relating to age restrictions for electrical epilation treatment. Signed consent is a requirement for the treatment of minors.

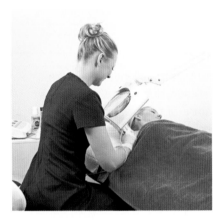

△ Therapist correctly seated for epilation treatment

- Advise the client which articles of clothing and jewellery they need to remove and, depending on the area to be treated, provide a gown for them to wear.

- Allow the client to undress in private and get onto the couch.

- Assist the client in getting comfortable: this may include using bolsters to support key areas of the body.

- Cover the client with a towel and only expose the area to be treated.

- Make sure they are warm and comfortable: before beginning the treatment.

Positioning of client and therapist

The therapist must maintain correct posture throughout the treatment to prevent repetitive strain injury and neuromuscular damage. You may find that you are working within a close proximity for a long period of time when performing electrical epilation, so a height-adjustable couch and chair to sit on is essential to ensure comfort. It is not appropriate to lean on your client throughout the treatment.

The client should be positioned on the couch to ensure a correct insertion can be achieved. This will very much depend on the area being treated and the direction of hair growth. The therapist may find they are working from the top or sides of the couch and moving about during the treatment to change their insertion position. Clients can be supported by the use of pillows and bolsters for comfort.

Safe and effective treatment

To perform electrical epilation safely and effectively the following requirements must be adhered to:

- techniques of probing/insertions

- angle of probe/insertions

- depth of probe/insertions

- timing of treatment

- effect of current on hair and skin

- probe size

- skin sensitivity.

These points will be discussed later in this chapter.

Consult, plan and prepare for treatment

Consultation techniques

Consultation techniques include:

- questioning techniques

- listening techniques

- body language

- visual assessment
- referral to client records
- visual aids.

See Chapter 6 Professional practices for more information on consultation techniques.

Communication and behaviour for therapists

Methods of communication and standards of behaviour during consultation for a beauty therapy can be found in Chapter 6 Professional practices. There are additional considerations for electrical epilation treatment and these are discussed below.

The consultation is always the initial point of contact between the client and the therapist. It provides an opportunity for the client to ask questions about the treatment and the therapist to find out information that will be essential for the client's treatment to go ahead. Consultation for electrical epilation should be undertaken without charge or obligation, as a large amount of business can be generated from effective consultations.

Many clients will feel embarrassed and apprehensive and so a caring and understanding approach by the therapist is essential. In addition, a client may have spent many years dealing with the superfluous hair using an unsatisfactory method of temporary removal; others may have heard that the treatment is painful and expensive which will heighten their apprehension.

The client should be taken to a private treatment room area and put at ease by the therapist's friendly and knowledgeable manner. The therapist must gain the client's trust and confidence by being professional at all times. This includes exhibiting a mature approach, being discreet, giving clear explanations as to the procedures, asking appropriate questions and allowing the client the opportunity to ask questions too. Do not make exaggerated claims but be honest as to the effectiveness in accordance with the client's circumstances and give an estimate as to the expense of the treatment by predicting an accurate treatment plan. The treatment plan should be discussed and likely costs made clear to the client.

The client should understand that with regular treatment and commitment the hairs will be permanently removed.

Remember that effective communication is about listening as well as talking and use your knowledge of non-verbal signs and body language to promote the treatment, the business and yourself. Explain how the treatment works using appropriate language and use diagrams to help the client to visualise what will happen. Choose words and phrases that will not alarm the client, for example say 'warmth' instead of 'hot', 'sting', 'heat' or 'current', and 'probe' rather than 'needle'.

Remember...

The probe is inserted into a hair follicle, which is a natural opening in the skin. You are not piercing the skin.

Questioning

Ensuring client suitability means that they will benefit from the treatment and that it may be performed in a safe manner. Information that must be elicited from the client before treatment can commence includes:

- personal details
- contraindications
- medical history
- cause of the hair growth
- hair and skin condition
- method of temporary removal used (if any)
- the client's emotional state and lifestyle
- previous electrical epilation treatments.

From the results of the consultation a treatment plan can be devised. This will include a period of intense treatment at first, usually every 7–14 days for a period of time. This period of time depends on the area being treated, the cause of the hair growth and the method of temporary removal employed by the client before epilation treatment began.

Hints and tips

Do not overtreat an area as time is needed for the skin to recover from the treatment or scarring and infection may result

The amount of time needed for each visit will largely depend on the area being treated. If the hairs are close together, as with the upper lip for example, it is possible that not all the hairs can be treated in one visit. The client should be given a follow-up appointment in 7–14 days in order for the area to rest before more treatment is given. It may mean more visits of a shorter time in order for the area to be cleared. The upper lip is a sensitive area and may require shorter treatments in accordance with the client's tolerance levels. Once the area is free from hair it is then wise to catch the regrowth as it appears to ensure treating the hairs in anagen. This may mean the client returns every week until the regrowth slows down, when fortnightly to monthly appointments can be made.

Table 10.2 shows a general treatment time guide for specific areas.

▽ Table 10.2 Epilation treatment guide

Service	Time
Upper lip	15 minutes
Chin	15 minutes
Bikini line	Up to 30 minutes each side
Eyebrows	10 minutes each eyebrow
Underarms	Up to 30 minutes each underarm
Neck	30 minutes
Breast	10 minutes

The price structure for epilation is determined according to the time spent performing the treatment. From the treatment plan an estimate as to the cost of the treatment can be forecast but it should be emphasised that this is only a guide.

A client may wish to know how many times each hair will need to be treated before the treatment is made permanent. This varies a great deal but a general guide is the coarser a hair is (and if the growth has been treated by waxing or tweezing prior to treatment) the more treatment will be needed to render the hair removal permanent. A fine, virgin growth will need much less treatment.

Contraindications

To ensure the suitability and safety of the client and to prevent cross-contamination, the therapist should question the client about possible contraindications for electrical epilation treatment. Contraindications fall into two categories: those that *prevent* treatment and those that may *restrict* treatment. If a contraindication is present the situation should be sympathetically explained to the client that either they may not have the treatment or that the treatment will need to be adapted to avoid making the condition worse.

Contraindications that prevent electrical epilation treatment

- Fungal infections
- Bacterial infections
- Viral infections
- Infestations
- Severe eczema
- Severe psoriasis
- Severe skin conditions
- During chemotherapy
- During radiotherapy
- Pace maker
- Haemophilia

Contraindications that restrict electrical epilation treatment

- Broken bones
- Recent fractures and sprains
- Cuts and abrasions
- Recent scar tissue
- Skin disorders
- Skin allergies
- Product allergies

- Epilepsy: electrical impulses to the brain may be disturbed which could result in a fit. Short-wave diathermy should be the only method of epilation given, particularly if the client suffers from anxiety. Seek GP referral.

- Diabetes: skin will be slow to heal and clients may have a low pain threshold. Give shorter treatments with long healing gaps in between. Seek GP referral.

- Undiagnosed lumps and swellings: GP referral is advised first to ensure client is safe for treatment.

- Pregnancy: hair growth due to pregnancy is advised to be left alone as often the hair falls out and does not return after the birth.

- Metal plates or pins in bone: may affect the choice of epilation method used.

- Heart disease/conditions: vascular disorders requiring anti-coagulant drugs. This is because coagulation of blood at the base of the follicle will be hindered. Seek GP referral.

- Respiratory conditions such as asthma: particular attention needs to be given to the positioning of the client due to possible breathing difficulties and stress of the treatment, which may trigger an attack.

- Dysfunction of the nervous system: the client needs to have suitable skin sensation to perceive discomfort and irritation.

- Piercings: need to be removed prior to treatment.

- Moles: must be checked for malignancy before any growing hairs from them can be treated. Seek GP referral.

- Endocrine disorders such as polycystic ovary syndrome will need correct medical treatment to work on the cause, which often results in hair growth in the male pattern. Treatment with electrical epilation can work well in conjunction with medication.

Necessary actions

The therapist should be aware of the possible actions to take if the client presents with a contraindication and these actions include:

- encouraging the client to seek medical advice

- explaining why the treatment cannot be carried out

- modifying the treatment.

Modification to electrical epilation treatment may include changing the length of service time to suit your client, working around moles and cuts or abrasions and altering the method used or probe size.

Skin sensitivity

The sensitivity of the skin varies from person to person and some clients will react badly to all types of current and probe; these clients are unsuitable for treatment. Others may show more sensitivity than is normal, which indicates that the skin has been pre-sensitised by an unknown factor, such as:

- heat treatments, either before or after epilation
- exposure to ultra-violet light, either the sun or sunbed treatments
- other beauty treatments such as glycolic peels, microdermabrasion and laser treatments; the skin will need to heal before epilation treatment can be performed
- products used on the skin may cause sensitivity when combined with epilation, for example perfume, deodorant, depilatory creams
- excessive use of abrasives and exfoliants
- some types of medication
- the menstrual cycle: the pain threshold is reduced around the time of menstruation.

> ☆ **Hints and tips**
> If you are concerned about your client's skin sensitivity always perform a patch test first. Remember to record the results on their record card.

Causes of hair growth

There are two classifications of increased hair growth:

1 Primary causes: these occur as a result of congenital influences or normal changes in hormone levels and include hereditary causes, ethnic differences, puberty, pregnancy and menopause.

2 Secondary causes: these include those brought about by illness and disease such as endocrine disorders, illness and stress.

Congenital causes

This refers to an inherited pattern of growth. Every child is born with a pre-determined pattern of hair growth, inherited from its parents' genetic structure. A congenital pattern of hair growth is influenced by hereditary factors, not environmental ones. Congenital hypertrichosis (excessive or abnormal hair growth) can appear at birth or later on in life. In extreme cases the whole body can be covered. This is the result of an unusual genetic structure.

> **Key terms**
>
> **Congenital hair growth** – refers to an inherited pattern of hair growth.
>
> **Topical hair growth** – this occurs in areas of skin as a result of local irritation, moles and birthmarks.

Topical cause

Topical cause refers to local areas of skin such as irritation, moles and birthmarks. Hair growth in a sustained area from irritation will become deeper and coarser to protect the epidermis. This occurs because the irritation causes increased blood supply to the follicle and the hair receives better nourishment. Other irritations that may increase hair growth include plasters, excessive scratching, X-rays, ultra-violet light and sunburn. Bandaging or plaster casts can often increase hair growth, although this usually disappears within 2–3 months. Hairs often protrude from moles and birthmarks because they have an unusual amount of capillaries close to the skin's surface, which provide extra nourishment.

> ☆ **Hints and tips**
> Tweezing is another topical cause that is capable of initiating hair growth from a resting follicle. When a club hair is lost there is a loosening of cells, which stimulate the new hair to be produced.

Systemic cause (normal and abnormal)

Systemic causes of hair growth relate to the endocrine system and its hormones. Some of the hormones produced by the endocrine system

Remember...

A basic knowledge of the endocrine system is necessary to recognise the disorders you may come across. However, you are not a member of the medical profession and it is unethical and unprofessional to diagnose your clients.

are responsible for normal hair growth in both males and females. With an abnormal systemic cause there is an imbalance of hormones that causes excess hair.

Endocrine disorders which affect hair growth

During the initial consultation you will establish the cause of the superfluous hair growth that is of concern to your client. The cause of the hair growth will be either primary or secondary in nature. If a primary cause is identified than epilation treatment can be carried out successfully. If secondary, a doctor's permission to treat may be needed and it should be explained that the treatment would not be successful until the underlying cause has been dealt with.

Normal hormonal stimulation includes puberty, pregnancy and the menopause. Abnormal hormonal stimulation is caused by a disorder of the endocrine system. The endocrine system consists of a series of hormone-secreting glands which are found throughout the body. Hormones are chemicals which cause changes within the body. The endocrine glands secrete hormones directly into the bloodstream. Under normal circumstances the endocrine system controls the correct amount of hormones in harmony with the body's needs.

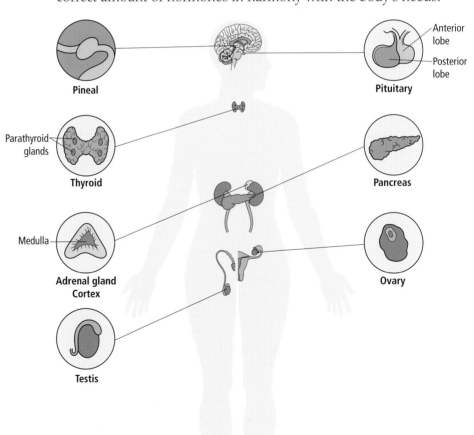

△ The endocrine system and identification of glands

The adrenal glands are situated one above each kidney. Each adrenal gland has two parts: the medulla and the cortex. The medulla produces adrenaline and the cortex produces hormones called steroids, corticosteroids and the sex hormones – androgens, oestrogen and progesterone.

The important point to remember about the adrenal glands is that in both male and female they are a source of androgens, which are capable of stimulating face and body hair. An excess of androgens can result in increased unwanted hair in females.

Hirsutism

This is the term used to describe a masculine pattern of hair growth that is normal in men but abnormal when found in women. Hirsutism is caused by increased androgen production by the adrenal glands and ovaries. It can be successfully managed with medical treatment, which will correct or control the endocrine disorder and prevent the development of new growth. Electrical epilation will eventually permanently remove the existing hair growth. However, it must be explained to the client that just as the established growth did not appear overnight, so time will be needed to permanently eliminate the problem. The fact that results are slow but certain should be emphasised.

> ☆ **Hints and tips**
> Some drugs that contain hormones such as cortisone and contraceptive pills may also lead to abnormal hair growth. Stress can also be responsible for increased hair growth because of the increase in adrenaline that is produced.

Adrenogenital syndrome

Usually caused by a tumour or an abnormality in the adrenal cortex, fortunately this condition is very rare. The adrenal cortex cannot use the chemical materials needed for manufacturing cortisones, but produces androgens instead. Adrenogenital syndrome is recognised by loss of menstrual cycle, development of a more masculine build and a deeper voice and male hair growth patterns including a receding hairline.

Cushing's syndrome

This syndrome may be caused by any prolonged medication which stimulates the adrenal cortex to produce an excessive amount of hormone including androgens, an excessive development of cells in the adrenal cortex and the presence of tumours in the cortex or pituitary gland. Symptoms include roundness of the face, neck and trunk (although limbs remain unaffected), cessation of menstruation in women and roundness of the shoulders. An abnormal amount of hair growth is produced, leading to hirsutism.

Polycystic ovary syndrome (Stein-Leventhal syndrome)

The development of ovarian cysts is thought to relate to the cause of this syndrome, which is fairly common. Polycystic ovaries are capable of secreting large quantities of androgens, which causes symptoms such as excessive bleeding or lack of menstruation, weight gain and the development of excessive hair growth leading to hirsutism.

Anorexia nervosa

Anorexia nervosa is an eating disorder where people lose more weight than is considered healthy for their age and height. It leads to muscle wastage and loss of body fat. Symptoms include dry skin that is covered with fine hair and loss of menstruation.

Gender differences

Generally, male clients are more hairy then females and male clients may seek to permanently remove hair for cosmetic reasons or because of irritation. You may also treat transgender clients who will want to permanently change a male pattern of hair growth. It is essential that you treat clients undergoing gender reassignment the same as other clients and that you maintain high levels of professionalism and confidentiality. The extent of hair growth will vary depending on their stage of treatment; initially the hair will be thick and dense in growth, which will require more frequent treatment over a longer period of time, usually at a higher intensity. As treatment progresses the hair should be finer and sparser, and therefore frequency, time and intensity of treatment can be adjusted. Neck and facial hair will be the most common area for permanent hair removal.

Visual assessment

The visual assessment of the area to be treated should be undertaken with consideration for the client's privacy and modesty at all times. A discrete observation maybe confirmed with a closed question, which will help the therapist to develop an effective treatment plan. The information gleaned will help determine the client's skin type, hair type and follicle size. This will assist the therapist in choosing which method of electrical epilation to use and which probe to select.

Skin type

The epidermis can vary in moisture content but the dermis is usually quite moist. The amount of moisture in the skin varies from person to person but there is always a moisture gradient, i.e. it will be moister in the deeper layers and drier on the surface. As the skin is moister around the base of the hair follicle than it is near the follicle opening, the current will be conducted better at the place where it is required. The current is available the full length of the needle but the dryness of the skin's surface helps to prevent the conduction of current that may result in blistering and discomfort due to the irritation of the sensory nerves. The effect is most intense in the moist areas near the base of the follicle and decreases as it reaches the drier surface.

The insulating properties of sebum are of benefit to the epidermis during electrical epilation. As the electrical current reaches the skin's surface, the sebum will act as an insulator, protecting the epidermis from the effects of the current. This insulation effect is only beneficial if the correct probing technique has been used.

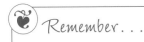 Remember...

The moisture gradient will only help to protect the skin if the correct probing technique is used, i.e. one that is not too shallow.

Because each of the main skin types differs in terms of its moisture content and sebum production, each will require a slightly different method of application to ensure safety and achievement of the desired result.

- Dry skin: this has a shortage of insulating sebum and may also be dehydrated. The intensity of the current must be at a suitable level to avoid burns at the epidermis. At times the dry skin of the stratum corneum make probing difficult. Dry skin may also lack sufficient moisture, making the chemical reaction that takes place under the galvanic current ineffective.

- Oily skin: extra sebum will only support the insulation effect of the current used and there is normally a higher moisture gradient in the skin, which will make the treatment more successful. Enlarged pores that are commonly found in oily skin will also make the treatment easier to perform.

Because any skin type can also have one or more of the skin conditions described below, they should also be taken into account when choosing the method of treatment.

- Sensitive skin: this has a high colour and is very fine and delicate. Galvanic or the blend technique is more favourable here as the heat produced from short-wave diathermy can cause a skin reaction.

- Mature skin: this can be oily, dry, sensitive and dehydrated. It is important to identify the skin type to treat accordingly. It is imperative to thoroughly stretch the loose skin during insertion and probing as the skin has a loss of collagen and elastin.

- Dehydrated skin: this can also be seen on different skin types and may present with other skin conditions. Dehydrated skin will have a low moisture gradient which may extend to the deeper layers of the skin. Care must be taken to set the intensity correctly to avoid causing burns to the skin.

Ethnic groups

- Caucasian skin: clients can suffer with facial hair; choose the method most suitable to the individual, based on skin type and sensitivity. Contra-actions can be more obvious due to the contrast on fair skin and heightened sensitivity.

- Olive skin: facial hair is darker, coarser and more obvious; skin tends to be less sensitive.

- Asian skin: facial hair is dark and long, yet fine. Follicles are generally shallower and hair reacts well to treatment. Can be prone to hyper-pigmentation as a contra-action to treatment.

- Black skin: hair is coarse, dark and curly, due to curved follicles. Skin is typically oily and can scar easily. Galvanic or blend method work well on these hairs. Can be prone to hyper-pigmentation as a contra-action to treatment.

Hints and tips

Electrical epilation should not be performed on damp skin as this can conduct the current to the surface of the skin and cause burning and scarring. Make sure you have thoroughly removed any pre-treatment products and if your client is sweating continue to blot the skin dry.

Health and safety

Non-pigmented hair or red hair should be treated with care. This type of hair can be difficult to see due to its light appearance and in many cases is coarser in texture. The latter means that you may require high intensities of current to successfully remove them and there is an increased risk of skin damage.

Health and safety

If micro-lancing an ingrown hair you must wear disposable gloves.

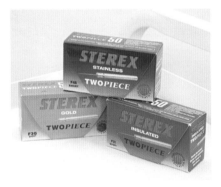

△ Box of probes and red dot of sterilisation

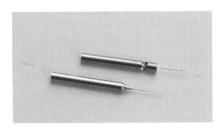

△ One-piece and two-piece epilation probes

Hair type

Hair is found all over the body, with the exception of the lips, eyelids, palms of the hands and soles of the feet. Various parts of the body have different types of hair growth which is divided into two main types:

1 Vellus hair: can originate from the sebaceous gland, not a follicle, and is nourished by connective tissue. Rarely exceeds 2 mm in length.

2 Terminal hair: these are deep-seated, strong hairs with a well-developed bulb and dermal papilla. They grow from deep follicles which can extend to the subcutaneous layer.

Types of follicle

Hair can be fine, coarse or curly and protrude from a number of different types of follicle.

- Compound: this is where two or more hairs grow out of the same follicle. Treat these separately as they have their own separate papillae.

- Curved follicles: these will produce a curly hair which may be fine or coarse. Treat with the galvanic or blend method.

- Ingrowing hair: this is when the hair has been unable to grow through the epidermis and instead cultivates underneath the skin. The area can become infected, red and sore. If possible the hair should be released by using a micro-lance to gently pierce the skin but the hair should not be removed until the skin has healed sufficiently.

Epilation needles

There are a number of needle types available for epilation work. Disposable epilation needles are sealed in an airtight packet then sterilised by gamma radiation. The probe then remains sterile until the packet is opened. There is a large red dot on each packet of probes to show that they have been through their sterilisation process. Epilation needles fall into two main categories:

- Two-piece probes: these are constructed of two pieces – a fine piece set into a thicker base. A two-piece probe is more flexible and it is easier to see the resistance in the follicle. Resistance occurs if the insertion is too long or at the wrong angle. The needle will bend slightly if the probing is incorrect and therefore the insertion can be altered.

- One-piece probe: these are constructed from just one piece – a fine piece graduating to a thicker base. They offer very little in terms of flexibility but may be used when your technique is very good and a sturdier probe is required.

Probes are generally made of stainless steel but they are also available in gold and insulated steel. If a client has very sensitive skin a gold or insulated probe should be used. Gold probes are plated with nickel-free, 24-carat gold and are recommended for clients who suffer from allergies and sensitive skin and whose skin reacts negatively to standard stainless steel probes. Redness and swelling are reduced after use.

If a client is diabetic then an insulated probe should be used. It is important to note that when using an insulated probe only the short-wave diathermy technique can be used. The insulated probe is coated with medical grade insulation. This special coating allows smooth insertions and stands up to the longest treatments. The insulated probe focuses the current at the base of the probe's shaft only and does not allow heat to be conducted up the length of the probe. Security from over-treatment is excellent and the sensitive surface layers of the skin are protected, enabling discomfort to be reduced and therefore minimising irritation.

The type and texture of the hair to be treated should be examined closely. Epilation needles come in varying diameters with the diameter of the probe chosen corresponding to the diameter of the hair that is to be treated. This will ensure that the probe tip is able to distribute sufficient current to the base of the follicle. A probe that is too large in diameter will stretch the follicle opening, which may result in bruising. There is also a risk of surface burns due to the probe being in contact with the skin at the follicle opening, which can also cause scarring. Table 10.3 shows the diameters for epilation needles.

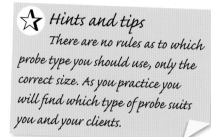

Hints and tips

There are no rules as to which probe type you should use, only the correct size. As you practice you will find which type of probe suits you and your clients.

▽ Table 10.3 Diameters for epilation needles

Diameter	Use
002	Used for very fine facial hair, e.g. upper lip
003	Used for fine hair, e.g. upper lip and face
004	Used for thicker facial hair and body hair
005	Used for body and leg hair
006	Used for very coarse hair

Finer probes should be used with a lower current intensity to achieve the same result as a higher current with a thicker probe.

 Health and safety

All probes are used only once and then disposed of in the sharps box. They are never re-sterilised. Disposable probes offer reassurance to clients that there is no risk of cross-infection.

Referral to client records

Refer to the client's record card for:

- an indication of their health and the presence of contraindications
- previous electrical epilation methods used, together with intensity and timings
- previous needles used, including size
- possible contra-actions to previous treatments and/or products
- possible photographs of the treatment area pre- and post-treatment to evaluate treatment effectiveness.

Contra-actions

It is important to explain the treatment and the possible contra-actions at the time of the consultation in order to gain the client's trust and to ensure their satisfaction with the treatment. The client can then ask questions to clarify and can make an informed decision as to whether to continue with the treatment. Adaptations to the treatment can also be put in place if necessary. The possible contra-actions to electrical epilation are:

- erythema: may be a normal contra-action or due to intensity or excessive service time

- irritation: due to the probe used or intensity or excessive service time

- bruising: over-insertion of the needle during treatment

- oedema: swelling of the tissues where treatment occurred

- blanching: high intensity of current and dry skin

- bleeding: incorrect probing or over-insertion

- pitting: over-treatment and too high intensity

- scarring: over-treatment and too high intensity

- weeping follicles: too high galvanic or blend current

- hyper- or hypo-pigmentation: intensity too high on all methods.

Contra-actions are symptoms your clients may experience and most should be considered as completely normal; not all clients will experience all the symptoms. Any contra-action should fade within 12 hours. If it does not dissipate, the salon and/or therapist should be contacted for advice. In the case of a severe reaction to electrical epilation treatment the client may need to seek medical advice.

  # Carry out electrical epilation treatment

All electrical epilation units are only as good as the therapist using them. There must be good insertions with the correct choice of current, intensities and timing.

Selection of current

The most important factors in selecting the current and intensity for a client are:

- the type of skin

- diameter of the hair

- nature of the hair (fine, coarse, curly)

- area to be treated

- their pain threshold

- size and choice of probe.

Timings

Timings refer to how long the intensity of current should run for in order to successfully epilate the hair. This will depend on the current you are using, the coarseness of the hair, the skin and hair type and the client's pain threshold. The aim is to remove the hair with no skin damage and the current intensity should be used at the minimum amount to successfully achieve this.

Probing techniques

The success of any type of epilation treatment relies on the accurate placement of the needle that is used to deliver the current. The insertion of the needle should cause the client no discomfort and should slide into the follicle to the base where the current is discharged. There should be no movement when the probe is in the correct position.

The depth of the hair follicle and therefore the needle insertion is the distance from the skin surface to the base of the follicle. This will depend on the hair type, stage of growth, area of growth, resistance felt in the base of the follicle and the appearance of the epilated hairs on removal.

With time an experienced therapist will be able to 'feel' the base of the follicle as the probe is inserted to the correct depth, but for students learning this treatment, care should be taken. Insert the probe slowly and gently and look out for a slight indentation of the skin surface around the follicle as the probe reaches the base of the follicle.

Steps for a good technique

- Use a three-way stretch to open the neck of the follicle to allow the needle to slide into it.
- Follow the direction of the hair into the follicle.
- Follow the angle of the hair with the skin into the follicle.
- Insert the needle on the underside of the hair.
- Allow the needle to slide until resistance is felt and then stop.

Incorrect probing

Incorrect probing includes inserting too deep, too shallow, at the wrong angle so the wall of the follicle is pierced, or movement of the probe while in position (either up and down or from side to side).

 Remember . . .

You do not need to use a higher intensity current than is required to release the hair.

⭐ *Hints and tips*

Another way of gauging the depth of the follicle is to tweeze a hair thought to be in anagen and hold it next to the skin surface. Compare it alongside the needle as this will give you the depth of similar hairs within an area being worked.

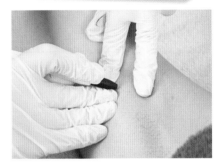
△ A three-way stretch

 Remember . . .

Hair grows at different angles depending on the body area. The probe should enter the follicle at the same angle as the hair to prevent piercing the follicle wall.

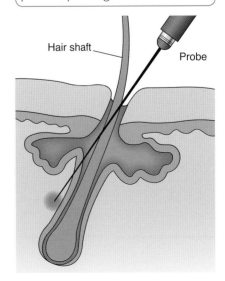

Hair shaft

Probe

△ Incorrect insertion in the follicle

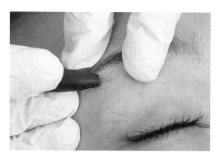

△ Insertion in eyebrow

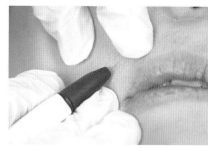

△ Insertion in top lip

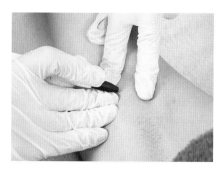

△ Insertion in underarm

Current sensations

It is important that as a therapist you have experienced all three methods of electrical epilation so you can describe the sensations that your client can expect to feel, as they may feel apprehensive about the treatment.

- Short-wave diathermy: this produces heat so the client may feel a warm, stinging sensation; this will pass very quickly

- Galvanic: this is a slower method with a chemical reaction so little should be felt by the client. They may feel some warmth as the current builds over the slow time process.

- Blend: this produces less heat than short-wave diathermy and is faster than galvanic treatment. Blend is therefore said to be the least uncomfortable method. Very little should be felt by the client.

Epilation procedure for short wave diathermy

1   Prepare working area and complete consultation checking for contraindications.

2   Prepare the client and ask them to remove outdoor clothes (as appropriate) and to remove glasses/contact lenses and jewellery once in the treatment area. Ensure that the client is comfortable in a semi-reclining position and protect with a robe or towel. If the body is to be worked on only expose the immediate area to be worked on. Consider client modesty at all times.

3   Wash hands and put on disposable gloves. Cleanse the client's skin to remove any make-up if working on the face. Prepare the area with a pre-epilation skin cleanser and blot dry.

4   Select needle and insert into the holder using tweezers.

5   Keep a pad of damp cotton wool close to the treatment area to collected epilated hairs.

6   Provide eye-pads if the client is sensitive to light and you are treating the facial area.

7   Switch on the magnifying lamp and examine the area (you may wish to do this in order to select a probe).

8 Turn the epilation unit on and set the machine accordingly. Start with a low intensity and build until you reach a suitable working point.

9 Ask the client to relax and remind them of the sensation they are going to feel.

10 Place tweezers in your left hand (if right handed) between forefinger and thumb, facing away from the client and support the skin firmly between the fingers using a three-finger stretch.

11 Hold the needle holder in your right hand (if right handed) like a pencil.

12 Insert probe into the follicle until you feel the resistance of the base of the follicle.

13 Release the current (either through a switch or a pedal) and then withdraw the probe making sure that you are not pressing the current.

14 Test the hair with the tweezers to see if it will release. Hold the hair close to the skin if hair does not remove easily and repeat probing. If it still does not remove return to it later – never pluck the hair out. The hair may be probed twice depending on the client's skin type.

15 Once the hair has been removed from the follicle it must be placed onto a piece of cotton wool. Continue to work through the area.

16 Conclude treatment by applying soothing antiseptic lotion on clean cotton wool. Turn the epilation unit down and off. Dispose of the probe directly into the sharps container.

17 Dispose of all epilated hairs in the contaminated waste bin.

18 Provide the client with the correct aftercare advice, update client records and book next appointment.

 Remember . . .

When performing short-wave diathermy treatment do not work on hairs too close together as heat can build up in the follicles and cause burning; instead spread your probing out.

With short-wave diathermy the client's pain threshold must be considered. If the intensity of current causes too much discomfort it may be reduced and the current allowed to run for a little longer to create the same result.

A popular method of treatment with short-wave diathermy is the 'flash' technique. This is where the current is allowed to run for a fraction of a second. This allows a high intensity of current to be used that is not long enough to stimulate the nerve endings and therefore useful for a client with a low pain threshold. This method is not without problems though, as it produces a heating pattern that is very narrow and may not cause enough destruction of the follicle to successfully remove the hair.

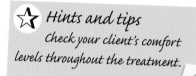 *Hints and tips*
Check your client's comfort levels throughout the treatment.

Epilation procedure for galvanic

1 Repeat steps 1–8 of the short-wave diathermy procedure.

2 Ensure any diathermy outlet is turned off. Set the timer to 10 seconds and put the galvanic intensity on 0.10 milliamps.

3 Repeat steps 9–18 of the short-wave diathermy procedure.

> ★ **Hints and tips**
>
> If your epilation unit allows, use a foot pedal when working with galvanic or blend to count the time. This is more accurate than counting for yourself with a switch on the needle holder.

Note: If there is tension when trying to remove the hair, increase the intensity if your client is comfortable, or lower the intensity and increase the time if they are uncomfortable.

Epilation procedure for blend

There are many treatment techniques available within blend. This is one of the reasons for its popularity as there is always a system to suit every client, although it takes a little time to get used to the choices. Although you will study the main techniques of blend, for techniques specific to your epilation unit you should consult the manufacturer's instructions.

The traditional technique is where the diathermy is kept to a minimum, the timer is set to 5 seconds and the direct current increased 5–10 digits after each follicle is treated until the hairs are removed from the follicle without traction.

Technique 1: Higher for shorter method

1 Repeat steps 1–8 of short-wave diathermy procedure.

2 Turn the direct current dial and the diathermy dial to minimum.

3 Turn the timer to 5 seconds.

4 Insert the probe and activate the current either by foot pedal or finger switch.

5 Wait for the timer to count down and then release the foot pedal or finger switch and withdraw the probe.

6 Try the hair to see if it will release without tension.

7 If the hair does not release increase the direct current by 5–10 digits.

8 Treat another follicle in the same way and then try the hair.

9 Repeat this procedure until the hairs epilate without traction.

Technique 2: Lower for longer method

1 Reduce the direct current intensity to the level your client finds acceptable.

2 Increase the time duration of follicle until the hairs epilate without traction.

The benefit of this technique is that it gives your client a more comfortable treatment, but because it is slower you will not normally be able to take out as many hairs in the normal treatment session. You will notice erythema and, on some areas, small white circles around the treated follicle. This is quite normal and a typical galvanic current reaction.

Technique 3: Treat and leave method

The benefit of the 'treat and leave' method is that it is a quicker way of working because you are not stopping after treating each follicle to remove the hair; instead you remove all hairs at the end.

This technique allows you to work at either a slightly lower intensity or in a slightly shorter time because the hairs get extra treatment by the lye while they wait for you to remove them. The traditional technique could be combined with 'treat and leave'. You could also combine Technique 2 with the 'treat and leave' method to hasten the slower treatment. Treat two groups of at least 10 hairs with the 'treat and leave' technique and ask your client for feedback. Even when using galvanic alone, you can work 'higher for shorter', 'lower for longer' or even 'treat and leave'.

Always start low and increase galvanic by 5–10 digits at a time until the hairs come out with ease. Remember if a client is uncomfortable turn the intensity down and increase the time.

On completion of your electrical epilation you should apply a soothing antiseptic lotion to the area. If you have been working on the face you can apply a tinted antiseptic lotion to give the client some coverage of any erythema.

Post-treatment cataphoresis

If your electrical epilation treatment consists of using either the galvanic or blend method then post-treatment cataphoresis is a successful technique in reducing skin irritation and redness. Cataphoresis uses a galvanic current on a positive polarity to return the skin to an acidic balance after the galvanic current has produced 'lye' in the follicles, which is alkaline.

Under a positive polarity a galvanic current will soothe the nerve endings and reduce erythema, as the blood vessels will constrict.

This method works in the same way as facial galvanic iontophoresis and facial machinery can be used if your epilation unit does not accommodate this technique.

Aftercare advice for electrical epilation treatment

There are a large number of common contra-actions following epilation. It is important that you conduct your treatment correctly and professionally to minimise these reactions.

After electrical epilation the skin will commonly appear red, with raised bumps, depending on the individual's skin sensitivity. The raised bump is due to the presence of lymph produced locally by the skin for protection. Providing after-care rules are observed no infection should result and the condition will subside in a couple of hours. Occasionally the skin will form scabs following treatment and the client must be advised not to pick them as scarring may occur.

Scabs may be an indication of incorrect treatment but this is not always so. Deep follicles such as those of the bikini line or sometimes when the flash technique is used can produce scabbing in its own right. Providing that the scabs are left alone and not picked they should heal safely with no scarring.

Remember...

All clients are different! You will notice that clients' hairs come out at different positions on the dial and with different meter readings. This is quite usual when working with galvanic current. Make sure you record their working intensity on each client's record card.

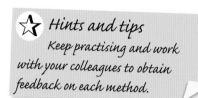

Hints and tips

Keep practising and work with your colleagues to obtain feedback on each method.

Health and safety

Post-treatment cataphoresis can often be performed using the aftercare lotion as the current conductor. However, you must check the manufacturer's instructions for the product to ensure it is suitable for use in this way.

Key term

Cataphoresis – a successful technique in reducing skin irritation and redness after galvanic or blend electrical epilation by using galvanic at a positive polarity.

Permanent scarring

Scarring may occur for the following reasons:

- Too high an intensity of current was used.

- Too much treatment in one area: approximately 3 mm must be left between each hair treated to prevent the heating patterns from joining up.

- No healing gaps left between treatments. Approximately 7–14 days must be left between treatments in an area for the skin to heal in the deeper layers. It is possible to work in a chess-board style on large areas if more frequent treatments are required, as long as a sufficient heat gap is left for each area.

- Releasing current while entering or withdrawing from the follicle – the skin can burn if this occurs.

- Incorrect probing: probing too deep – when going past the hair bulb, deep tissues can be burned; probing too shallow – this is likely to burn the hair shaft and result in the surrounding tissues being burned; wrong angle – this causes a release of current and the formation of heat in the wrong area.

- Picking off scabs.

- Poor or incorrect aftercare.

Aftercare advice

Aftercare advice should be given following every electrical epilation treatment. Ideally, aftercare advice should be written in the form of a leaflet and handed to the client with explanations after the treatment has been performed. The client should be advised:

- to not touch the area and not pick scabs if any occur

- to avoid tweezing out the hair between treatments as this encourages the blood supply and will not only make the problem worse but will work against the treatment

- to not wax the hairs between treatments as the skin may be sensitive and react to waxing; as with tweezing it may encourage hair growth and work against the treatment

- to avoid bleaching the hair between treatments due to skin sensitisation; if it is absolutely essential for them to bleach the hair then they should avoid epilation treatments both before and after for as long as possible; always inform the client of the risks of bleaching

- to avoid heat and UV light, particularly sun beds, for 24 hours before and after treatment

- to avoid tight clothing if epilation was performed on the body

- not to wear make-up for 24 hours after treatment, if treatment was on the facial area

- not to apply deodorants or perfumed products in the area treated for 24 hours after treatment.

The client should be encouraged to:

- trim hairs with fine-pointed scissors if they are conscious of them between treatments. Shaving can coarsen the skin and cause skin sensitivity and should be discouraged at all times

- moisturise their skin well in between treatments to keep the moisture gradient high in the skin to promote an effective treatment.

Future treatment needs

The client should be advised:

- to return for further electrical epilation treatment after 7–14 days as necessary

- of the correct method of hair growth management between treatments.

Methods of evaluation

To be an effective therapist it is useful to reflect on the electrical epilation treatment to ensure client satisfaction, promote good client relationships and encourage the client's return of custom.

The therapist should consider the short- and long-term effects of the treatment to evaluate the effectiveness of their choice of current and probe and whether it has been beneficial to the client and the condition they presented for treatment.

Methods of evaluating an epilation treatment include visual and verbal assessment and written feedback.

Visual assessment

Visual assessment of the area should be performed after the treatment to ascertain the immediate effects. The therapist should note a difference in hair reduction to the area and any contra-actions that may be apparent. Making accurate notes on the client's record card can enable a comparison to be made at the beginning of the next treatment. You can also use photographs to track the effectiveness of the treatment.

Verbal assessment

Asking the client how they feel immediately after treatment can give an insight into their view of the treatment. Periodically remind the client of the benefits of the treatment because it can be an uncomfortable treatment to have performed.

On the client's return visit ask a few probing questions of how they felt several hours after the treatment and what the area looked like. This can reveal useful information and help shape the follow-up treatment.

Written feedback

The client can be asked to provide written feedback about their treatment. In order to obtain useful information it is a good idea to ask some simple questions with a choice of possible answers, otherwise the information obtained may be quite bland and for not useful the next treatment.

 Want to know more?

Sterex are world leaders and experts in hair removal. They distribute a wide variety of epilation equipment to the beauty and medical industry in over 30 countries worldwide. They have a training academy in Birmingham where they offer training courses, including the advanced electrolysis course. You can access their website at www.sterex.com.

NVQ assessment checklist

To complete this unit you must have the following theoretical and practical skills. Check against the list below and refer back to the relevant section for information on anything you are unsure about.

1. **Be able to maintain safe and effective methods of working when providing electrical epilation treatments**

❑ **1.1** Prepare and monitor the treatment area, according to organisational procedures and manufacturers' instructions

❑ **1.2** Maintain personal standards of hygiene, protection and appearance, according to industry and organisational requirements

❑ **1.3** Use personal protective equipment to avoid cross-infection and exposure to hazardous waste

❑ **1.4** Position the client and themselves to minimise fatigue and risk of injury to meet the needs of the service

❑ **1.5** Disinfect or sterilise all reusable tools and equipment using the suitable methods

❑ **1.6** Position equipment and products for safety and ease of use

❑ **1.7** Position the client comfortably to respect modesty, privacy and sensitivities to personal appearance

❑ **1.8** Check the client's wellbeing at regular intervals, according to organisational policy

❑ **1.9** Dispose of single use items, hazardous waste and waste materials safely

❑ **1.10** Complete the treatment within a commercially viable time

❑ **1.11** Leave the treatment area in a suitable condition for further treatments

❑ **1.12** Keep records up to date, accurate, easy to read and signed

2. **Be able to consult, plan and prepare**

❑ **2.1** Use client questioning to identify contraindications to treatment, recording the for electrical epilation treatments with clients client's responses

❑ **2.2** Provide advice to the client without causing concern or referring to specific medical conditions

❑ **2.3** Refer clients with contraindications

❑ **2.4** Obtain signed, written, informed consent prior to carrying out the treatment from the client or parent/guardian if the client is a minor

❑ **2.5** Check that a parent or guardian is present throughout the treatment for minors

❑ **2.6** Use consultation techniques to identify the client's treatment needs

❑ **2.7** Encourage clients to ask questions to clarify any points

❑ **2.8** Record the client's past and present hair management techniques and the implication for treatments

❑ **2.9** Take photographs of the area(s) to be treated, with the consent of the client

❑ **2.10** Use visual aids to inform the client about the treatment process and the physical sensation it creates

❑ **2.11** Prepare the area to be treated and carry out a patch test to establish suitability for treatment

❑ **2.12** Provide written aftercare procedures to the client following the patch test

❑ **2.13** Recommend alternative treatments or products which are suitable for the client, if contraindicated for electrical epilation treatment

❑ **2.14** Confirm the projected cost, likely duration, frequency, types of treatment and client commitment

❑ **2.15** Document the area(s) to be treated, client expectations and treatment objectives

❑ **2.16** Select and prepare equipment to meet legal and safety requirements and treatment objectives

3. **Be able to carry out electrical epilation treatments**

❑ **3.1** Clean and dry the area to be treated prior to treatment

❑ **3.2** Load and use the size and type of needle which is suitable to meet the client's hair and skin needs, avoiding contamination

❑ **3.3** Illuminate and magnify the treatment area to create maximum visibility during treatment

❑ **3.4** Stretch and manipulate the skin to meet the needs of the area being treated

❏ **3.5** Use the needle holder at the proper angle, direction and needle depth for the hair follicle and the area to be treated

❏ **3.6** Adapt the intensity and duration of current flow to ensure hair release, taking account of client tolerance, sensitivity and safety

❏ **3.7** Remove the hair from the treated follicle without traction

❏ **3.8** Use systematic techniques to remove hair within the area(s) to be treated

❏ **3.9** Stop treatment when contra-actions occur, in accordance with manufacturer's instructions and recommend suitable alternative treatment, if required

❏ **3.10** Sooth the treated area using suitable techniques and products

❏ **3.11** Take treatment progress photographs of the area(s) treated, with consent of the client when required

❏ **3.12** Confirm the clients satisfaction of the finished result

❏ **3.13** Provide suitable aftercare advice to the client

4. **Understand the organisational and legal requirements of providing electrical epilation**

❏ **4.1** Explain personal and salon responsibilities under relevant health and safety legislation, local authority licensing regulations, standards and guidance

❏ **4.2** Justify the importance of the Disability Discrimination Act in relation to the salon

❏ **4.3** Clarify the age at which an individual is classed as a minor and how this differs nationally

❏ **4.4** Justify the importance of checking current insurance guidelines and age-related restrictions for electrical epilation treatment

❏ **4.5** Explain why minors should only be treated with the informed consent and presence of a parent or guardian

❏ **4.6** Explain the legal significance of gaining signed, informed consent to treatment

❏ **4.7** Explain local authority and organisational requirements for waste disposal

❏ **4.8** Explain the importance of storing client records in accordance with the Data Protection Act

❏ **4.9** Explain how to maintain the client records in the salon and its importance

❏ **4.10** Explain own responsibilities and reasons for maintaining personal hygiene, protection and appearance, according to accepted industry and organisational requirements

❏ **4.11** Explain the organisation's requirements for client preparation

❏ **4.12** Clarify the organisation's service times for electrical epilation treatments

❏ **4.13** Explain the organisation's requirements for client preparation, treatment area, equipment maintenance and equipment cleaning regimes

5. **Understand how to work safely and effectively when providing electrical epilation treatments**

❏ **5.1** Explain how to safely prepare the work area for electrical epilation treatments

❏ **5.2** Explain the environmental conditions for make-up application and their importance

❏ **5.3** Explain the types of personal protective equipment that should be worn for electrical epilation treatments and why

❏ **5.4** Explain the condition contact dermatitis and how to avoid developing it whilst carrying out electrical epilation treatments

❏ **5.5** Clarify the causes and condition of repetitive strain injury (RSI) and how to avoid developing it when delivering electrical epilation treatments

❏ **5.6** Explain the causes and hazards of accidental exposure to clinical waste

❏ **5.7** Explain how to disinfect hands and its importance

❏ **5.8** Explain how to prepare and position themselves and the client for electrical epilation, avoiding potential discomfort and injury

❏ **5.9** Explain the principles of avoiding cross-infection and the importance of maintaining standards of general hygiene

❏ **5.10** Explain the reasons for maintaining client modesty, privacy and comfort during the treatment

❏ **5.11** Explain why it is important to monitor the client's wellbeing at regular intervals

6. **Understand the use of client consultation for electrical epilation treatments**

❏ **6.1** Explain how to use consultation techniques to meet the needs of different client groups

❏ **6.2** Explain how to give advice and make recommendations to clients

❏ **6.3** Justify the importance of effective communication and discussion

❏ **6.4** Justify the importance of providing time and encouragement for client's to ask questions

❏ **6.5** Justify the importance and legal significance of questioning clients and recording responses about contraindications to electrical epilation

❏ **6.6** Justify the importance of explaining the commitment required to maintain optimum results

❏ **6.7** Explain why it is advisable to take photographs of the treatment area(s) pre and post treatment and how they should be taken to maintain client confidentially

❏ **6.8** Explain how to recognise skin types, conditions and their response to treatment

❏ **6.9** Explain how to carry out a patch test to identify skin allergies, reactions and issues

❏ **6.10** Justify the importance of providing clients with written aftercare instructions immediately after the test patch and reinforcing this on subsequent visits

❑ **6.11** Explain why it is important to maintain client confidentiality

❑ **6.12** Explain the types of alternative treatments to recommend if contraindications to electrical epilation treatments are identified

❑ **6.13** ustify the importance of providing information to assist the client's understanding of the treatment

❑ **6.14** Clarify the constraints surrounding electrical epilation treatments

❑ **6.15** Clarify the physical sensation of the treatment and how pain threshold and sensitivity varies

❑ **6.16** Explain how sensitivity is affected by other skincare treatments which may inhibit electrical epilation

❑ **6.17** Justify the importance of consulting previous record cards

7. Understand anatomy and physiology relevant to electrical epilation

❑ **7.1** Explain the structure and functions of the skin

❑ **7.2** Compare the skin characteristics and skin types of different ethnic client groups

❑ **7.3** Explain the principles of skin healing

❑ **7.4** Explain the structure of the hair and hair follicle

❑ **7.5** Explain the growth pattern of the hair and how this influences present and future treatments

❑ **7.6** Explain the hair growth cycle, hair types and causes of hair growth

❑ **7.7** Explain the structure and function of the endocrine system

❑ **7.8** Explain the effects of malfunctions of the endocrine system on hair growth

❑ **7.9** Explain the principles of the blood and lymphatic system

❑ **7.10** Explain the principles of lymph circulation and the interaction of lymph and blood within the circulatory system

❑ **7.11** Explain how the hormones are circulated via the blood stream

8. Understand the contraindications and contra-actions of electrical epilation

❑ **8.1** Clarify the contraindications that prevent treatment and why

❑ **8.2** Clarify the conditions that require medical approval and why

❑ **8.3** Clarify the conditions that restrict treatment and why

❑ **8.4** Explain the potential consequences of carrying out electrical epilation on a contra-indicated client

❑ **8.5** Explain potential contra-actions which may occur during the treatment and how to resolve them

❑ **8.6** Explain the reasons for not naming specific contraindications and the importance of encouraging clients to seek medical advice

9. Understand the use of equipment and materials in electrical epilation

❑ **9.1** Explain the types and uses of equipment, materials and products for electrical epilation

❑ **9.2** Explain how to prepare and use equipment and materials for electrical epilation treatments, and the importance of following manufacturer's instructions

❑ **9.3** Explain how to recognise equipment, products and materials which are unsuitable for use

❑ **9.4** Explain methods of disinfecting, sterilising and maintaining equipment

❑ **9.5** Classify the available types and sizes of needles for electrical epilation

10. Understand how electrical epilation treatments are used

❑ **10.1** Describe the importance of magnifying and lighting the treatment area

❑ **10.2** Describe the importance of reassuring the client during the treatment

❑ **10.3** Describe how to work systematically and methodically with dense and scattered hair growth

❑ **10.4** Describe the principles, uses and benefits of galvanic and alternating currents

❑ **10.5** Describe the principles, uses and benefits of blending the galvanic and alternating current

❑ **10.6** Describe how to select the type and size of needle to suit the hair type, skin type and area(s) to be treated

❑ **10.7** Describe why and how you stretch and manipulate the skin

❑ **10.8** Describe needle angle and depth of insertion into the hair follicle and the consequences of inaccuracy

❑ **10.9** Describe the causes of skin sensitivity

❑ **10.10** Describe how to adapt electrical epilation methods to suit different skin condition, hair type and treatment area(s)

❑ **10.11** Describe how to adapt electrical epilation methods to client's emotional state and physical condition

❑ **10.12** Describe how to remove hairs from different types of follicle

❑ **10.13** Describe the importance of recognising and treating unusual hair growth

❑ **10.14** Describe the benefits and effects of post-treatment cataphoresis

❑ **10.15** Describe the signs, causes and treatment limitations of erythema and oedema

❑ **10.16** Describe the importance of knowing how to treat the follicles of red and non-pigmented hair

❑ **10.17** Describe why moisture affects the electrical epilation treatment

❑ **10.18** Describe the importance of providing aftercare advice to clients relating to product use, hygiene and hair management in-between treatments

11. Understand how to provide aftercare advice following electrical epilation

❏ **11.1** Explain the normal reactions which occur after treatment and how to resolve abnormal reactions

❏ **11.2** Explain the lifestyle factors and changes that may be required to improve the effectiveness of the treatment

❏ **11.3** Explain post-treatment restrictions and future treatment needs

❏ **11.4** Explain the reasons for avoiding different post-electrical epilation activities

❏ **11.5** Clarify beneficial and unsuitable products for the client's home use

❏ **11.6** Explain suitable methods of dealing with regrowth between treatments

Test yourself

1. The best stage of hair growth to epilate is:

a) anagen

b) catagen

c) telogen

d) faradic

2. Scarring can be caused by:

a) suitable intensity

b) incorrect probing

c) regular treatments

d) stretching the skin

3. The moisture gradient is important to the therapist because:

a) the client wants supple skin

b) the hairs are easier to remove if the skin is drier

c) the conduction will determine the current level

d) the moisture insulates the skin

4. The probe angle when treating a client depends on:

a) the client's pain threshold

b) the area of the body you are treating

c) the type of skin the client has

d) the type of probe being used

5. When performing blend epilation the client holds an indifferent electrode because:

a) it completes the circuit for the treatment to work

b) it helps to prevent further discomfort during the treatment

c) the client would suffer an electrical shock

d) it has no effect on the treatment

6. Lye is:

a) sodium hydrogen

b) sodium chloride

c) sodium hydroxide

d) sodium oxide

7. Electrical epilation should be performed on
   a) vellus hair
   b) terminal hair
   c) moles
   d) lanugo hair

8. Cross-infection can be avoided by:
   a) using a new probe for every client
   b) wearing a new pair of gloves each day
   c) using tweezers that are sterilised every week
   d) using a new probe every day

9. In between epilation treatments unwanted regrowth should:
   a) be shaved so it is short enough to epilate
   b) be trimmed with scissors
   c) tweezed to stimulate the blood supply
   d) be waxed to encourage hair growth

10. If hairs are difficult to remove you should:
    a) probe the follicle as many times as necessary
    b) tweeze the hairs to clear the area
    c) probe twice only
    d) turn up the intensity

11. To soothe the skin after treatment:
    a) tinted aftercare lotion should be applied
    b) cold cotton wool should be applied
    c) the area should be massaged
    d) heat should be applied to the area

12. How do you judge how long to perform the epilation treatment?
    a) how much time the client has
    b) skin reaction
    c) type of hairs you are treating
    d) how much the client can afford

13. The hair has been correctly treated if:
    a) it slides out of the follicle
    b) there is a slight pull but it comes out with a bulb
    c) the client can feel the hair coming out
    d) the client cannot feel the current

Chapter **11**
BODY MASSAGE TREATMENTS

This chapter covers the following units:

NVQ unit B20 Provide body massage treatments

City & Guilds VRQ unit 305 Provide body massage

VTCT VRQ unit UV30424 Provide body massage

LEARNING OBJECTIVES

This chapter is about providing manual and mechanical body massage treatments.

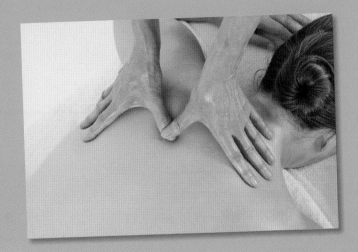

The learning outcomes for NVQ unit B20 are:

1 Be able to maintain safe and effective methods of working when providing body massage treatments

2 Be able to consult, plan and prepare to provide body massage treatments

3 Be able to perform manual massage treatments

4 Be able to perform mechanical massage treatments

5 Understand organisational and legal requirements for protecting body massage treatments

6 Understand how to work safely and effectively when providing body massage treatments

7 Understand how to consult with clients

8 Understand how to prepare to provide body massage treatments

9 Understand anatomy and physiology related to body massage treatments

10 Understand contraindications and contra-actions that affect or restrict body massage treatments

11 Understand how to carry out body massage treatments

12 Understand how to provide aftercare advice

You will need to be competent in all of these outcomes to be competent in body massage treatments, qualify for insurance and perform the treatments on members of the public.

NVQ evidence requirements

For the NVQ your assessor will need to observe you perform these treatments successfully on at least four occasions, each involving a different client. This includes:

- Two full body massage treatments including the face.
- One of the full body massages must include the use of mechanical massage and infra-red.

You must practically:

1 Demonstrate the use of all these types of equipment on suitable treatment areas:
- gyratory massage
- audio sonic
- infra-red

2 Demonstrate the use of all these massage mediums:
- oil
- cream
- powder

3 Demonstrate the use of all these consultation techniques:
- questioning
- visual
- manual
- reference to client records

4 Deal with all these client physical characteristics:
- weight
- height
- posture
- muscle tone
- age
- health
- skin condition

5 Take one of the following necessary actions:
- encourage the client to seek medical advice
- explain why the treatment cannot be carried out
- modify the treatment

6 Meet all these treatment objectives:
- relaxation
- sense of wellbeing
- uplifting
- anti-cellulite
- stimulating

7 Use all these massage techniques:
- effleurage
- petrissage
- tapotement
- vibration
- friction

8 Massage all these treatment areas:
- face
- head
- chest and shoulders
- arms and hands
- abdomen
- back
- gluteals
- legs and feet

9 Provide all these types of advice:
- avoidance of activities which may cause contra-actions
- future treatment needs
- modifications to lifestyle patterns
- healthy eating and exercise advice
- suitable homecare products and their use.

VRQ practical evidence requirements

There are different evidence requirements for the VRQ qualifications dependant on the awarding body.

City & Guilds unit 305 Provide body massage

- A minimum of four body massage treatments should be carried out before a final observation in front of an assessor
- These four massage treatments should meet four of the following objectives
  - relaxation
  - stimulation
  - invigoration
  - sedation
  - assist in weight reduction
- Mechanical massage and infra-red must each be carried out at least once.

One of the four massage treatments must be carried out on a client over the age of 55.

VTCT unit UV30424 Provide body massage

- Four occasions covering the following range:

Massage mediums:
- oil
- cream
- powder

Consultation techniques:
- questioning
- visual
- manual
- reference to client records

Physical characteristics:
- weight
- height
- posture
- muscle tone
- age
- health
- skin condition

One necessary action:
- encourage the client to seek medical advice
- explain why the treatment cannot be carried out
- modify the treatment

Treatment objectives:
- relaxation
- sense of well being
- uplifting
- anti-cellulite
- stimulating

Treatment areas:
- face
- head
- chest and shoulders
- arms and hands
- abdomen
- back
- legs and feet

Massage techniques:
- effleurage
- petrissage
- tapotement
- vibration
- friction

Types of advice:
- avoidance of activities which may cause contra-actions
- future treatment needs
- modifications to lifestyle patterns
- healthy eating and exercise advice
- suitable homecare products and their use

In all cases, simulation is NOT allowed.

VRQ knowledge requirements

City & Guilds unit 305 Provide body massage	VTCT unit UV30424 Provide body massage	Page no.
Learning outcome 1: Be able to prepare for a body massage treatment		
Practical skills/observations		
Prepare themselves, client and work area for body massage		366–8
Use suitable consultation techniques to identify treatment objectives		359
Advise the client on how to prepare for the treatment		367–8
Provide clear recommendations to the client		363
Select products and tools to suit client treatment needs, skin types and conditions		372
Underpinning knowledge		
Describe salon requirements for preparing themselves, the client and work area		366–8
Describe the environmental conditions suitable for body massage treatments		366–7
Describe the different consultation techniques used to identify treatment objectives		359
Describe how to select products and tools to suit client treatment needs, skin types and conditions		372
Describe the different skin types and conditions		217–223
Explain the contraindications that prevent or restrict body massage treatments		360–1
State the objectives of massage treatments		368–71
State the benefits derived from massage treatments		368–71
Identify general body types		224–5
Describe the different types of body fat		233–4
Outline common postural faults		226–31
Learning outcome 2: Be able to provide for a body massage treatment		
Practical skills/observations		
Communicate and behave in a professional manner		183–4
Follow health and safety working practices		355–7
Position themselves and client correctly throughout the treatment		357–8
Use products, tools and techniques to suit clients treatment needs, skin types and conditions		372
Complete the treatment to the satisfaction of the client		391
Record and evaluate the results of the treatment		391–2
Provide suitable aftercare advice		390–1
Underpinning knowledge		
Explain how to communicate and behave in a professional manner		183–4
Describe health and safety working practices		355–7

City & Guilds unit 305 Provide body massage	VTCT unit UV30424 Provide body massage	Page no.
Explain the importance of positioning themselves and the client correctly throughout the treatment		357–8
Explain the importance of using products, tools and techniques to suit clients treatment needs, skin types and conditions		372
Describe the benefits and uses of mechanical massage and pre-heat treatments		384
Describe how treatments can be adapted to suit client treatment needs, skin types and conditions		382–3
State the contra-actions that may occur during and following treatments and how to respond		365
Explain the importance of completing the treatment to the satisfaction of the client		391–2
Explain the importance of completing treatment records		363; 391–2
Describe the methods of evaluating the effectiveness of the treatment		391–2
Describe the aftercare advice that should be provided		390–1
Describe the structure and the main functions of the following body systems in relation to massage: • skin • skeletal • muscular • cardio-vascular • lymphatic • nervous • digestive • urinary • endocrine		369–71
Describe the main diseases and disorders of body systems		71–7; 98–9; 114–5; 121–2; 131; 135–6; 139; 148; 150
Describe the effects of massage on the body		371–2
Describe the uses of the five classical massage movements		374–80
Describe the uses of different massage mediums		372–4
Describe the legislation relating to the provision of massage treatments		357

Introduction

Massage is a term used to describe the manipulations of the soft tissues of the body. These manipulations are traditionally performed with the hands but can also be performed using the forearms, elbows and even the feet.

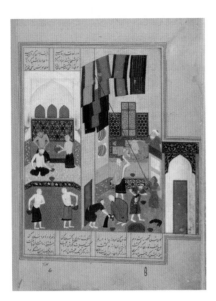

△ Massage in ancient times

History of massage

Massage is an ancient art. Its presence has been recorded throughout history, from the earliest of cave paintings that show people massaging each other. The word 'massage' is thought to be derived either from the Arabic 'mass' or 'Mas'h' meaning to press softly, or from the Greek 'massō' for 'knead'.

The use of massage as a cure for ill health has been recorded in Ancient China as early as 3000 BC where the techniques centred on pressure along certain points of the body for their effect, a practice which was also developed in Japan and India.

The Egyptians and Persians used massage, not only for its therapeutic effects but also cosmetic ones. In 51 BC Cleopatra became the queen of Egypt when her father died. She is reported to have bathed in asses' milk and to have been massaged with highly scented aromatic oils. The art of massage then spread to Europe, possibly with Cleopatra's help, when she made an alliance with Julius Caesar in Rome in 48 BC. Probably the most commonly known use of massage was recorded in Roman times where, combined with steam baths and hot rooms, it became very much a part of everyday life.

Modern massage techniques were developed in the early nineteenth century by a Swede named Henrik Ling. This system of massage is still in use today and is called 'Swedish massage'. Although Ling died in 1839 his system of massage lived on in the Royal Central Institute of Sweden. In 1899 Sir William Bennett inaugurated a massage department at St George's Hospital in London.

In recent times massage has taken on a greater scientific meaning and movements are studied for their effect on the various systems of the body.

LO9 Anatomy and physiology

Massage over an area directly affects the underlying structures of the body. A sound knowledge of the anatomy body systems shown below will improve the safety and effectiveness of massage for the client.

- Structure and function of cells and tissues
- Structure and function of the skin
- Structure and location of the adipose tissue
- Skin characteristics and types of ethnic client groups
- Primary bones and joints of the skeleton
- Types of muscle tissue
- Structure and function of muscles
- Position and action of the muscles of the body
- Structure, function and location of the blood vessels of the body
- Principles of blood circulation, blood pressure and pulse
- Interaction of lymph and blood circulation
- Structure and function of the lymphatic system

- Position and function of the sinuses
- Basic principles of the central nervous system and autonomic nervous system
- Basic principles of the endocrine system
- Basic principles of the respiratory system
- Basic principles of the digestive system
- Basic principles of the excretory system

For the structure and functions and main diseases and disorders of these body systems please refer to Chapter 4 Anatomy and physiology. The effect of massage on the underlying structures of the body is described later in this chapter.

Maintain safe and effective methods when providing body massage treatments LO1 LO5 LO6

Hygiene procedures

Back to basics personal appearance and hygiene checklist

Personal appearance and hygiene checklist:

1. A high standard of personal hygiene.

2. Fresh breath, free from cigarette or food odours.

3. A clean, pressed overall.

4. Clean, low-heeled shoes.

5. Arms and hands free from jewellery (plain wedding bands are acceptable).

6. Any earrings or necklaces are discreet.

7. Make up is discreet and expertly applied.

8. Long hair is tied neatly away from the face and shoulders.

9. Nails are short, smooth, clean and free of nail enamel.

10. Tights, or socks with trousers, are worn.

11. Any cuts are covered with a clean plaster.

12. Hands are washed immediately before and after physical client contact.

Hygiene of the treatment area and client

To avoid cross-infection from one client to another or to the therapist the following precautions should be taken:

1 Wipe down surfaces such as the couch and trolley with a low-odour, non-irritant chemical sterilising agent. Use a spray to deliver the product and wipe with a clean cloth or disposable paper such as couch roll.

2 Use clean laundered towels for each client. Wash laundry in the hottest water possible using a detergent containing anti-bacterial agents.

3 Use disposable couch roll on all client contact surfaces.

4 Check clients for contraindications. Never treat a client who has a contagious condition unless very minor, in which case it should be covered with a waterproof dressing.

5 Any cuts, abrasions or other small open wounds on the therapist's hands or in the treatment areas should be covered with a sterile waterproof dressing

6 The client should shower if the facilities are available.

7 Always use a 'cut out' technique when handling products.

8 Sanitise hands before and after treatment. Washing hands in hot soapy water or the use of an antibacterial wipe is advised.

9 Cleanse the client's feet before beginning the treatment with a suitable antiseptic, using a clean piece of cotton wool for each foot to avoid the possibility of cross-contamination from one foot to another.

10 During the massage treatment wipe your hands with anti-bacterial wipes when passing from feet to body or body to face.

11 Dispose of waste material correctly, immediately after treatment.

For more information on suitable sterilising methods, see Chapter 6 Professional practices.

Health and safety practices

Under the legislation of the Health and Safety at Work Act therapists have a duty of care to others as well as themselves to work safely and cooperate with employers to maintain safe working practices. These practices are centred on the treatment environment and hygiene practices as outlined above while working within the requirements of the law.

The main pieces of legislation that a therapist works under are shown in Table 11.1 below. Others are discussed within Chapter 1 Monitoring health and safety.

▽ Table 11.1 Relevant legislation

Area	Act	Areas covered by Act
The treatment room	Health & Safety at Work Act 1974	General safety of staff and visitors to the salon including clients
	Workplace (Health, Safety & Welfare) Regulations 1992	Governs the working environment including ventilation, temperature and lighting, etc.
	Regulatory Reform (Fire Safety) Order 2005	The safe evacuation of the building in an emergency such as a fire
Massage equipment	Provision and Use of Work Equipment Regulations 1998	Governs the acquisition of safe and reliable equipment
	Electricity at Work Regulations 1989	Governs the regular maintenance of electrical equipment including the recording of such
Massage products	Control of Substances Hazardous to Health 1988	Governs the exposure of persons to substances likely to cause harm including flammability and the effect on the tissues
	Cosmetic Products (Safety) Regulations (2008)	Requires cosmetics to comply with correct labelling, to have safe formulation and be fit for the purpose intended
Disposal of waste	Controlled Waste Regulations 1992	Governs the correct disposal of contaminated waste, i.e. that contaminated with blood or other bodily fluids

Local bylaws

Locally there may be additional bylaws which a therapist must comply with regarding the provision of massage treatments. For example, the London Local Authorities Act 2007 requires local councils to provide improvement and development of local services in a variety of areas, one of which is for the licensing of businesses that carry out treatments on the general public. This kind of bylaw is intended to protect the general public from bad practitioners and supports the membership of a professional body to ensure safe practice.

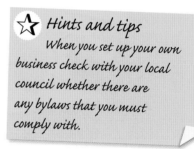

⭐ *Hints and tips*
When you set up your own business check with your local council whether there are any bylaws that you must comply with.

Positioning of client and therapist

The position of the client to ensure their comfort and complete relaxation during a massage service is paramount. The use of 'props' or 'bolsters' correctly positioned to maintain the natural curvature of the body provides the ultimate in support and comfort. These bolsters can be made by simply rolling towels tightly and covering with disposable couch roll for hygiene or can be purchased, in which case they are usually made of firm foam rubber with a vinyl cover that can be sprayed with a suitable disinfectant between uses.

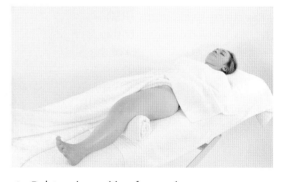

△ Bolsters in position for use in massage

The key areas for the use of bolsters are as follows.

In a supine position:

- the neck
- the lower back
- behind the knee.

Key terms

Prone – client lying on their front, face down.

Supine – client lying on their back, face up.

☆ Hints and tips

Height adjustable couches are 'hydraulic' and either require the application of a pumping action to a lever to raise the couch or use electricity. The latter provide a 'smoother ride' for the client when altering the position of the couch during the treatment.

In a prone position:

- the head (with use of a face hole to keep the spine straight)
- the hips
- the ankle.

Attention to the posture and position of the therapist in relation to the client is also important to prevent work-related health conditions such as fatigue and/or back pain and posture faults. The height of the treatment couch is important and one that adjusts to suit the height of the therapist and any variation in massage technique required is ideal.

There are two main standing positions that should be used by the therapist when performing massage treatments:

1. walk standing: used when massaging along the length of the body where travelling may be necessary
2. stride standing: used when massaging an area and travelling is not needed.

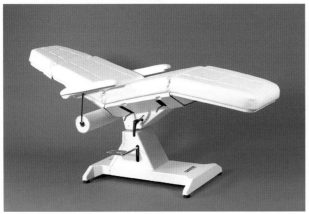
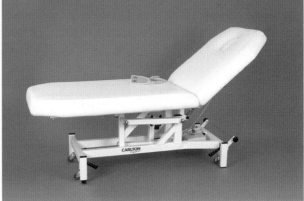

△ Hydraulic and electric-action treatment couches

Key term

Repetitive strain injury (RSI) – a condition where pain and other symptoms occur in an area of the body which has carried out repetitive tasks over a period of time.

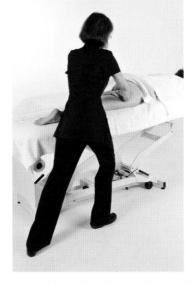
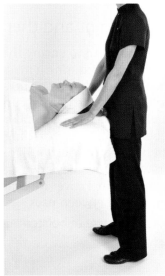

△ Stride and walk standing positions during massage

The therapist's back should be kept straight and the body weight rather than the arms used where more depth or pressure is required in the massage routine. This reduces the risk of fatigue and protects the therapist's hands and wrists are from repetitive strain injury.

Consult, plan and prepare for treatment

Consultation techniques

Consultation techniques include:

- communication and behaviour
- questioning and listening techniques and appropriate body language
- visual assessment
- manual assessment
- referral to client records
- visual aids.

Health and safety

Always bend your knees and not your back when performing massage or any other treatment on a client to protect against back pain and postural faults.

Communication and behaviour

The appropriate methods of communication and standards of behaviour and the consultation techniques for before a beauty therapy treatment are dealt with in detail in Chapter 6 Professional practices. There are, however, additional considerations for a massage therapist. To be successful, a massage therapist must have a strong belief that whatever she is doing is right. This involves a deep and sincere interest in the treatments and clients and colleagues. The therapist should treat each client as an individual case, even though the treatment procedures and techniques for some may be similar. Massage therapy is a personal business and the therapist must have the ability to concentrate on the special requirements necessary for each case in hand to obtain the best possible result for the client's total benefit and well-being.

Sensitivity and respect for the body is vital. Personal consideration when moving, massaging and manipulating the client should not be overlooked, especially when the client is dressing and undressing.

Rapport with each client must remain professional. It is up to the therapist to judge each situation and control the conversation accordingly. There will be times when silence must be respected by the therapist if the client wishes to relax.

Questioning

Effective questioning of the client during a consultation will elicit the required information to assess the suitability of the client for the treatment. Asking questions about the client's health, their needs and requirements of the treatment (also known as the treatment objectives) as well as details of the client's lifestyle will enable you to make suitable recommendations and design a treatment plan.

Contraindications

To ensure the safety of the client and the prevention of cross-contamination of infectious diseases and disorders, the therapist should question the client about the possible contraindications for massage treatment. These contraindications fall into two main categories: those that *prevent* and those that may *restrict* the treatment (see Table 11.2). If a contraindication is present the situation should be sympathetically explained to the client that either they may not have the treatment or that the treatment needs adapting in some way to avoid making the condition worse.

▽ Table 11.2 Contraindications to body massage treatment

Conditions that prevent treatment	Conditions that restrict treatment
• Fungal infections such as Tinea corporis • Bacterial infections such as impetigo • Viral infections such as herpes zoster • Infestations such as Pediculosis corporis • Severe non-infectious disease and disorders such as psoriasis and eczema • Severe skin conditions that to a lesser degree would normally restrict treatment such as bruising, sunburn, loss of tactile sensation, etc. • Dysfunction of the muscular and nervous systems • Deep vein thrombosis and embolism • During chemotherapy and/or radiotherapy • Heart disease and circulatory disorders	• Broken bones • Recent fractures and sprains • Cuts and abrasions • Recent scar tissue • Skin disorders • Skin allergies • Product allergies • Epilepsy • Diabetes • High/low blood pressure • Undiagnosed lumps and swellings • Recent haemorrhage • Warts or moles • Areas of recent scar tissue • Abdominal area during pregnancy or menstruation • Recent operations • Recent fractures • Metal plates or pins in bone • Electronic implants • Oedema (swelling) • Back pain or injury

For additional information on specific skin diseases and disorders see Chapter 4 Anatomy and physiology.

The contraindications that prevent treatment fall into two categories: those that lead to a risk of cross-infection and those of a medical nature. All types of skin diseases present a risk of cross-infection and contact should be avoided. The client should be advised to seek medical advice from their doctor or chemist as appropriate and return for treatment when the disease has cleared.

The contraindications that restrict treatment may also involve a dialogue with an appropriate medical practitioner, for example, conditions such as epilepsy, diabetes, high/low blood pressure, undiagnosed lumps and swellings, electronic implants, oedema (swelling) of a systemic cause and back pain or injury. This is to ensure the safety of the client. Once permission has been granted there should be adaptation of the treatment in terms of the position in which the client lies (e.g. legs raised in the case of oedema), the massage movements/ manipulations used (e.g. omit deep petrissage on the feet of diabetics), adaptation to the routine (e.g. omitting the lower back in the case of back pain) or raising the head of the couch at the end of the massage to allow the client to sit up to receive aftercare advice (e.g. for a client suffering with low blood pressure).

Contraindications of a medical nature may mean that to continue with the massage treatment may cause the client serious harm. In some instances it may be appropriate to ask a medical practitioner if treatment can go ahead but details of the effects of the treatment must be fully explained so that the client can make an informed judgement.

Necessary actions

The therapist should be aware of the possible actions to take if the client presents with a contraindication:

- encourage the client to seek medical advice
- explain why the treatment cannot be carried out
- modify the treatment.

Assessing lifestyle patterns

The increasing popularity of massage as a treatment may be because of an increase in stress levels caused by our lifestyles. Long working hours, families and worries about finances all increase a person's perceived stress levels and many are resorting to the use of therapies such as massage for relief of these stresses. When questioning your client you should consider their:

- occupation
- diet
- exercise levels
- alcohol consumption
- smoking
- stress levels.

Treatment objectives

The client should be questioned about the reasons for their visit and why they have chosen a massage treatment. By checking the client's needs the therapist can ensure she meets their objectives they will be satisfied with the massage treatment. Massage treatment can be used to provide:

- feelings of relaxation/sedation
- a sense of well being
- an uplifting feeling
- anti-cellulite treatment
- assistance with weight reduction
- feelings of stimulation/invigoration

Suitable adaptations to the massage treatment for these individual objectives are given below under the heading 'Planning treatment'.

Remember . . .

If a client presents with a contraindication that prevents the treatment, explain clearly why the treatment cannot go ahead. Use a suitable tone of voice so as not to cause the client alarm and do not diagnose the condition but recommend they see a doctor or other medical practitioner.

Visual assessment

The visual assessment of the client should be undertaken with consideration of the client's privacy and modesty at all times. A discreet observation maybe confirmed with a closed question that will help the therapist to develop an effective treatment plan. The information gleaned will help determine which type of massage medium and movements to use as well as the depth, rate and use of massage movements. The visual assessment can be used to ascertain information on the following:

- Skin type: this is defined by the activity of the sebaceous glands in the skin and is described as normal, dry, oily or combination.

- Skin condition: this is a result of internal influences such as health and external influences such as sun exposure.

- Differences related to gender: generally male clients are more hairy than females and have more muscle bulk. This will affect the choice of massage medium as well as the depth and type of massage movement used. Female clients have a different body fat distribution from males – commonly fat deposits are likely to be found from the waist to the knee in women, including the hips and thighs, whereas men can accumulate fat around the abdomen and trunk area. This may influence the time spent in these areas, especially if assisting in weight loss is one of the treatment objectives.

- Differences related to age: as the body tissues age they go through a series of changes that need to be taken into account when performing massage on middle-aged and older clients. The skin thins as it ages and loses elasticity. The muscular system can diminish with age, resulting in less bulk and poor muscle tone may result from a lack of exercise and/or use. The skeletal system gives up its calcium deposits, especially in women as a result of reduced oestrogen production through menopause, which may result in brittle bones or osteoporosis.

- Body type: also known as 'soma type', this is the classification of the shape of the body, considering the natural skeletal structure, musculature and weight distribution. There are three types: ectomorph, endomorph and mesomorph.

- Fat deposits and type of fat: the position of fat deposits can influence body shape. There are three main types of fat: hard, soft and cellulite. Cellulite can be improved by a strict regime of a toxin-free diet, increased water intake and salon treatments including lymph drainage massage and applications of lotions. It is a four-pronged attack on the problem that will gain satisfactory results; the application of a cream alone will not rid the body of the toxins.

- Posture: this is maintained by the action of the anti-gravity muscles found in the front and back of the legs, trunk and neck. Poor posture is gained through a lack of muscle tone through little exercise and age but can also develop through incorrect standing, walking and sitting positions. Poor posture leads to back and neck pain which may be an indication for massage treatment, but can also indicate the following conditions: kyphosis, lordosis, winged scapulae,

⭐ *Hints and tips*
The medical profession say there is no such thing as cellulite as it appears as normal adipose tissue within the skin. Yet women do not need convincing of its existence. Cellulite is a skin condition where there is a build up of waste products in the tissue fluid surrounding the fat cells which has a progressive action on the fat cells and the surrounding connective tissues.

unbalanced pelvis, short limbs, scoliosis, knock knees, bowlegs, flat feet, 'dowager's hump' or 'pigeon chest'. Generalised lower back pain that is not the result of an injury is caused by poor muscle tone in the abdominal muscles resulting in a forward hip tilt.

More information on all these aspects of body analysis can be found in Chapter 7 Skin and body analysis.

Manual

Physical characteristics: in addition to those discussed above, other aspects of the client's physical appearance relate to their weight, height and muscle tone. Weight and height are largely used to predict and indicate the health of the client in terms of weight loss or gain; this is a simple measure but is not always an accurate one.

Muscle tone is a subjective measure and difficult to determine. Generally, those that do little exercise and/or are middle aged or older have poor muscle tone, while the young and those that exercise will exhibit good muscle tone. The degree of muscle tone will again influence the type and depth of massage movements used during the treatment.

Referral to client records

Refer to the client's record card for:

- an indication of their health and the presence of contraindications
- their preferred massage medium and any potential allergies
- the massage movements used and their depth and rate of rhythm; find out whether these were successful and the long term effects
- possible contra-actions to previous treatments and/or products.

Planning treatment

The massage treatment and techniques should be adapted to suit the client's needs and treatment objectives. The considerations for adaptation to the treatment include:

- the environment
- the massage routine
- type of movement
- depth of movement
- speed of movement.

Relaxation/sedation treatment

A calm and quiet atmosphere should be created with the careful use of soft lighting and slow, rhythmical music. The client should be kept warm as the body temperature lowers as the body relaxes. It is usual to omit tapotement movements from the massage routine as these movements are invigorating. The remainder of the massage movements should be performed slowly and rhythmically with light to medium depth and the transitions between movements imperceptible. Work in a procedure from an extremity towards the heart.

Sense of well-being

For this treatment objective the treatment room and its environment can be similar to that of a relaxation treatment to promote the release of stress and promote self healing. There are some circumstances where tapotement movements should be included, especially if the client is suffering from fatigue, as the stimulation received from the movements can invigorate the client.

Uplifting

A client requiring an uplifting massage may be suffering from depression or have been through a prolonged period of stress. They may be feeling tired and run down and may fall asleep during the treatment. In this case it may be detrimental to resort to adaptations that sedate the client further. Instead, promote energy levels and lift the spirits with inspirational music and slightly brighter but not strong lighting. Perform brisk, rhythmical massage movements and complete the massage with brisk effleurage movements. Allow time during the consultation for the client to unload their problems while remaining professional and supportive. The therapist should offer lifestyle advice and, if necessary, encourage the client to seek medical assistance if deemed necessary.

Anti-cellulite

The adaptations for this type of massage relate to the routine as the therapist may be performing the techniques as part of a full body massage treatment or as a part body treatment that concentrates on the areas affected by cellulite. The client should be warned that this can be an uncomfortable process. The movements used should encourage an increase in blood circulation and lymph drainage to promote the removal of the tissue fluid containing the high degree of toxins. Begin the massage of the area below the appropriate lymph node closest to the heart and use deep effleurage movements in a pumping action towards the heart before deeper petrissage movements are used. Repeat the movements so that the area is drained into the now clear lymph nodes. Work in areas further from the heart, keeping the pressure of the movements towards the heart.

Assist in weight reduction

Massage can assist in weight loss by making the stored adipose tissue deposits available as a source of energy by breaking them down and encouraging them to be deposited into the bloodstream via the lymphatic system. Tapotement movements such as pounding and beating to break down fatty deposits and the use of deep effleurage and petrissage to drain the area are effective. The massage is really quite stimulating and the treatment environment should reflect this. The massage routine may include relaxing and weight reduction aspects on the different areas of the body.

Stimulation/invigoration

The environment should reflect the type of massage and not be too sedating. The routine includes all areas of the body being massaged as it will be less effective if only done on parts of the body. The purpose of the massage is to invigorate where the client is mentally or physically fatigued and should have a general effect on raising the blood pressure and pulse rate of the client. The movements used should be performed briskly and at a fast rate; an increased depth should be aimed for and the use of tapotement movements are important for this type of massage.

Treatment times for massage

The times shown in Table 11.3 have been determined by the industry as standard commercial timings for body massage services and should be used during the practical assessment.

▽ Table 11.3 Treatment times for massage

Service	Time
Back massage	30 minutes
Full body manual massage	60 minutes
Full body including head and face massage	75 minutes

Contra-actions

It is important to explain the treatment and the possible contra-actions at the time of the consultation to gain the client's trust and to ensure their satisfaction with the treatment. The client can then ask questions to clarify and can make an informed decision as to whether to continue with the treatment. Adaptations to the treatment can be put in place if necessary. The possible contra-actions to massage are:

- lethargy
- headache
- muscle ache
- nausea
- increased emotions
- frequent urination
- bruising
- allergy to the massage medium.

Contra-actions are symptoms your clients may experience and most should be considered as completely normal; not all clients will experience all the symptoms. Any contra-action should dissipate (fade) within 12 hours. If they do not dissipate the salon and/or therapist should be contacted to gain advice. In the case of a severe reaction to the massage cream the client may need to contact a doctor.

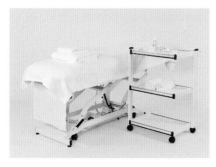

△ Preparation of the treatment couch and trolley

Equality and diversity

Electric couches that can adjust to a low height are invaluable when dealing with clients who use a wheelchair as this enables them to transfer to the treatment couch more easily.

Prepare for treatment

Environmental conditions

Treatment rooms should be clean, adequately lit, properly ventilated and in a good general state of repair. A wash basin with hot and cold water supply should be located in the treatment area and antiseptic soap and some means of drying the hands should be available.

- Warmth: the treatment room should be warm but not stuffy. Although the therapist may get hot during the massage treatment the client may feel cold as they have less clothing and the temperature of the body lowers as it relaxes.

- Ventilation: this should be sufficient to allow a steady exchange of air as this will prevent fatigue in the therapist. It should not cause a drop in temperature as this will result in the client feeling chilled and reduce their enjoyment of the treatment.

- Lighting: could be soft and minimal to aid relaxation or brighter if stimulation or invigorating massage is being performed. A treatment room with a variable light control is preferable.

- Privacy: a quiet, private treatment room is essential for body massage treatment. The client is asked to remove their outer clothing and may feel vulnerable and unable to relax if the treatment area is in a busy area of the salon.

- Volume and type of music/sounds: soft background music creates a peaceful ambience.

- Pleasant aroma: the use of aromatic oils in an oil burner or an aromatic candle can create a pleasant aroma and can be adapted to suit the type of client or their treatment objectives.

Take care not to use flowery feminine oils when treating male clients. Aromas such as sandalwood and peppermint are more suitable for a male client.

The trolley should be prepared with:

- clean bedroll
- bowls
- cotton wool
- massage mediums
- medicated swabs/wipes
- bowl or bin in with disposable bin liner for waste.

Treatment couches should be sturdy, safe, clean and hygienic and should be prepared with:

- freshly laundered towels
- clean bedroll
- bolsters or supports
- headband.

After the consultation, keep conversation polite and brief so that full relaxation can be experienced by the client. Make the client feel special as she is likely to return to the salon if she feels she has been well treated. A happy client will tell others of your professional approach and expertise.

Preparation of the therapist

The massage therapist's hands should be warm, relaxed and smooth. At first the hands may ache after performing massage, but as the muscles in the hands strengthen with practice this feeling will fade.

The therapist should also undertake a level of mental preparation before beginning a massage. It is poor practice to bring personal stress or anxiety to a massage treatment and so the therapist should relax and become calm, shutting out any incidents that may have occurred before the treatment.

The ability to be kind, comforting and sympathetic, to be tactful and reassuring, to be cheerful and optimistic, are qualities every beauty therapist should possess. Consecutive massages on different clients however can leave the therapist physically and mentally drained. It is important that the therapist protects themselves by mentally distancing themselves from the client's problems, by listening but not becoming emotionally involved. In this way the therapist is more able to help the client with relevant and appropriate advice.

Preparing the client

1. When the client arrives for treatment they should be treated with courtesy and respect.

2. Always address the client by their name and inform them of yours.

3. Take the client to the treatment area and briefly explain the treatment procedure.

4. Carry out a thorough consultation and discuss the aims of the treatment.

5. Ask the client to shower if the facilities are available.

6. Advise the client which articles of clothing and jewellery they need to remove and provide a gown that they may wear if they prefer.

7. Allow the client to undress in private.

8. Help the client onto the couch and allow them to get comfortable. This should include the placement of bolsters to support key areas of the body.

9. Cover the client with towels and ensure that they are warm and comfortable before beginning the treatment.

Activity

Hand exercises will prepare your hands for massage treatments. Before you begin a massage try these simple hand exercises. They will help you to relax and prepare your hands to give a more effective treatment.

1. Circle hands round and round from the wrist.
2. Quickly make a fist, clenching and stretching out the fingers.
3. Roll the thumbs round and round first one way and then the other.
4. Stretch each finger separately and then together.
5. Flap the wrist up and down, side to side and in a circle until they feel relaxed.
6. Shake the whole arm and shoulder.

Do your hands feel more relaxed now?

⭐ *Hints and tips*

During the treatment the therapist should focus solely on the client and the treatment. They should not allow themselves to be distracted with noise or other disturbances that might break the flow of the massage.

Health and safety

The development of repetitive strain injuries or RSIs in therapists has been well documented by the Health and Safety Executive (HSE) and the industry lead body Habia. Conditions such as 'carpel tunnel syndrome' and 'tennis elbow' are occupational health conditions and can prevent a therapist from working or indeed give up beauty therapy altogether. As you embark on your career please be aware of these conditions and put in place procedures to minimise your risk of developing them. During massage, for example, use the forearm rather than the hand, the elbow instead of the thumbs, or use mechanical massage equipment such as audio sonic when you can.

⭐ **Hints and tips**
The receptionist should be encouraged not to book a therapist with consecutive manual Swedish massage treatments and to vary the bookings to alleviate the physical stresses placed on the body.

Removal of accessories

In order to facilitate a free-flowing massage without disruptions the removal of the client's outer clothing and jewellery that may break the flow of the massage strokes is essential.

The client should be asked to remove all outer clothing and to keep on only lower under-clothing for a massage treatment. Clothing should be folded and placed in a safe place away from the treatment area to avoid damage from spillage of the massage medium.

All jewellery should be removed if possible including earrings, necklaces, bracelets, anklets, body piercings, etc. This will also avoid accidental breakage or damage by the oil or the action of the massage movements, as well as promoting a flowing undisrupted massage treatment. Where piercings are new and/or cannot be removed they should be avoided during the massage routine.

Perform manual massage treatment

Benefits of massage

The benefits and uses of body massage are:

- relaxation/pleasure
- to treat muscle aches and pains
- as a treatment after exercise
- as part of a 'detox' programme
- to relieve stress, anxiety and tension
- to disperse fibrous adhesions
- to improve general health and well-being.

The effects of a massage can be categorised under two main headings: psychological and physiological.

Psychological

The giving and receiving of a massage treatment is in itself a very personal experience. The physical touch of another person can have amazing results on the mental state of a client, especially if they do not usually spend any time on themselves or are feeling neglected, lonely or unloved. The close contact and personal attention and the psychological benefits obtained from touch can then have a healing effect on physical conditions that the client may present for treatment, such as headaches.

The client is made to feel special because they receive individual attention. This can create a sense of well-being because they feel someone cares and is dedicating their time to them. The relief from pain after massage can produce an uplifting feeling for the client. Maybe an aching shoulder is relieved or a headache soothed. This can produce a boost to the client's morale and general feelings.

Occasionally, following a massage, the client can feel tearful. This is not a sign of a failure, simply a release of emotions. The physical

⭐ **Hints and tips**
Client's jewellery should be placed safely in a tissue-lined bowl and returned to the client after the treatment or placed in a small plastic bag and given to the client to put with their belongings so as not to leave it behind after the treatment.

⭐ **Hints and tips**
It is important to give the client clear instructions surrounding the items of clothing to be removed so as to avoid embarrassment later in the treatment. Jewellery should be removed so as not to disrupt the flow of the massage treatment.

contact may have triggered off a reaction that has been building up inside the client. It is important that this is dealt with carefully and tactfully in order that more psychological damage is not done. Being a good listener is another important part of the treatment. The client may need to talk and share things with an outsider – someone not in their immediate circle of associates – and you could provide that 'ear'. After a massage a therapist can feel physically and emotionally drained; some clients seem to sap all your energy – they leap off the couch revitalised and raring to go, while you are left feeling drained!

A body massage can have a very positive effect on how the client feels about their own body. By touching areas that perhaps they are not fond of (large hips, flabby tummy, rough skin) and not saying anything negative to the client, while skilfully applying the massage movements over the 'problem', you can help to soothe away their negative thoughts. This can in itself have incredible results. A massage can help clients to cope with the general day-to-day running of their lives, to increase their self esteem and boost their ability to cope with the pressures of modern day life.

> ☆ **Hints and tips**
> It is vital to remember not to slip into a counselling role. Do not to be tempted to give advice that may be inappropriate. Instead, simply listen and allow the client to 'unwind' through you.

Physiological

To study the physiological effects of a massage it is necessary to look at all the systems of the body. Many of these systems are inter-linked and the effect on one automatically affects another. Chapter 4 Anatomy and physiology gives more detail on the systems of the body but below is a summary of the effects of massage on these systems.

Skin

The effect of the massage medium on the skin and the increased desquamation from the massage movements leaves the skin feeling smoother and softer. The skin benefits from a massage in lots of other ways, too. The temperature of the skin is raised, thus bringing blood to the area, supplying fresh nutrients and removing waste products. This helps cell regeneration and speeds up the skin's metabolism. With regular massage the texture and appearance of the skin will definitely improve.

The skin's excretion mechanism is increased, the sudoriferous glands are stimulated, therefore ridding the body of waste materials and 'cleansing' the pores. The sebaceous glands increase sebum activity keeping the skin soft and supple.

The underlying subcutaneous tissue is manipulated and this can help to loosen blockages, release tension and mobilise stubborn fatty deposits. The skin's sensory nerve endings register the effects of physical contact and this has an effect on the nervous system, both physically and psychologically, as described above.

Skeletal system

When carrying out a massage, the pressure exerted when a bone is near to the surface is usually minimal and effleurage movements tend to glide over bony prominences. However, with careful use of thumb circles or finger kneading, a lot of benefit can be gained around joints. The knee, elbow, wrist, ankle and vertebrae are examples. Cellular regeneration is encouraged, helping to alleviate stiff, aching joints, releasing tension in the area, dissipating waste products, dispersing fluid that may have collected and generally lubricating and loosening the joints.

Muscular system

A massage can have amazing effects on the muscular system of the body. Petrissage movements remove tension by increasing the local blood circulation and encouraging lymphatic flow to remove waste product accumulations. Deep petrissage movements move the muscle against bony structures and in this way underlying cells and tissues are stimulated. With regular massage the tone of a muscle can be improved.

Professional sports people have a pre-sport massage to warm the muscles beforehand and post-sport massage to remove waste products afterwards. If a muscle is massaged immediately after exercise, the increased blood flow will help remove the lactic acid and other waste materials that have built up as a by-product of the exercise. By doing this, stiff aching muscles can be avoided.

Nervous system

The surface of the skin is rich in sensory nerves and as the massage strokes are carried out these nerve endings are affected. With soft effleurage strokes the nerve endings will be soothed, while hacking, cupping and tapotement movements will stimulate the nerve endings. The effects of the nervous system can be adapted to suit the client's requirement. Frictions performed along the spine can have the effect of stimulating a nerve and the area of the body it serves, creating a temporary increase in muscle tone, which then dissipates to leave the muscle in a more relaxed state.

Circulatory system

The body has two circulatory systems: the blood and the lymph. Both of these systems are affected by a massage. Massage movements are generally performed towards the heart, thus aiding venous return. The strong strokes go up the limbs, with soft gliding movements back down to link movements together.

Any movement that improves the flow through blood vessels will increase the lymphatic drainage from that area too. Whenever the blood supply is stimulated this has a wide range of beneficial effects on all the tissues of the body. The metabolism of the cells is increased and fresh oxygenated blood flows into the area, bringing nutrients and removing waste products. Certain movements produce a surface erythema, which indicates the blood supply has been stimulated.

Respiratory system

During a body massage the client's breathing slows down and deepens as the body relaxes. This increases the efficiency of the lungs because more oxygen is taken in and more carbon dioxide is expelled from the body. All the bodily functions are closely linked. As more oxygen is inhaled, the blood supply is speeded up and therefore more oxygen is taken around the body, creating a positive effect on all the body systems.

Quite often clients will relax so much that they lapse into semi- or complete sleep. With experience the practitioner and client will breathe in unison – thus aligning the bodies and minds of the two people.

Digestive system

It is unwise to perform a massage immediately after a heavy meal or if a client has not eaten at all for a few hours. Gentle abdominal massage is excellent for increasing the process of digestion. The movements are performed clockwise – thus going with the digestive tract and aiding peristalsis. A mild case of constipation may in fact be relieved by a skilful massage.

The whole process of massage speeds up the journey of food through the digestive tract. It helps with the release of enzymes, aids the breakdown of food and helps the absorption of nutrients.

Urinary system

It is quite normal for a client to need to visit the toilet straight after a massage. The movements performed on the body increase metabolic rate, aid digestion and improve the blood and lymph, all of which leads to an increase in urine output. It is good practice to offer the client a drink of mineral water immediately after the massage to further help the detoxification of the body.

Endocrine system

This is a system of ductless glands that control the internal chemical environment by the release of hormones into the blood stream. As the blood supply is stimulated, the hormones are distributed faster and this will have a feedback effect on the glands.

Some of the endocrine glands are also greatly influenced by the autonomic nervous system and therefore affected by the psychological state of the person. As the body relaxes and succumbs to the effects of the massage, so the balance of hormones may be affected.

Effects of massage

The physiological, psychological and physical effects of massage are shown in Table 11.4.

▽ Table 11.4 Effects of massage

Physiological	Psychological	Physical
• Improves skin texture • Aids blood circulation in the skin • Aids desquamation • Aids circulation in veins and indirectly aids arterial circulation • Improves lymphatic drainage so hastening removal of waste products • Increases deep muscular circulation avoiding lactic acid build-up • Helps prevent hardened nodules (fibrosis) forming in muscle tissue • Helps improve muscle tone • Stimulates nerve endings • Aids absorption of fluid around joints • Improves metabolism and aids breakdown of adipose tissue • Improves joint mobility • May loosen and stretch scar tissue • May prevent skin adhesions	• Sedative and relaxing to the client • Brings about general feeling of well-being • Relieves feelings of fatigue • Relieves stress and anxiety	• Introduces therapist's hands to the client • Applies the massage medium • Produces an erythema • Produces a local rise in skin temperature • Skin feels softer due to the action of the massage medium • Improves skin colour • Newly formed milia may be reabsorbed if firmly massaged

Massage mediums

> **Key term**
>
> **Emollients** – creams, ointments and oil moisturisers which reduce water loss from skin and provide protection.

If a therapist can perform a massage with no form of lubrication, the massage technique will have been perfected. However, emollients such as oils and creams are often used as lubrication from which the client gains both physical and psychological benefit. The most suitable massage medium should be chosen and then used only sparingly.

Whichever lubricant is used it should always be applied to the therapist's hands first and not directly onto the client. Remove the product from its container using the appropriate cut-out technique to maintain the hygiene of the product and the container. Any product left over after the massage should be discarded. Table 11.5 gives details of the appropriate cut-out techniques for each type of product.

▽ Table 11.5 Cut-out techniques for massage products

Product	Cut-out technique
Oil should be stored in an opaque, plastic bottle to minimise degrading through light exposure. The bottle should have a 'flip' top which should be closed immediately after dispensing the oil	Oil should be placed into a clean plastic bowl or dispensed directly into the hand of the therapist. No contact should be made with the bottle
Cream is stored in a tub with a screw lid which should be replaced immediately after dispensing the product	Use a sterile spatula to lift from the pot and place into a clean plastic bowl
Powder/talc is usually stored in a sealed container with a perforated top to enable the product to be shaken and dispensed. Occasionally powder can be found in a pot or tub-type container	The powder can be used either directly from the 'shaker' style container onto the therapist's hands or dry cotton wool
Gel can be stored in a tub or pot or in a sealed bottle with a pump action top	Use a sterile spatula to lift from the pot or pump directly into a clean plastic bowl or the product can be dispensed directly into the hand of the therapist as long as there is no contact made with the bottle
Emulsion is stored in a sealed bottle with a pump action top	Either pump directly into a clean plastic bowl or the product can be dispensed directly into the hand of the therapist, as long as there is no contact made with the bottle

Oil

Oil used for massage should be of vegetable origin because unlike mineral oil, vegetable oil is absorbed more readily by the skin. This is because it is very close in composition to the body's natural oil, sebum. Vegetable oils allow the massage movements to be performed more deeply and also help nourish the skin, with each having its own beneficial effect. A disadvantage is that the basic oils can have a characteristic smell, although this can be disguised by adding essential oils such as lavender.

Mineral oil and baby oil are very rich and are not easily absorbed, making the hands slip and not facilitating depth of pressure for massage movements.

If treating someone with a nut allergy, care must be taken when choosing the massage oil. The therapist should take an active interest in the manufacturer's processes.

Table 11.6 gives some examples of oils suitable for massage.

▽ Table 11.6 Massage oils

Type of oil	Description
Grapeseed	Seed-based oil that is quickly and deeply absorbed by the skin. It is suitable for delicate or oily skins
Avocado	Fruit-based oil that is dark green in colour. The oil is obtained from the dehydrated or dried fruit and contains vitamins A, B and D, protein, lecithin and fatty acids. It is especially good for dry and dehydrated skins because it is highly penetrative. It keeps for up to two years as it contains natural antioxidants. Used to nourish and restore the skin and to penetrate adipose tissue
Sweet almond	Sweet almond is a very pale yellow oil which is obtained from the kernel of the nut. It contains glycosides, minerals, vitamins A, B1, B2, B6 and E. It keeps reasonably well for up to two years. Used where itching, eczema, soreness and inflammation are present on the skin; it is ideal for use with babies and children. Do not use if nut allergies suspected

Cream

Creams are usually absorbed into the skin more readily than any other medium and can be used where the client's skin is oily and where oil would add to the problem. Cream may be needed in greater quantity than oil and can be easier for a student of massage to master the technique with. Usually lanolin-based with eau-de-cologne added to perfume. Cream is suitable for massage for a client with a hairy body.

Powder/talc

Only the finest of powder should be used and preferably one with a mild smell. Fine French chalk or the brand name baby powders are suitable. Talc must never be applied to the client in a shaking motion. The powder is of no benefit to the client and is purely to prevent the therapist's wet or sticky hands from ruining the massage. This method is not to be used on dry skin or with a client with known allergies. Powder is a suitable medium for clients with a hairy body.

Gel

Gel massage mediums rely on natural or synthetic slipping agents such as silicone to provide the slip needed for massage. Gel absorbs easily into the skin and is good for normal to dry skin types. The gel can have added ingredients for additional benefit such as collagen and is cooling on the skin.

Emulsion

This is a lotion containing a mix of oil and water to provide a lighter product than a cream. It is suitable for combination skin types and can be scented with essential oils which provide additional therapeutic benefits.

Massage techniques

Effleurage

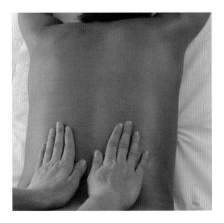

△ Effleurage on the back

The term effleurage comes from the French 'effleurer' which means to 'skim over' and can be defined as the passage of the palm of the hand over the body. There are two types of stroke: effleurage and stroking. The pressure for each may vary from very light to very deep.

Effleurage is always performed in the direction of the venous return of the local blood supply and towards the nearest lymph node and the stroke ends with an increase in pressure. The hands remain in contact with the skin and with reduced pressure skim over the skin to return to the starting point of the movement.

Superficial effleurage is performed with light pressure, using the entire palmer surface of the hands. The fingers are held together and the thumb is open (abducted) or closed (adducted) as necessary to increase or lessen the area of surface to fit the part of the body being massaged. One or both hands may be used at the same time; the rhythm is even to secure relaxation and at a rate of 15 strokes per minute or 7 inches per second.

Deep effleurage is performed with sufficient pressure to produce both mechanical and reflex effects. It is performed with any part of one or both hands depending on the area being massaged, but for the body it is normal to use the palmer surface of the whole hand, fingers and thumb. One hand can be placed on top of the other to reinforce the stroke and create more concentrated pressure. The part of the hand used is kept in contact with the skin at the end of the stroke and returned over the same area with a superficial stroke. The purpose of maintaining contact with the skin is to avoid the reflex stimulus to the nerve endings caused by breaking and again making contact with the skin. It is essential that the client's muscles are relaxed when performing these movements.

Stroking remains at a constant pressure once chosen and can be light, moderate or deep. Unlike effleurage, stroking can be performed in any direction and not only towards a lymph node. The hands can be lifted from the skin to return to the beginning of the movement.

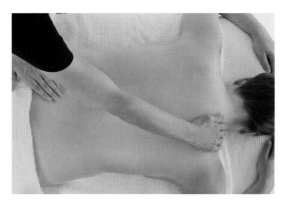

△ Stroking on the back

The benefits of effleurage are:

- stimulation of sensory nerve endings promoting relaxation

- venous circulation is increased as a mechanical response to the physical pressure placed on the veins

- arterial circulation is aided by removal of congestion in the veins

- increased blood circulation brings nutrients and oxygen to the tissues, increasing cell metabolism and improving the functioning of the tissues

- the venous and lymphatic circulations are increased locally, removing waste products

- an increase in lymph drainage and the subsequent removal of tissue fluid prevents stagnation and oedema

- muscle tension is relieved by the removal of waste products, relieving muscle stiffness and pain

- relaxation of contracted, tense muscle fibres is obtained through the reflex response to deep effleurage

- increased blood flow and the action of the hands over the skin creates warmth which promotes relaxation.

- the action of the hands promotes desquamation of the epidermal cells, improving skin appearance.

- generally a feeling of relaxation is accomplished, which can be very sedative in effect.

Uses of effleurage:

- Stroking is used to apply and spread the massage medium at the beginning of the routine.

- Superficial effleurage is used at the beginning of the routine to introduce the client to the touch of the therapist.

- Effleurage is used within a routine between other types of movement to drain an area and to link the routine together.

- Brisk, deep effleurage is used to stimulate an area, promoting warmth and improving.

- Deep effleurage is used to reduce swelling and promote healthy tissues.

- Stroking is used at the end of a massage routine to conclude and to inform the client the therapist is about to break contact.

Key terms

Distal – point furthest away from the body.

Proximal – point closest to the body.

Anterior – front of body.

Posterior – back of body.

Medial – towards the middle/centre of the body.

Lateral – away from the middle/outside of the body.

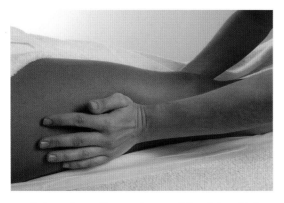

△ Palmer kneading to the outside of the thigh

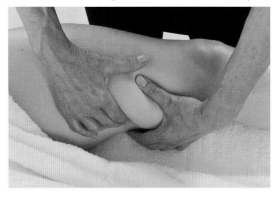

△ Wringing to the medial aspect of the thigh

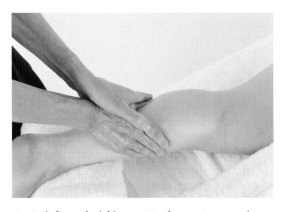

△ Reinforced picking up to the gastrocnemius

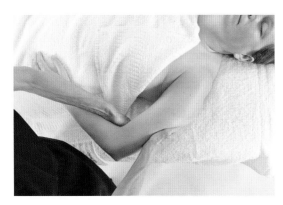

△ Rolling to the posterior aspect of the upper arm

Petrissage

Petrissage comes from the French 'petrir' which means to knead. Petrissage is a compression movement performed using intermittent pressure, either with one hand, both or part of the hands. It consists of grasping or compressing the skin, a muscle group, a muscle or part of a muscle and applying pressure, then releasing the pressure, before progressing to an adjacent area and repeating the process.

Kneading movements are generally described by the part of the hand used to accomplish the massage, i.e. palmar or thumb kneading, and rely on the compression of the tissues onto the underlying bony structures. Others such as wringing, picking up and rolling rely on the tissues being lifted away from the bone and being manipulated by squeezing and then releasing for their effect.

Although the pressure in petrissage is intermittent, great care must be taken to avoid pinching the skin and the superficial tissues. To avoid this, pressure should be gradually reduced as the bulk of tissues diminish under the hand. The pressure used must vary according to the purpose of the massage and the bulk of the tissues under treatment.

The direction of the petrissage movements depends on the purpose for which the massage is being given, for example when massaging a limb the massage may be started at the proximal part and each succeeding movement performed more distally, providing the heavy pressure is applied centrally to aid venous and lymphatic flow.

An even rate and rhythm should be established and can mimic effleurage movements, i.e. 15 strokes per minute to maintain the rhythm of the massage routine.

For effective kneading it is essential that:

- the client is in a comfortable relaxed position with the area being massaged supported with bolsters if necessary
- the movements are performed slowly, gently and rhythmically
- the hand performing the movement conforms to the contour of the area being treated
- effleurage is used freely to link the petrissage movements and afterwards to drain the area.

The effects and benefits of petrissage:

- the compression and relaxation of muscle tissue, which causes veins and lymphatics to be filled and emptied, thus increasing their circulation and the removal of waste products
- an increase in deep muscular circulation, which removes lactic acid, eliminating fatigue and muscle stiffness

- hard, contracted muscles are relaxed and softened, preventing the formation of fibrosis nodules (tension) in the tissue

- the skin, superficial and deep tissues are all stimulated to improve their function and activity

- petrissage movements produce a toning effect on muscular tissue, which can act as a reinforcement to natural exercise

- increased lymphatic and blood circulation

- increased venous return

- helps to soften and mobilise fat

- more effective than deep effleurage in aiding the absorption of substances within the tissues.

Uses of petrissage:

- To improve poor blood circulation in areas indicated by cold skin.

- To prevent or relieve oedema.

- To improve muscle condition and function.

- To maintain muscle tone and elasticity.

- To remove fibrous adhesions and tension in the muscles.

- To provide relaxation and act as a sedative when performed slowly or to stimulate and invigorate to combat fatigue when performed briskly.

Tapotement

These movements may be referred to as percussion manipulations. They consist of a series of brief, rapidly applied contacts of the hand or hands in alternating movements. The hands must be kept loose and mobile so that all the movements produced are light, springy and stimulating.

Types of tapotement movements:

- hacking

- cupping/clapping

- beating

- pounding.

Hacking

The technique for hacking is performed with the elbows bent and arms abducted. The hands should be at right angles to the wrists, the palms facing but not touching. The movement is of pronation and supination of the forearm allowing the ulna side but dorsal surface of the 5th, 4th and 3rd fingers to strike the area being treated. First one hand then the other is used in quick succession. The wrists should be extended with the fingers slightly flexed, yet fairly relaxed. This movement must produce a quick, springy flick, not a dull, heavy blow.

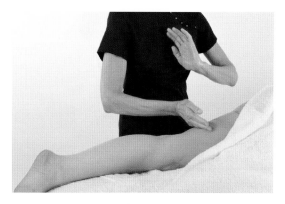

△ Hacking to the hamstrings of the thigh

377

Key terms

Dorsal – back/topside of the body.

Plantar – underside of the body.

If a deeper effect is required where there is more tissue bulk, such as on the gluteals in the buttocks, then the ulna border only of the hands and fingers can be used. Hacking can be performed with the tips of the fingers for more delicate areas such as the face; this movement consists of flexion and extension of the wrists. This is referred to as point hacking, tapping or digital tapotement. Hacking is always performed across the muscle fibres.

The effects and benefits of hacking:

- If light hacking is used across the muscle fibres it can cause them to contract momentarily as a response to the stimuli. Nerve paths become clearer and muscle tone improves.

- There is a local rise in skin temperature and an erythema is produced due to the increased blood supply. Therefore hacking can be used to warm up cold areas.

- A very stimulating effect is produced on the circulatory and muscular systems. The client will experience a glowing and tingly sensation due to the increased flow of blood to the muscles, which is good for sluggish circulation.

- Light hacking may be used over the abdominal organs as it helps to stimulate their action and to aid digestion.

- Light hacking may be used down either side of the spine, which will stimulate the spinal nerves.

- Stimulates sensory nerve endings.

- Adipose tissue can be picked up and hacked with one hand, which will aid its combustion within the system; this helps to reduce obesity.

- Helps to loosen mucus in chest conditions.

- Improves blemished skin.

Contraindications to hacking:

- Never use over bony areas.

- Never use over painful or sore areas.

- Never use if the client is nervous, excitable or if a more relaxing and sedative effect is desired.

Cupping

The technique involves the palms of the hands contracting to form a hollow cup shape. The fingers are closed and the thumbs abducted. The wrists must be flexible and the movements of flexion and extension take place in the wrist. The hands endeavour to form a suction effect as they strike the area under treatment. The hands must spring off the part lightly and quickly, creating a hollow, cupping sound. The hands are used alternately.

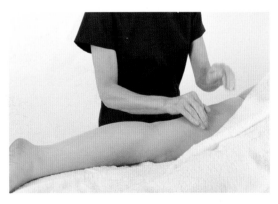

△ Cupping to anterior hamstrings of the thigh

The effects and benefits of cupping:

- Blood flow is increased to the skin, a local erythema is evident and skin condition improves.
- Local rise in skin temperature and sensation of warmth.
- Nervous system is stimulated.
- Tissue activity is increased; useful over areas of adipose tissue.

Beating

In this technique the hands are formed into loose fists and either the back of the hand is allowed to strike the area or the back of the fingers with the heel of the hand. The movement comes from the elbow with a kind of flick from the wrist while the hands are circling each other. It is performed in a quick manner and can be made heavy for areas of increased tissue bulk.

The effects and benefits of beating:

- Very stimulating to the blood circulation.
- A local erythema is produced.
- Local rise in skin temperature.
- Sensory nerve endings are stimulated.
- Reflex contraction of underlying muscle tissue.
- Breakdown of adipose tissue.

Pounding

The technique requires the hands to form into loose fists and the ulnar border of the hand is used to strike the area. The hands are allowed to drop from shoulder height to strike the area. The movement comes from the elbow and uses gravity to assist and not the strength within the arms. It is a heavy percussion movement and is performed rhythmically, either quickly or slowly depending on the effect required.

The effects and benefits are similar as for beating.

Vibration

Vibrations are shaking or fine trembling movements performed with one or both hands. The tips of the index fingers, the first two fingers or the distal phalanx of the thumb may be used. The muscles of the forearm are contracted and relaxed rapidly, so a fine, rapid trembling is produced.

Vibrations are always applied to a nerve or a nerve pathway. The vibrations can be static, i.e. performed in one place, or if the fingers are run along the course of the nerve they are known as running nerve vibrations. They can be fairly gentle or more vigorous.

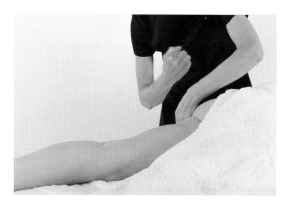

△ Beating to the lateral aspect of the thigh and gluteals

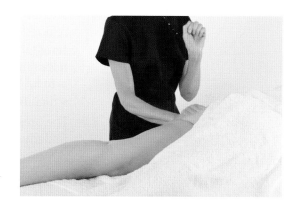

△ Pounding to the gluteals

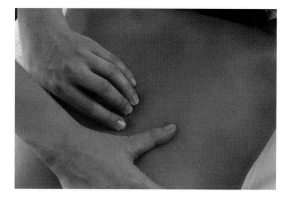

△ Vibrations along the spine

The effects and benefits of vibrations:

- Stimulates the nerves and clears nerve paths.
- Relieves pain as they have a sedative effect.
- Can be used to help to loosen old scar tissues and to stretch adhesions.
- Relieves tension in the neck and long muscles of the back.
- Increases the action of the lungs.

Frictions

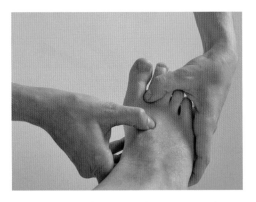

△ Frictions to between the metatarsals

Although frictions are classified within the petrissage group they do have a different purpose and effect from the kneading movements. Frictions are stationary pressure manipulations; they are concentrated movements exerting deep, controlled pressure on a small area of the surface tissues, moving them over the underlying structures.

The movements are applied in a circular manner, using the pad of the thumb, fingers or thumb pad of the palm. Several small circles are completed over a limited area, with a gradual increase in pressure to achieve a maximum depth into the muscle or structures being treated. It is important to release the pressure completely before moving onto an adjacent area but contact should not be lost.

Friction movements may also be applied along a muscle and are then referred to as transverse frictions. A steady, even pressure is maintained across the muscle fibres and its purpose is to produce a stretching, releasing effect on the tissues. The purpose of the friction movements is to loosen adherent skin, loosen scars, free adhesions of deeper structures and to aid in the absorption of fluid around the joints.

The pressure is firm and deep but not so heavy as to cause injury to underlying structures. The movement is usually applied in a circular direction and the pressure of the movement must be applied in the direction that will produce tension on the involved structures in order to strengthen and loosen them. The movement, when applied along a muscle, should follow the muscle fibres and it is usual to perform linking deep effleurage movements during and after frictions.

When applying frictions care must be taken not to cause a deadening sensation with too much pressure, unless specifically required.

One or two hands may be used to perform friction movements:

- two thumbs alternately
- one thumb supporting and the other thumb working against it
- over larger flatter surfaces one palm does the friction movement, reinforced by the other hand.

The effects and benefits of frictions:

- Adhesions are broken down and freed, improving stiff joints. A localised erythema is produced, which brings nourishment to the area and softens the adhesion.

⭐ *Hints and tips*
It is important to refrain from hyper-extending the fingers, particularly when working deeply, as this places strain on the joints of the therapist's fingers.

- Can prevent the formation of fibrositis in muscular tissue if regularly applied and will aid the dispersal of fibrous nodules.

- Can loosen and stretch scar tissue.

- Can prevent the formation of skin adhesions and newly formed milia will often be taken back into the system if firmly massaged.

- By producing a localised erythema it is possible to nourish joint structures and by so doing help to prevent arthritic conditions developing and increase and maintain mobility of joints.

- Spinal frictions can be very invigorating as they stimulate the spinal nerves. This leaves the client with a 'glowing' feeling.

- Frictions aid the absorption of fluid around the joints, particularly oedema in the ankle area. This may only be applied if the condition is not systemic, has been medically checked and is simply caused by poor circulation, tiredness, etc.

Massage routine

A massage routine can vary greatly from the area of the body on which to start the routine to the movements/manipulations to include, as well as the order in which the movements are performed. Before the routine begins it may be necessary to cleanse the client's face of make-up using appropriate cleanser and toner for their skin type if the face is to be included in the routine. The feet may need cleaning with eau de cologne or a sterilising agent if a shower is not available for the client to use.

Below is a suggested routine but other routines may have their individual benefits and preferences.

Massage procedure for a full body massage with client in a supine (face up) position:

- Left foot (2 minutes)

- Right foot (2 minutes)

- Front of right leg (4 minutes)

- Front of left leg (4 minutes)

- Left hand and arm (4 minutes)

- Right hand and arm (4 minutes)

- Abdomen (4 minutes)

- Neck and chest (5 minutes)

Massage procedure for a full body massage with client in a prone (face down) position:

- Back of right leg and gluteals (5 minutes)

- Back of left leg and gluteals (5 minutes)

- Back massage (15 minutes)

If the face and scalp are included a further 15 minutes is added to the length of the routine.

Manual massage treatment procedure

- Greet the client and introduce yourself.

- Carry out a full consultation.

- Inform the client which clothing to remove and how they should lie on the massage couch.

- Offer to help the client onto the couch and place support bolsters, for example at the neck and back of knees.

- Choose correct massage medium.

- Wash your hands.

- Ensure client is comfortable and warm.

- If you are carrying out a face and scalp massage you will need to cleanse the face at this point.

- Wipe over client's feet with steriliser (e.g. virkon) and if necessary rewash your hands.

- Apply massage medium using the procedure as outlined, ensuring client comfort and privacy at all times.

- At the end of the treatment offer the client a glass of water while you go through the homecare advice, for example, using oils in the bath or on a pillow, and asking how they feel. Ask they client if they have any queries.

- Assist the client getting off the couch.

- Tell client where you are going and leave them to dress in privacy.

Adaptation of manual massage treatment for male clients

Ideally, if male clients are to be a regular clientele of the salon it would be wise to decorate the salon in neutral colours. During the massage treatments consider making the heating slightly lower than for female clients as men generally do not feel the cold so readily. If a scent is used in the form of an essential oil try peppermint or tea tree but nothing 'flowery'. Ask the client what kind of music he would enjoy.

Changes to the routine include more pressure and depth to the movements as generally males have more muscle bulk and less adipose tissue; use your body weight to gain more depth rather than the strength in the arms as this is more likely to cause repetitive strain injuries in the hands, wrist and arms.

Stroking movements can be performed in the same direction of hair growth to avoid any discomfort by inadvertently pulling the hair. Do not work too close to the groin area by finishing movements low, particularly on the inside of the leg, and do not massage the lower abdomen and inner thigh. If the body is hairy oil or powder will need to be used.

⭐ *Hints and tips*

To avoid breaking the continuity of the routine and perhaps disturbing the client's enjoyment of the massage, it is important to consider the sequence in which the parts of the body are massaged. Your routine should consider the cleansing of the feet and the turning of the client to massage the reverse side.

 Health and safety

If a client of the opposite gender is booked for treatment, do not be alone in the salon or make the appointment for the very end of the day, to minimise the risk of encouraging inappropriate behaviour from the client. Always be professional.

Pregnant clients

A pregnant client should not receive massage in the first trimester but once this has passed it is perfectly safe to receive massage, as long as there are no further complications such as high blood pressure.

Prepare the massage environment with soothing, relaxing music and have additional pillows for support. Prop up the client if lying on their side or sitting on a chair. The head of the massage couch can be slightly raised and/or the legs, especially if the feet or ankles are swollen.

Concentrate the routine on the back, especially if there is lower back pain. After the first trimester the abdomen can be massaged using effleurage only. If the ankles are swollen, use effleurage movements on the calf and upper leg to help drain the fluid, massaging above the swelling.

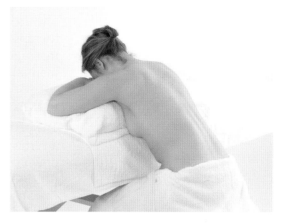

△ Client in a sitting position for massage treatment

Elderly clients

Elderly clients may be less mobile and may need you to be present to help them on and off the massage couch. Electric couches that can be adapted to a very low level can assist in getting the client onto the couch.

As many elderly clients lose muscle bulk as well as tone they may feel the cold more and so a higher room temperature may be appropriate. Additional blankets for warmth and pillows and/or bolsters for support are advisable.

Many elderly clients suffer from osteoarthritis so avoid joint manipulations and use light pressure on reduced tissue bulk. You may use more effleurage than petrissage movements and avoid the heavier tapotement movements such as beating and pounding; hacking can be used successfully however.

If the client has high or low blood pressure and following medical referral, adapt the procedure for getting them off the massage couch by raising the head of the couch and sitting them up while they drink water and you offer aftercare advice. Slowly get the client to their feet and place a chair for them to sit on while they get dressed. Avoid over-relaxing or stimulating massage to keep the blood pressure more stable.

Disabled clients

Medical permission should be obtained before massaging a disabled client. It may be necessary to have a carer present during the treatment to answer questions if the client is considered to be a vulnerable adult. The carer may also need to help the client dress and undress. In such cases the carer should remain throughout the massage treatment. For a physically disabled client an electric couch that can go quite low and assistance out of a wheelchair may be necessary. Additional pillows and bolsters may be required to provide extra comfort.

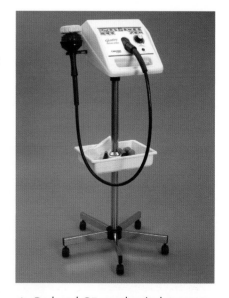

△ Pedestal G5 mechanical massage unit

Perform mechanical massage treatment

The use of mechanical massage adds another dimension to the therapist's skills. It provides the opportunity for deep and lasting massage effects without the strain and risk of injury to the therapist if manual techniques were used to achieve the same effects.

Gyratory massage

The pedestal gyrator such as the G5 is floor standing and works in a vertical and horizontal plan, i.e. circular (horizontal) and up and down (vertical).

Types of applicator

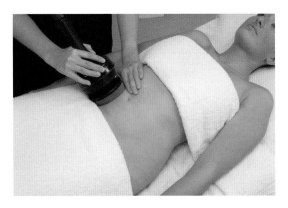

△ G5 sponge applicator

- The smooth-surfaced or sponge applicator is used at the beginning and end of the treatment and is a strong version of effleurage movements used in manual massage. As with effleurage, the applicator should be used in one direction towards the lymph node and following the venous return of blood. Two shapes exist: flat and moulded.

- The ball-studded applicator gives deep, penetrating effects, similar to petrissage in manual massage. There are many variations of this applicator, some with as few as two ball shapes to those with numerous shapes. All produce the same effects but your choice of which to use is determined by the size and part of the body you are working on. The applicators should be used in a rotary fashion to emulate petrissage movements.

- The brush or spiked applicator gives effects similar to tapotement in manual massage with the improvement of skin tone and texture. A high degree of desquamation can be achieved with this applicator.

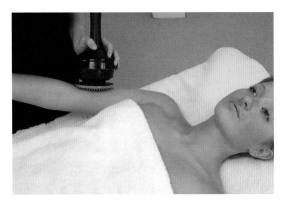

△ G5 spiked applicator

The applicators should not be used with oil or cream as a massage medium, as this will lead to them perishing. Instead a powder such as talc should be used. After use they should be washed in warm soapy water. They should then be sterilised in a chemical sterilising agent, rinsed and dried thoroughly. As with all electrical equipment, the vibratory unit should be serviced regularly to maintain its working life.

Hand-held gyrator

A hand-held gyratory massager produces similar effects to the pedestal version but for a lower cost. They are more tiring to the therapist as they must hold the weight of the machine. The equipment cannot be used for more than 15 minutes at one time as the powerful motor is encased in a small compartment and it may overheat.

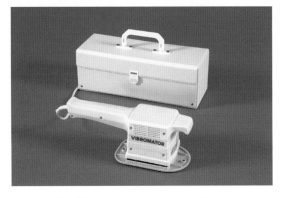

△ Hand-held gyratory massage unit

Audio-sonic massager

As the name implies, audio-sonic massager uses sound waves to create the vibration, a little like a tuning fork which, when tapped causes vibration.

It is a hand-held device which is really suitable only for treatment on localised areas. Sound waves are used to create the effects by putting the air-filled cavities of the body and the soft tissues through sound vibrations, which brings about gentle stimulation and relief of tension. The sound vibrations travel through soft tissue, such as muscle, easily relieving discomfort caused by fibrositis and other fibrous adhesions. Although the surface skin reaction is only slight, making it suitable for hypersensitive skins, the depth of vibratory effects can penetrate as much as two inches. The same intensity is obtained at that depth as at the skin surface.

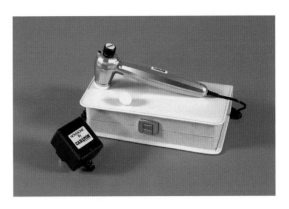

△ Audio-sonic massager

△ Comparison of depth of vibration between gyratory and audio-sonic

The vibrations are able to penetrate further at the same intensity, which means that fibrous nodules can be relieved. The action of the vibrations appears to 'shake' or vibrate the nodules loose. It is also useful in the treatment of deep, soft, fat deposits where the skin is sensitive or a vascular condition exists, a condition common in older clients on legs, upper arms and abdomen.

Audio-sonic can also be used for a longer period of time than a gyrator over the buttocks and thighs to break down adipose tissue, where excessive irritation or erythema may cause a premature halt to the treatment before results can be obtained.

Relief from migraine can be obtained with use along the trapezius muscle to the occipital.

Audio-sonic is not, however, suitable for use over bony areas or over the abdominal area due to the vibrations penetrating into the deeper tissues.

Types of applicator

- The flat disc head is used for general face, neck and body massage (localised areas), directly or indirectly (over the hand).

- The round, hard head is used when an intensified action is required, for example fibrous adhesions in the trapezius.

Table 11.6 summarises the differences between audio-sonic and gyratory massagers.

▽ Table 11.6 Differences between audio-sonic and gyratory massagers

Audio-sonic massager	Gyratory massager
Penetrates at equal intensity	Gets weaker the deeper the penetration
Penetrates to a depth of 6 cm or 2.5 inches	Less penetration
Less reaction on skin surface due to sound waves	Tapping movements create advanced skin reaction (erythema)
Can be used on sensitive and loose skin conditions	Not advisable for sensitive or loose skins
Less likely to cause broken capillaries, bruising, etc.	Liable to cause broken capillaries and bruising
Do not use on bony or abdominal areas due to the depth of sound waves	Areas can be treated indirectly (over the hand)

Contraindications for mechanical massage:

- Very thin clients
- Very loose, crêpey skin
- History of slipped disc (avoid the back area)
- Areas of extreme hair growth (use the spiked applicator)
- Pregnancy (avoid the abdomen)
- During menstruation (avoid the abdomen)
- Care should be taken when treating the abdomen with poor muscle tone as there is no supporting tissue.

Table 11.7 summarises the effects and uses of mechanical massage treatment.

▽ Table 11.7 Effects and uses of mechanical massage treatment

Physiological, psychological and physical effects	Treatment uses
• Increases blood circulation • Increases lymph drainage • Improves skin metabolism • Improves skin texture • Relaxes muscles • Aids desquamation so skin feels smoother • Breaks down fatty tissue • Breaks down fibrous thickenings in muscle tissue • Tones muscles • Soothes nerve endings (audio-sonic only) • Relaxing	• To maintain a client's interest in figure reduction (swifter results) • Relax muscles and relieve stiffness after physical exertion (exercise) • Aids a slimming diet by making adipose tissue more available as a source of energy • Skin types requiring stimulation, e.g. sluggish, mature and dehydrated skin • Relaxation • Audio-sonic is indicated on sensitive skins or those that redden easily • Cellulite

Mechanical massage treatment procedure

1 Prepare the client as for normal body treatments.

2 Decide on which applicator heads are to be used. If relaxation only is required then the smooth, soothing aspects of the equipment combined with manual massage should be considered. A combined treatment should last 30–40 minutes and be a general application to the whole body. If weight loss and figure reduction are required then the stimulating applicators can be used in a more localised fashion.

3 Apply talc to the area being treated with light, stroking manual massage movements.

4 Using the smooth-surfaced applicator (sponge) apply long, sweeping upward strokes towards the heart. Follow the natural contours of the body and use your free hand to support the area being worked.

5 Follow the sequence of full body manual massage for a general, relaxing application, i.e. right leg, left leg, left arm, chest, right arm, abdomen, shoulders and back, buttocks and thigh, and back.

6 For a more stimulating massage, the sponge applicator is used first, then kneading with ball-studded applicator. The spiked or brush-type applicator follows in areas of adequate subcutaneous fat. All are interlinked with effleurage manual massage. A good sequence to follow is:

 a) the legs

 b) the abdomen (more lightly and controlled)

 c) the arms and chest (avoid ball-studded applicator as there is not enough flesh)

 d) the back

 e) the buttocks and back of thighs.

7 Always finish each area with manual massage effleurage to reinforce relaxation by maintaining client contact. Finally, cover the area worked to maintain and prolong the effects of the massage.

The above is a guideline for application and the sequence can be altered to benefit client needs. The treatment can be combined with manual massage, heat treatments such as infra-red or on its own for localised treatment of the back, buttocks or thighs.

Hand-held gyrators are used in a similar way but are not used to treat the whole body, as it is tiring for the therapist and could cause the motor of the machine to burn out if used for a prolonged period. It is useful to treat specific areas and for localised treatment.

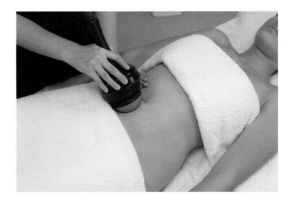

△ The gyratory massager in use

Adaptations for treatment

Generally, mechanical massage gives a deeper and more therapeutic massage than can be achieved by manual massage but it should not replace the use of manual massage entirely. A mechanical massage on its own can be very impersonal and cannot replace the therapist's touch and the benefits and sense of well-being that brings. Always introduce the client to massage with manual techniques, introducing the mechanical massage later into the routine, and complete the massage with manual techniques so they are the lasting memories that the client experiences.

Pre-heat treatments

Pre-heat treatments involve the use of sources of heat to intensify the effects of massage on the body's tissues. The types of heat treatment available are:

- infra-red heat lamps
- hot towels
- paraffin wax
- hot stones
- sauna
- steam room or bath
- spa-pool.

The latter three forms may not be readily available for use in a high-street salon but infra-red and hot towels can easily be utilised in most salon environments.

The benefits of such heat treatments are:

- increases body temperature
- induces perspiration
- eliminates waste products
- increases blood circulation
- produces an erythema
- lowers blood pressure
- raises pulse rate
- increases metabolic rate
- induces weight loss
- improves lymph flow
- warms the tissues
- relaxes muscles
- relieves minor pain and stiffness
- gives a feeling of relaxation and well-being (but may also induce fatigue or exhaustion).

Infra-red

Luminous infra-red lamps are known as radiant heat lamps. They emit infra-red light rays through an infra-red treatment bulb to produce a red-coloured light that is visible. They are safer than the non-luminous type, which produce light rays invisible to the human eye and so cannot be detected. More information on infra-red lamps can be found in Chapter 5 Theory of electrical currents.

Both luminous and non-luminous types of lamp have a heating and therapeutic effect on the body's tissues. The skin becomes warmer, sweating increases and blood circulation will increase locally in the area as the blood vessels dilate. The subsequent reddening of the skin is called hyperaemia. The infra-red rays have a soothing effect on the sensory nerve endings, promoting relaxation and a sense of well-being and relieving localised pain. The underlying muscle tissue relaxes due to the heating action of the lamp and the local increase in blood circulation. Muscle stiffness is relieved and fibrous adhesions are relaxed by the action of the heat. Popular areas for using this service are the lower back, shoulders, legs and buttocks.

As a pre-heating treatment, infra-red is usually applied 10 minutes before massage application. The infra-red lamp does have its disadvantages, however. For example, heat can only be applied to localised areas because of the limitations of the arc of light from the lamp.

Procedure for infra-red treatment

1. The infra-red lamp is heated in advance of the treatment.

2. Prepare the client comfortably on the couch.

3. Check lamp.

4. Cover areas not to be exposed with towels.

5. While the lamp is heating the area can be prepared with manual effleurage movements.

6. Position the lamp so the skin feels comfortably warm (a distance of 45–90 cm) and so that it is parallel to the skin's surface. The arm of the lamp should be over a leg of the stand for stability.

7. Stay in close attendance to check the skin reaction.

8. Treatment can last 10–30 minutes, depending on skin sensitivity, the body part being treated and the distance of the lamp from the skin.

9. Remove lamp, switch off and allow to cool in a safe place.

10. Deep, penetrating massage can follow to relieve tension.

11. The client may be left warmly covered for complete relaxation.

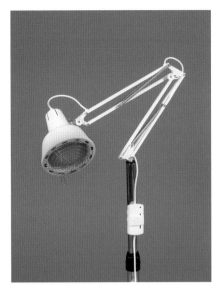

△ Infra-red lamp

Key term

Hyperaemia – The increase of blood flow to different tissues in the body.

Health and safety

Infra-red is applied to skin that is clean from products and free from jewellery. It is important that a tactile and thermal skin sensation test is performed before the treatment. Ensure no contraindications are present. As a precaution it is good practice for the client to wear protective eye shields to prevent injury to the eyes.

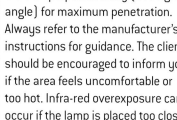

Health and safety

The rays from the bulb must strike the skin perpendicularly (at a right angle) for maximum penetration. Always refer to the manufacturer's instructions for guidance. The client should be encouraged to inform you if the area feels uncomfortable or too hot. Infra-red overexposure can occur if the lamp is placed too close or the duration of the treatment is too long. This could result in burns, headaches or fainting.

Remember...

As a reminder, the contra-actions to massage are:

- lethargy
- headache
- muscle ache
- nausea
- increased emotions
- frequent urination
- bruising
- allergy to the massage medium.

 LO12 # Aftercare advice for massage treatment

The aftercare advice for massage treatment can be considered under the following headings:

- avoidance of activities which may cause contra-actions
- future treatment needs
- modification of lifestyle patterns
- healthy eating and exercise advice
- suitable homecare products and their use.

Avoidance of activities which may cause contra-actions

For 12–24 hours following treatment the client should be advised to:

- rest, to give the tissues time to recover/heal
- drink plenty of water to rid the body of toxins that have been released into the blood stream
- avoid physical exercise as the muscles need to rest to recover
- ensure light food intake; indigestion is likely if a heavy meal is eaten as the blood supply has been diverted to the muscles, etc.
- avoid alcohol as this will add more toxins to the body
- deal with an allergic reaction by washing off the massage medium with warm water and seeking medical advice if necessary.

Future treatment needs

The client should be advised to:

- return for further massage treatment about once per week or more frequently if needed
- consider the use of heat therapy such as infra-red if appropriate
- consider the use of mechanical massage if appropriate.

Modification of lifestyle patterns

The client should be advised to:

- perform relaxation techniques such as deep breathing exercises
- allocate time for self and take up a hobby or interest that is absorbing
- monitor sleep patterns, avoid alcohol in the evening and go to bed at a reasonable time if sleeping is a problem
- promote sleep by the use of essential oils on the pillow
- have a relaxing bath before bedtime to induce sleep
- avoid stimulants such as cola drinks, tea, coffee and alcohol after 6pm

- give up smoking or at least cut down on the number of cigarettes smoked in a day

- eat regularly and healthily.

Healthy eating and exercise advice

The client should be advised to:

- perform postural exercises to help relieve aches and pains

- perform stretching exercises for those muscles that have shortened and toning exercises for those that have lengthened

- walk briskly for 30 minutes a day

- eat light meals frequently

- eat five portions of fruit and vegetables per day

- reduce sugar intake as this gives a 'sugar high' followed by an extreme low and can lead to low metabolism and diabetes

- reduce alcohol levels and have at least three days per week that are alcohol free

- drink plenty of water and fruit juice

- reduce the intake of coffee and other high-caffeine drinks

- avoid low-calorie diets as they lower the metabolism.

Suitable homecare products and their use

The client should be advised to:

- purchase a natural bristle body brush to perform dry brushing as a detox aid for the treatment of cellulite

- use scented candles to aid relaxation.

Methods of evaluation

To be an effective therapist it is beneficial to reflect on the massage treatment to ensure client satisfaction, promote good client relationships and encourage the client's return of custom.

The therapist should consider the short- and long-term effects of the treatment to evaluate the effectiveness of their choice of product, massage technique or equipment and to judge whether it has been beneficial to the client and the condition they presented for treatment.

Methods of evaluating a massage treatment include:

- visual assessment

- verbal assessment

- written feedback.

 Remember...

The benefits of a change in lifestyle include sleeping well and waking refreshed. This will lead to less fatigue during the day and an increased ability to cope with stressful situations.

Visual assessment

Visual assessment of the area should be performed after the treatment to ascertain the immediate effects. The therapist may note a change in skin colour or temperature, or the client's posture may have improved immediately after the treatment. Making accurate notes on the client's record card will mean a comparison can be made at the beginning of the next treatment.

Verbal assessment

Asking the client how they feel immediately after the treatment can give insight into the effectiveness of the treatment. The client may complain of headache or even nausea but these are signs that the treatment has been effective and the appropriate aftercare advice should be given to prevent these contra-actions becoming worse.

On the client's return visit a few probing questions of how they felt several hours and then days after the treatment can reveal useful details and can shape the follow-up treatment.

Written feedback

The client can be asked to provide written feedback. For this to be of real use they should be given some simple questions and a choice of possible answers otherwise the information obtained may be quite bland and ineffective.

 Want to know more?

For more information on massage and its professional implementation go to the website of the General Council for Massage Therapy: www.gcmt.org.uk

---

NVQ assessment checklist

To complete this unit you must have the following theoretical and practical skills. Check against the list below and refer back to the relevant section for information on anything you are unsure about.

1. **Be able to maintain safe and effective methods of working when providing body massage treatments**

☐ **1.1** set up and maintain the treatment area to meet legal, hygiene and service requirements

☐ **1.2** maintain personal hygiene, protection and appearance that meets accepted industry and organisational requirements

☐ **1.3** clean all tools and equipments using the correct methods

☐ **1.4** position equipment and massage mediums for safety and ease of use

☐ **1.5** position the client and themselves to minimise fatigue and risk of injury and and for the treatment

☐ **1.6** use industry hygiene and safety practices throughout the treatment to minimise the risk of cross-infection

☐ **1.7** adopt a positive, polite and reassuring manner towards the client throughout the treatment

☐ **1.8** maintain the client's modesty, privacy and comfort throughout the treatment

☐ **1.9** complete the treatment within a commercially viable time

☐ **1.10** keep the records up to date, accurate, easy to read and signed by the client and practitioner

☐ **1.11** leave the treatment area and equipment in a suitable condition for future treatments

2. **Be able to consult, plan and prepare to provide body massage treatments**

☐ **2.1** use consultation techniques to determine the client's treatment needs

☐ **2.2** obtain signed, written and informed consent prior to carrying out the treatment from the client or parent/guardian if the client is a minor

☐ **2.3** question the client to identify the client's medical history, physical characteristics and lifestyle pattern

☐ **2.4** consult with the client to identify any contraindications to facial electrical treatments, recording the client's responses, taking any necessary action

❏ **2.5** provide client advice without referring to a specific medical condition and without causing undue alarm and concern

❏ **2.6** explain and agree the projected cost, likely duration, frequency and types of treatment needed

❏ **2.7** agree in writing the client's needs, expectations and treatment objectives, ensuring they are realistic and achievable

❏ **2.8** clean and prepare the client's skin to suit the type of massage to be given

❏ **2.9** protect the client's clothing, hair and accessories prior to beginning massage

❏ **2.10** select equipment and related products to suit the treatment objectives

3. Be able to perform manual massage treatments

❏ **3.1** check that the client's body is suitably supported prior to and during the treatment

❏ **3.2** adapt massage techniques, sequence and massage mediums to meet the client's physical characteristics and treatment area(s)

❏ **3.3** vary the depth, rhythm and pressure of massage movements to meet treatment objective, treatment area(s) and client's physical characteristics and preferences

❏ **3.4** apply and use massage oil medium to minimise waste

❏ **3.5** take prompt remedial action if contra-actions or discomfort occur during the course of treatment

❏ **3.6** give the client sufficient post-treatment recovery time

❏ **3.7** consult with the client to confirm the finished result is to the client's satisfaction and meets the agreed treatment objectives

❏ **3.8** provide aftercare advice specific to the client's individual needs

4. Be able to perform mechanical massage treatments

❏ **4.1** explain to the client the sensation created by the equipment used

❏ **4.2** explain the treatment procedure to the client in a clear and simple way at each stage in the process

❏ **4.3** check the client's body is suitably supported prior to and during the treatment

❏ **4.4** use safely the correct treatment settings, application and applicator heads on the body throughout the treatment to meet manufacturers' instructions

❏ **4.5** adjust the intensity and duration of the treatment to suit the client's physical characteristics and the treatment area(s)

❏ **4.6** vary the sequence, depth and pressure of massage movements to meet treatment objectives and treatment area(s)

❏ **4.7** check the client's wellbeing throughout the mechanical massage treatment

❏ **4.8** take prompt remedial action if contra-actions or discomfort occur during the course of treatment

❏ **4.9** give the client sufficient post-treatment recovery time

❏ **4.10** check the finished result is to the client's satisfaction and meets the agreed treatment objectives

❏ **4.11** provide aftercare advice specific to the client's individual needs

5. Understand organisational and legal requirements for protecting body massage treatments

❏ **5.1** explain own responsibilities under relevant health and safety legislation, standards and guidance

❏ **5.2** explain own responsibilities under local authority licensing regulations for themselves and the premises

❏ **5.3** explain the importance of not discriminating against clients with illnesses and disabilities and why

❏ **5.4** state the age at which an individual is classed as a minor and how this differs nationally

❏ **5.5** explain why it is important, when treating minors under 16 years of age, to have a parent or guardian present

❏ **5.6** explain why minors should not be given treatments without informed and signed parental or guardian present

❏ **5.7** explain the legal significance of gaining signed, informed consent to treatment

❏ **5.8** explain own responsibilities and reasons for maintaining personal hygiene, protection and appearance according to accepted industry and organisational requirements

❏ **5.9** explain the manufacturers' and organisational requirements for waste disposal

❏ **5.10** explain the importance of the correct storage of client records in relation to the Data Protection Act

❏ **5.11** explain how to complete the client records and the reasons for keeping records of treatments and gaining client signatures

❏ **5.12** explain the organisation's requirements for client preparation

❏ **5.13** explain the organisation's service times for body massage treatments and the importance of completing the service in a commercially viable time

❏ **5.14** explain own responsibilities and reasons for keeping own nails short, clean, well-manicured and free of polish for massage treatments

❏ **5.15** explain the organisation's and manufacturers' requirements for treatment area, equipment maintenance and equipment cleaning regimes

6. **Understand how to work safely and effectively when providing body massage treatments**

❏ **6.1** explain how to set up the work area for body massage treatments

❏ **6.2** explain the necessary environmental conditions for body massage treatments (including lighting, heating, ventilation, sound and general comfort) and why these are important

❏ **6.3** explain the reasons for disinfecting hands and how to do this effectively

❏ **6.4** explain how to position themselves and the client for body massage treatments taking into account individual physical characteristics

❏ **6.5** explain what repetitive strain injury (RSI) is, how it is caused and how to avoid developing it when delivering massage treatments

❏ **6.6** explain the importance of adopting the correct posture throughout the treatment an the impact this may have on themselves and the outcome of the treatment

❏ **6.7** explain the reasons for maintaining client modesty, privacy and comfort during the treatment

❏ **6.8** explain why it is important to maintain standards of hygiene and the principles of avoiding cross-infection

❏ **6.9** explain how to minimise and dispose of waste treatments

❏ **6.10** explain why it is important to check the client's wellbeing at regular intervals during mechanical massage

7. **Understand how to consult with clients**

❏ **7.1** explain how to use effective consultation techniques when communicating with clients from different cultural and religious backgrounds, ages, disabilities and genders for this treatment

❏ **7.2** explain why it is important to encourage and allow time for clients to ask questions

❏ **7.3** explain the importance of questioning clients to establish any contraindications to head and body massage treatments

❏ **7.4** explain why it is important to record client responses to questioning

❏ **7.5** explain the legal significance of client questioning and the recording of client responses

❏ **7.6** explain how to give effective advice and recommendations to clients

❏ **7.7** explain how to assess posture and skeletal conditions that may be present and how to adapt and change the massage routines

❏ **7.8** explain how to recognise different skin types and conditions

❏ **7.9** explain the reasons why it is important to encourage clients with contraindications to seek medical advice

❏ **7.10** explain the importance of and reasons for not naming specific contraindications when encouraging clients to seek medical advice

❏ **7.11** explain why it is important to maintain the client's modesty and privacy

❏ **7.12** explain the relationship between lifestyle patterns and effectiveness of treatment

❏ **7.13** explain the beneficial effects which can result from changes to the client's lifestyle pattern

8. **Understand how to prepare to provide body massage treatments**

❏ **8.1** explain the importance of giving clients clear instructions on the removal of relevant clothing, accessories and general preparation for the treatment

❏ **8.2** explain why it is important to reassure clients during the preparation for the treatment

❏ **8.3** explain how to select the appropriate massage medium suitable for skin type and condition

❏ **8.4** explain how to cleanse different areas of the body in preparation for treatment

9. **Understand anatomy and physiology related to body massage treatments**

❏ **9.1** explain the structure and function of cells and tissues

❏ **9.2** explain the structure and function of muscles, including the types of muscle

❏ **9.3** explain the positions and actions of the main muscle groups within the treatment areas of the body

❏ **9.4** explain the position and function of the primary bones and joints of the skeleton

❏ **9.5** explain how to recognise postural faults and conditions

❏ **9.6** explain the interaction of lymph and blood within the circulatory system

❏ **9.7** explain the structure and function of the lymphatic system

❏ **9.8** explain the basic principles of the central nervous system and autonomic system

❏ **9.9** explain the basic principles of the endocrine, respiratory, digestive and excretory systems

❏ **9.10** explain the structure and function of skin

❏ **9.11** compare the skin characteristics and skin types of different ethnic client groups

❏ **9.12** explain the structure and location of the adipose tissue

❏ **9.13** summarise the effects of massage on the individual systems of the body

❏ **9.14** explain the function of blood and the principles of circulation, blood pressure and pulse

❏ **9.15** summarise the physical and psychological effects of body massage

❏ **9.16** explain how to recognise erythema and hyperaemia and their causes

10. Understand contra-indications and contra-actions that affect or restrict body massage treatments

❏ **10.1** explain the contraindications that prevent treatment and why

❏ **10.2** explain the contra-indications which may restrict treatment or where caution should be taken, in specific areas and why

❏ **10.3** explain the possible contra-actions which may occur during and post-treatment, why and how to deal with them

11. Understand how to carry out body massage treatments

❏ **11.1** explain the preparation and application of the massage equipment

❏ **11.2** explain the benefits of using the massage equipment

❏ **11.3** explain the different types and uses of massage mediums

❏ **11.4** explain the types and benefits of pre-heat treatments which can be used prior to massage

❏ **11.5** explain why it is important to maintain correct posture during massage and complete their own stretching exercises to prevent repetitive strain injury

❏ **11.6** explain the correct use and application of massage techniques to meet a variety of treatment objectives

❏ **11.7** explain how to adapt the massage sequence, depth and pressure to suit different client physical characteristics, areas of the body and client preferences for manual massage

❏ **11.8** explain how to adapt the massage sequence, depth and pressure to suit different client physical characteristics and areas of the body for mechanical massage

❏ **11.9** explain how to adapt massage treatments for male and female clients

❏ **11.10** explain the areas of the body and body characteristics needing particular care when undertaking mechanical treatments

❏ **11.11** explain the advantages of mechanical and manual massage

❏ **11.12** evaluate the advantages of combining mechanical and manual massage

❏ **11.13** explain how to select and utilise massage equipment, media and techniques to achieve maximum benefits to the client

❏ **11.14** explain how and why support and cushioning would be used during the treatment

12. Understand how to provide aftercare advice

❏ **12.1** explain the lifestyle factors and changes that may be required to improve the effectiveness of the treatment

❏ **12.2** explain post-treatment restrictions and future treatment needs

❏ **12.3** explain products for home use that will benefit and protect the client and those to avoid and why

❏ **12.4** explain how eating and exercise habits can affect the effectiveness of treatment

Test yourself

1. Why is the use of 'props' or 'bolsters' necessary in a massage treatment?

2. What is the correct action to take if a client presents for massage treatment with a contraindication that prevents treatment?

3. What adaptations can be made to a massage treatment?

4. Which massage movement or manipulation is capable of loosening scar tissue, breaking down adhesions and increasing joint mobility?

   a) Effleurage
   b) Petrissage
   c) Frictions
   d) Percussion

5. Which massage movement or manipulation is not a tapotement or percussion movement?

   a) Hacking
   b) Cupping/clapping
   c) Stroking
   d) Pounding

6. State the effects and benefits of vibration massage movements or manipulations.

7. Which one of the following is the best direction to apply massage?

   a) Towards the lymph nodes
   b) Along the muscle fibres
   c) Towards lower limbs
   d) Pressure towards the heart

8. Which one of the following is not a contraindication to gyratory massage?

   a) Varicose veins
   b) Broken capillaries
   c) Cellulite
   d) Bruising

9. Name three sources of heat that can be used prior to a manual or mechanical massage treatment.

10. Which one of the following determines the distance of the lamp from the skin's tissues?

    a) Cosine law
    b) Grotthus law
    c) IInverse square law
    d) Hertz law

11. What are the contra-actions of overexposure to the use of infra-red lamps?

Chapter **12**

INDIAN HEAD MASSAGE TREATMENTS

This chapter covers:

NVQ unit B23 Provide Indian head massage

City & Guilds VRQ unit 311 Provide Indian head massage

VTCT VRQ unit UV30574 Provide Indian head massage

LEARNING OBJECTIVES

This chapter is about providing Indian head massage treatments.

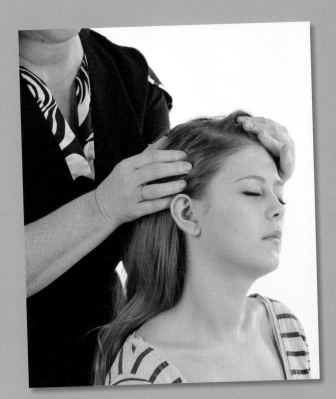

The learning outcomes for NVQ unit B23 are:
1 Be able to maintain safe and effective methods of working when providing Indian head massage
2 Be able to consult, plan and prepare for treatments with clients
3 Be able to perform Indian head massage
4 Understand how to work safely and effectively when providing Indian head massage
5 Understand how to consult with clients
6 Understand how to prepare for providing Indian head massages
7 Understand anatomy and physiology related to Indian head massages
8 Understand contraindications and contra-actions that affect or restrict body massage treatments
9 Understand different Indian head massage mediums
10 Understand the principles of Indian head massage
11 Understand how to provide aftercare advice

You will need to be competent in all of these outcomes to be competent in Indian head massage treatments, qualify for insurance and perform the treatments on members of the public.

NVQ evidence requirements

For the NVQ your assessor will need to observe you perform these treatments successfully on at least three occasions, each involving a different client. This includes:

- One massage treatment incorporating the use of massage oil.
- One massage which excludes the use of oil.

You must practically:

1 Demonstrate the use of all these consultation techniques:
  - questioning
  - visual
  - manual
  - reference to client records.

2 Deal with all these client physical characteristics:
  - posture
  - muscle tone
  - age
  - health
  - skin condition
  - hair condition
  - scalp condition.

3 Take one of the following necessary actions:
  - encourage the client to seek medical advice
  - explain why the treatment cannot be carried out
  - modify the treatment.

4 Meet all these treatment objectives:
  - relaxation
  - sense of well-being
  - uplifting
  - improvement of hair and scalp condition.

5 Use all these massage techniques:
  - effleurage
  - petrissage
  - tapotement
  - friction
  - Marma (pressure) points.

6 Massage all these treatment areas:
  - face
  - head
  - chest and shoulders
  - arms and hands
  - back
  - chakras.

7 Provide all these types of advice:
  - avoidance of activities which may cause contra-actions
  - future treatment needs
  - modifications to lifestyle patterns
  - suitable homecare products and their use.

VRQ practical evidence requirements

There are different evidence requirements for the VRQ qualifications dependant on the awarding body.

City & Guilds unit 311 Provide Indian head massage

- A minimum of two Indian head massage treatments should be carried out on two separate occasions before one final observation in front of an assessor.
- Each of these three occasions should be accompanied with a treatment plan that includes the client's history, lifestyle and treatment requirements; products used to suit skin type and condition; massage techniques selected and their adaptation to suit the client and contra-actions to the treatment and the correct response.

VTCT unit UV30574 Provide Indian head massage

- Three occasions covering the following range:

Consultation techniques:
- questioning
- visual
- manual
- reference to client records

Physical characteristics:
- posture
- muscle tone
- age
- health

- skin condition
- hair condition
- scalp condition

All the necessary actions:
- encourage the client to seek medical advice
- explain why the treatment cannot be carried out
- modify the treatment

Treatment objectives:
- relaxation
- sense of well-being
- uplifting
- improvement of hair and scalp condition

Massage techniques:
- effleurage
- petrissage
- tapotement
- friction
- Marma (pressure) points

Treated all areas:
- face
- head
- chest and shoulders
- arms and hands
- back
- chakras

In all cases simulation is NOT allowed.

VRQ knowledge requirements

City & Guilds unit 311 Provide Indian head massage	VTCT unit UV30574 Provide Indian head massage	Page no.
Learning outcome 1: Be able to prepare for Indian head massage		
Practical skills/observations		
Prepare themselves, client and work area for Indian head massage		415–7
Use suitable consultation techniques to identify treatment objectives		409–10
Provide clear recommendations to the client		433
Select products, tools and equipment to suit client treatment needs		418–20
Underpinning knowledge		
Describe salon requirements for preparing themselves, the client and work area		415–7
Describe the environmental conditions suitable for Indian head massage		415–6

City & Guilds unit 311 Provide Indian head massage	VTCT unit UV30574 Provide Indian head massage	Page no
Describe the different consultation techniques used to identify treatment objectives		409–10
Describe the importance of assessing the hair and scalp for any diseases and disorders prior to treatment		85
Explain how to select products, tools and equipment to suit client treatment needs		418–20
Explain the contraindications that prevent or restrict Indian head massage		410–11
Learning outcome 2: Be able to provide Indian head massage		
Practical skills/observations		
Communicate and behave in a professional manner		183–4
Follow health and safety working practices		407–8
Position themselves and client correctly throughout the treatment		409
Use products, tools, equipment and techniques to suit clients treatment needs		418–20
Complete the treatment to the satisfaction of the client		434
Record and evaluate the results of the treatment		436
Provide suitable aftercare advice		434–6
Underpinning knowledge		
Explain how to communicate and behave in a professional manner		183–4
Describe health and safety working practices		407–8
Explain the importance of positioning themselves and the client correctly throughout the treatment		409
Explain the importance of using products, tools, equipment and techniques to suit clients treatment need		418–22
Explain the effects and benefits of Indian head massage		417–8
Describe how treatments can be adapted to suit client treatment needs		433
State the contra-actions that may occur during and following treatments and how to respond		414–5
Explain the importance of completing the treatment to the satisfaction of the client		434
Explain the importance of completing treatment records		207
Explain the methods of evaluating the effectiveness of the treatment		436
Describe the aftercare advice that should be provided		434–6
Describe the structure and functions of the skins		64–70
Describe skin types, conditions, diseases and disorders		71–77
Describe the structure and function of the hair		82–83
Describe the structure of the neck, upper back and arms		91–95
Explain the position and action of the muscles in the upper back, neck and arms		105–9
Describe the structure, function and supply of the blood and lymph to the head		124–5; 127–9
Describe the location and function of chakras		405–7

Introduction

Westernised Indian head massage uses the manipulations or movements of Swedish massage combined with techniques based in ancient philosophies such as Marma points and chakras to bring about therapeutic effects on the shoulders, upper arms, neck, head, scalp, ears and face.

History and origins of Indian head massage

Indian head massage (IHM) originates from old Ayurvedic texts from the Hindu religion and written over 4,000 years ago. At this time, 'Ayurveda', which means 'the science of life', was used as a traditional form of medicine and practitioners prepared medical preparations, such as herbs, spices and aromatic oils and performed surgical procedures for the prevention and treatment of disease. This form of medicine can be found in the culture of many countries in Asia including India, Bangladesh, The Maldives, Pakistan and Sri Lanka and still remains an influential system of medicine in South Asia. It is also found further afield in Greek and Islamic medicine.

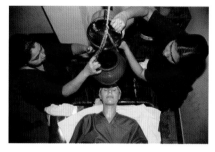

△ An Ayurvedic treatment

Ayurveda is considered in Western countries to be a form of complementary and alternative medicine but it is classed as the 'traditional' form of medicine by its practitioners in South Asia; in Sri Lanka there are more Ayurvedic practitioners than modern medicine professionals.

The ancient Ayurvedic texts state not only the use of preparations and surgical procedures but other treatments such as yoga, meditation and massage to balance the body and bring about equilibrium to the body's energy. This will then bring about self-healing as it is believed that body in a balanced state will be healthy, whereas an imbalanced body will be diseased. It is believed by practitioners of Ayurveda that the body has seven energy centres called 'chakras' which, when blocked, are the cause of imbalance in the body, resulting in disease.

Practitioners and followers of Ayurveda also believe in the 'maintenance' of the physical, emotional and spiritual health through the nourishment of the 'root of life'. In Ayurveda, there are three principles or 'doshas' for maintaining a healthy physical, mental and spiritual life: 'Dosha Vata', 'Dosha Pitta' and 'Dosha Kapha'. Each dosha is associated with the five elements: ether (space), air, fire, water and earth which, in turn, are associated with the health and maintenance of systems and organs of the body and mind.

Dosha Vata is associated with the elements ether and air and the movement and space within the body. The blood circulatory and nervous and endocrine systems are governed by Dosha Vata, as are conscious mental activities and the process of elimination. A person with excess 'vata' will tend to have dry hair and skin, a tendency to constipation, have poor blood circulation with cold feet and hands and have high energy levels so cannot stay still for very long. When the vata is low, a person is sluggish, can be prone to indigestion, diarrhoea and have general fatigue and a lack of enthusiasm. When in balance the mind and body work together and there is an easy flow of movement within the body and out of it. When out of balance, there are problems with the throat and a loss of speech, an increase in fear, anxiety and any artistic tendencies diminish and the person will become forgetful.

Dosha Pitta is associated with the element of fire which affects body temperature, digestion, absorption and elimination (so primarily the digestive system) and water which affects the conscious and unconscious thought and is essential in the homeostatic functioning of the body. A 'pitta' person will have a warm heart and oily skin, a good appetite and a moderate frame. When balanced, the person is cheerful and content but when out of balance feelings of anger, aggression and resentment set in and ailments associated with fire (heat and inflammation) such as heartburn, rashes, fever, diarrhoea and cystitis may occur.

Dosha Kapha is a combination of water and earth and is associated with growth and protection, with the balance of body structure and fluid. 'Kapha' people are prone to weight gain with a slow metabolism. Generally kapha is responsible for the stability of the mind and body. When balanced the person is strong and kind with an even temperament; when unbalanced the person is depressed and lethargic and develops physical complaints such as colds, coughs, allergies and asthma.

Indian traditions regarding the use of IHM

Traditionally, there is a 'whole family' approach to the receiving and the giving of Indian head massage in India and this tradition has been ongoing for the last 1,000 years. Massage is a weekly event for the majority of people in India and continues throughout life.

The treatment was used by Indian women to maintain the health and strength of their long hair and utilised vegetable-based oils that were in season and therefore easily available and cheap. Oils such as coconut, mustard, almond and olive oil were used depending on their availability. They are, however, not the only users of Indian head massage; children and babies traditionally also receive the treatment, as do the male members of the family.

From birth, babies receive daily massages from their mothers to stimulate their body systems, soothe temperament and to keep them in good health. From the ages of three until six years, a massage is given once or twice a week. After six the children are encouraged to participate in the family culture of receiving and giving massage.

Male members of the Indian family largely receive their head massage called a Champissage from their spouse or another family member at home or at the barbers while having a haircut. This is not a barbershop as we know it in the UK but a place where the men meet and debate. It may also have a religious or spiritual function, including the spiritual side of having massage using scented oils as part of male grooming and the cutting of hair.

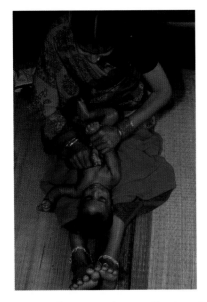

△ Family approach to Indian head massage

This spiritual side of the massage also comes into importance during ceremonial rituals such as a wedding, for example. Before a wedding both the bride and groom will receive a massage to achieve both physical and psychological effects. The psychological effect is to calm the nerves and provide a meditative state to prepare them for the sober nature of the vows they are about to make. The massage includes the use of oils scented with herbs and spices and the physical effects are designed to prepare the couple for married life, providing health and stamina as well as promote fertility for the procreation of many children.

Indian head massage was bought to Europe by an Indian man called Narendra Mehta, a massage therapist and osteopath, who came to England in 1973 to study physiotherapy. He was horrified to find that when he went to the barbers all he got was a haircut! When he returned to India as a qualified physiotherapist he began to research the treatment that was such a normal and integral part of family life in India. He travelled all over India to study the different techniques because they varied from place to place, barber to barber and from family to family. With all that he learnt he put together his own massage style and brought it to England.

Mehta developed the treatment to increase the area covered by the treatment and tried to find a way for Europeans to accept the more spiritual aspect of the massage. Eventually he decided upon the balancing of the three upper body chakras: the crown, the brow and the throat. It is less aggressive than the Champissage the barbers perform in India but incorporates some vigorous movements and with a good therapist provides a relaxing or invigorating massage. Although it may not be the traditional Champissage, it is a variation of techniques used all over India.

In the early 1990s Narendra Mehta opened a school in London for the teaching of a 'new' or Westernised Indian head massage or Champissage, which included the massage of the shoulders, upper arms, neck, scalp, ears and face with chakra balancing.

The treatment has developed primarily to treat stress, although it does have other beneficial effects and has become a popular professional treatment in salons including hairdressing salons, spas, cruise liners, airports and even within the workplace.

Cultural differences between the Western and original use of IHM

As stated earlier, Ayurveda and Indian head massage are considered by the western world to be a form of complementary and alternative medicine (CAM) rather than a traditional or conventional medicine. Conventional medicine centres on the elimination of symptoms of disease or disorder which may involve the prescription of drugs. With conventional medicine there is a similar regime for treatment for patients with the same disease or disorder.

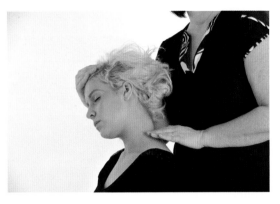

△ Western approach to Indian head massage

Complementary and alternative therapies rely on a 'holistic' approach where the patient is treated as a 'whole', with little distinction between the body, mind and spirit. The CAM therapist stresses that these three human dimensions should be considered together, with a combination of treatments to provide a treatment plan to promote a cure.

The term 'alternative medicine' implies that the therapies are used as a substitute for conventional medicine whereas 'complementary therapies' implies that the therapies are used alongside conventional medicine. These terms, however are not definitive and are often used interchangeably. Table 12.1 summarises the differences between the Western and traditional use of IHM.

▽ Table 12.1 Cultural differences between Western and traditional use of IHM

Traditional use	Western use
Babies, small children and adults treated as regularly as daily within a family	No cultural use of IHM or any other form of massage on children
IHM is used as part of Indian ceremonies such as weddings to prepare the couple physically and psychologically for married life	No cultural use of IHM in wedding or other ceremonies
Massage is performed by family members or as part of a male grooming routine	Massage is performed by trained professionals under self-regulation values and constraints
The massage is performed at home on family members, in barber shops but also more recently on beaches, market places and street corners	The treatment is available in salons including barbers and female and unisex hairdressing salons, spas and sometimes within the workplace
The treatment is restricted to the head and scalp	The treatment has been extended to include the shoulders, upper arms, neck, head, scalp, ears and face
The use of locally available and common oils is used to promote health of the hair and scalp	A wider variety of oils are available due to the commercial availability of oils from around the world. Some of these are expensive due to their rarity. Often the use of oil is avoided during the scalp massage due to a culture of appearance and cosmetic concerns
Additionally, herbs and spices are added to the massage oil	Essential oils can also be added to the massage base oil. These are derived from a variety of sources such as flowers and resins as well as herbs and spices
Spiritually, IHM plays an important part in Indian culture, being based on ancient principles of Ayurveda	The majority of Western spirituality is based on Christian principles which are only 2010 years old and in which treatments such as IHM play no part
Ayurveda promotes the importance of balance for the body and the equilibrium of the body's energy to bring about self healing through the chakras and Marma points (see later in this chapter)	Although there is still a strong cultural use of conventional medicine techniques and principles based on scientific evidence for their effectiveness, there is an increased interest in ancient philosophies as dissatisfaction with Western medicine has led to an increase in the availability and participation in IHM
Holism is an important part of the implementation of the treatment under Ayurvedic principles, where the body, mind and spirit are considered equally	Reductionism is the approach applied to conventional Western medicine where the emphasis is placed on the relief of symptoms of a disease/disorder
Performed as a daily or at least regular treatment to bring about spiritual and physical benefits	Performed as a weekly treatment (depending on the treatment plan) to bring about stress relief

Location of the chakras and their function in IHM

The term 'chakras' refers to the centres, wheels or vortexes of energy which have no physical form but are found in certain positions on the body and are the focal point for restoring balance to the body in Ayurveda and other ancient treatment philosophies. There are seven major chakras, which equate to the position of the main glands of the endocrine system. The endocrine system secretes hormones, which are chemical messages that control the functioning of the human body.

In ancient philosophy, the chakras affect the physical, emotional and spiritual aspects of the human body and when they are free-flowing equilibrium is reached and the person is free from physical illness and is happy and contented. Spiritually, the chakras are intricately linked to the person's 'aura' or energy field.

A blockage within one or more chakra is when illness and emotional upset occurs. The illness may not manifest itself in the physical body for some time, however, and the manifestation may appear emotionally as a disturbance in behaviour or feeling, long before any physical symptoms are apparent. To further complicate the issue, disturbed emotions of the mind can cause blockages in the chakras, also leading to illness.

Key terms

Chakra – the seven spinning wheels of energy. They are non-physical and located centrally within the body.

Marma points – pressure points on the body that stimulate life force.

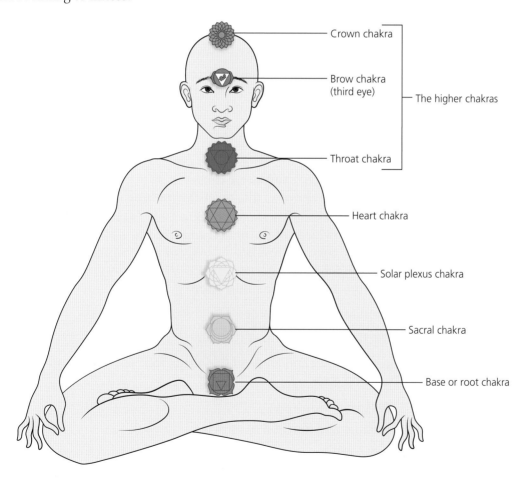

Crown chakra

Brow chakra (third eye)

The higher chakras

Throat chakra

Heart chakra

Solar plexus chakra

Sacral chakra

Base or root chakra

△ The seven major chakras and the colours associated with them

Indian head massage involves the three higher chakras: the crown, the brow and the throat chakras.

Crown chakra

The crown chakra in connected with the endocrine gland and the pineal gland. A stagnant or blocked crown chakra will exhibit itself as migraine, epilepsy, neuritis or even brain tumours or diseases such as Parkinson's. Psychologically, an imbalance will exhibit a closed mind, fear, nightmares and gullibility.

Brow chakra

The brow chakra is associated with the master endocrine gland, the pituitary gland. An imbalance will result in physical conditions such as headaches, sinus problems, visual and memory disorders and dizziness. Psychological problems associated with this gland are depression, confusion, identity crisis, mood swings, inability to focus and daydreaming.

Throat chakra

The throat chakra is associated with the thyroid gland, with physical imbalances showing themselves as neck and shoulder problems, throat problems, non-stop talking and thyroid and parathyroid problems. Psychological problems include stuttering, a negative attitude, self destruction and an inability to express oneself verbally.

Benefits of IHM

Indian head massage is of such enormous benefit as first it relaxes the mind and when the mind is still the body can go about healing itself. Second, the massage works on the upper chakras which helps to clear the blockages in these areas, further increasing energy flow and allowing the body to heal.

The chakras are worked from the upper chakras to the lower or 'root' chakra. If the upper chakras are cleared first, the released energy eventually filters down to the lower chakras unblocking them too.

Indian head massage can have profound effects on the systems of the body and knowledge of the underlying structures of the body and a sound knowledge of the anatomy body systems shown below will improve the safety and effectiveness of IHM for the client.

- Structure and function of the skin
- Skin diseases and disorders
- Structure and function of the hair
- Primary bones and joints of the head, neck, shoulders and upper back and arms
- Types of muscle tissue
- Structure and function of muscles
- Position and action of the muscles of the head, neck, upper back and arms
- Structure, function and location of the blood vessels of the head, neck, upper back and arms
- Principles of blood circulation, blood pressure and pulse

- Interaction of lymph and blood circulation
- Structure and function of the lymphatic system
- Position and function of the sinuses
- Basic principles of the central nervous system and autonomic nervous system
- Basic principles of the endocrine system
- Basic principles of the respiratory system

For the structure and functions and main diseases and disorders of these body systems please refer to Chapter 4 Anatomy and physiology.

Maintain safe and effective methods of work

Hygiene procedures

High levels of personal hygiene and presentation are expected for the performance of Indian head massage on clients. Use the following checklist to check the industry's expectations.

Back to basics

Personal appearance and hygiene checklist:

1. A high standard of personal hygiene.
2. Fresh breath, free from cigarette or food odours.
3. A clean, pressed overall.
4. Clean, low-heeled shoes.
5. Arms and hands free from jewellery (plain wedding bands are acceptable).
6. Any earrings or necklaces are discreet.
7. Make up is discreet and expertly applied.
8. Long hair is tied neatly away from the face and shoulders.
9. Nails are short, smooth, clean and free of nail enamel.
10. Tights, or socks with trousers, are worn.
11. Any cuts are covered with a clean plaster.
12. Hands are washed immediately before and after physical client contact.

Hygiene of the treatment area and client

To avoid cross-infection from one client to another or to the therapist the following precautions should be taken:

1 Any surfaces within the work area should be wiped down with a suitable chemical disinfectant, including the treatment stool, chair and trolley. Use a spray to deliver the product and wipe with a clean cloth or disposable paper such as couch roll.

2 Laundry such as gowns or towels should be fresh for each client and washed on the hottest wash after use.

3 Disposable paper should be used to cover surfaces such as the floor and the trolley.

4 Check the client for contraindications at the consultation. Never treat anyone with an infectious disease.

5 The client should shower if the facilities are available.

6 Always use a 'cut out' technique for Indian head massage oils and other products.

7 The therapist should wash their hands thoroughly before and after treating the client

8 Any cuts, abrasions or other small open wounds on the therapist's hands or in the treatment areas should be covered with a sterile waterproof dressing.

9 Wipe your hands with anti-bacterial wipes during the Indian head massage treatment if necessary.

10 Dispose of waste material correctly, immediately after treatment.

For more information on suitable sterilising methods, see Chapter 6 Professional practices and for the disposal of contaminated waste see Chapter 1 Monitoring health and safety.

Health and safety practices

The main pieces of legislation that a therapist works under are shown in Table 12.2 below. Others are discussed within Chapter 1 Monitoring health and safety.

▽ Table 12.2 Relevant legislation

Area	Act	Areas covered by Act
The treatment room	Health & Safety at Work Act 1974	General safety of staff and visitors to the salon, including clients
	The Workplace (Health, Safety & Welfare) Regulations 1992	Governs the working environment including ventilation, temperature and lighting
	Regulatory Reform (Fire Safety) Order 2005	The safe evacuation of the building in an emergency such as a fire
Indian head massage equipment	Provision and Use of Work Equipment Regulations 1998	Governs the acquisition of safe and reliable equipment
Indian head massage products	Control of Substances Hazardous to Health 1988	Governs the exposure persons to substances likely to cause harm including flammability and the effect on the tissues
	Cosmetic Products (Safety) Regulations (2008)	Requires cosmetics to comply with correct labelling, to have safe formulation and be fit for the purpose intended
Disposal of waste	Controlled Waste Regulations 1992	Governs the correct disposal of contaminated waste, i.e. that contaminated with blood or other bodily fluids

Positioning of client and therapist

As the client will be sitting for the duration of the treatment it is important that they are comfortable. Provide a chair with a supporting back and one that is of the correct height so that their feet can be placed flat on the floor with the knees and hips at right angles. The small of the back should be placed into the back of the chair and the arms allowed to rest naturally in their lap.

The use of pillows and bolsters may be needed to support clients that have a physical disability, are elderly or pregnant.

The therapist should be able to move around the client without fear of falling over an obstruction or disturbing the treatment by asking the client to move. The client should be positioned so that the therapist need not bend or stretch to perform the treatment. This will avoid fatigue and the possibility of postural faults occurring or the development of back or joint pain.

Consult, plan and prepare for treatment

Consultation techniques

Consultation techniques include:

- communication and behaviour
- questioning and listening techniques and appropriate body language
- visual assessment
- manual assessment
- referral to client records
- visual aids.

Communication and behaviour

A mature approach is needed by the therapist when dealing with clients for complementary therapies such as Indian head massage. The client may exhibit irrational feelings and behave unpredictably or have an emotional response to the treatment and it is part of the therapist's job to handle these difficult situations in a professional manner.

Questioning

Details of questioning techniques including the use of open and closed questions, listening and recognising body language can be found in Chapter 6 Professional practices.

For Indian head massage the client should be asked questions regarding:

- personal details that will identify a client from another of a similar name, such as name, address, telephone number, date of birth
- general and specific health problems if relevant and including contraindications; this will determine whether the client is safe to treat and identify techniques that might be of benefit

> ☆ **Hints and tips**
> Because it is usual to accept a range of reactions from a client when dealing with physical feelings, such as individual pain threshold, so it should be accepted that emotional feelings may also vary when exposed to the same stimuli. What one client perceives as stressful, another may find a positive challenge. It is important for the therapist to recognise these differences in their clients and to respond to them appropriately.

- lifestyle, including occupation, stress levels, diet and eating habits, exercise habits, smoking, sleep patterns, hobbies and interests and methods used to relax, as these will help in the development of the treatment plan.

Contraindications

To ensure the safety of the client and the prevention of cross-contamination of infectious diseases and disorders, the therapist should question the client about the possible contraindications for massage treatment. These contraindications fall into two main categories: those that *prevent* and those that may *restrict* the treatment (see Table 12.3).

▽ Table 12.3 Contraindications to Indian head massage

Conditions that prevent treatment	Conditions that restrict treatment
<ul><li>Fungal infection such as Tinea capitis</li><li>Bacterial infection such as impetigo</li><li>Viral infection such as herpes simplex</li><li>Infestations such as Pediculosis capitis</li><li>Severe non-infectious disorders such as eczema and psoriasis</li><li>Skin conditions such as bruising</li><li>Eye infections such as conjunctivitis</li><li>During chemotherapy and/or radiotherapy</li></ul>	<ul><li>Broken bones</li><li>Recent scar tissue</li><li>Skin allergies</li><li>Cuts and abrasions</li><li>Sebaceous cysts</li><li>Epilepsy</li><li>Diabetes</li><li>Heart disease/conditions</li><li>High or low blood pressure</li><li>Skin disorders</li><li>Recent fractures and sprains</li><li>Undiagnosed lumps and swellings</li><li>Product allergies</li><li>Respiratory conditions</li><li>Circulatory conditions</li><li>Dysfunction of the nervous system</li><li>Dysfunction of the muscular system</li><li>Osteoporosis</li><li>Whiplash</li><li>Pregnancy</li></ul>

For additional information on specific skin diseases and disorders see Chapter 4 Anatomy and physiology.

Those contraindications that are infectious and prevent Indian head massage treatment do so because there is a risk that the disease may be spread to another client or the therapist. In most cases the client should be referred to a medical practitioner such as their doctor or a pharmacist who will be able to provide suitable medication to rid them of the condition. Once the infection has gone the client can safely return for treatment.

Severe skin conditions including psoriasis and eczema can be made worse by Indian head massage treatment and therefore continuing with the treatment is not advisable. There is no risk of cross-infection as these skin disorders are not infectious but when severe there can be cracking of the epidermis and the possible transference of blood or serum, which is of concern. The client should be encouraged to return when the condition has cleared up sufficiently. However, being stress-related, mild psoriasis can be improved by regular Indian head massage treatments and from the therapeutic effects of certain oils.

If a client is undergoing radiotherapy or chemotherapy they will be under the care of an oncologist and they should be consulted before any massage treatment is performed as there is a risk of spreading cancerous cells around the body to other tissues. Generally, do not treat clients with cancer as the treatment they are receiving is usually aggressive and can result in side effects which can be worsened by massage treatments.

Contraindications that *prevent* treatment should be considered as those that need medical referral to ensure the safety of the client and to abide by professional codes of practice; those that need treatment *adaptations* will ensure that the condition is not aggravated or made worse.

A client presenting with a medical condition such as epilepsy, diabetes, heart disease/conditions, high or low blood pressure, respiratory conditions, circulatory conditions, dysfunction of the nervous system, dysfunction of the muscular system, undiagnosed lumps and swellings, whiplash and osteoporosis should consult their doctor before treatment. Appropriate adaptations can then be made during the IHM treatment. Possible adaptations are dealt with in more detail later in this chapter.

Conditions such as cuts and abrasions, broken bones, skin disorders, recent sprains, sebaceous cysts and recent scar tissue need to be avoided during the treatment by either omitting the affected area of the body or, if minor, avoiding the area while the surrounding tissue is treated.

To avoid exacerbating skin and product allergies a sensitivity test should be performed 24 hours before treatment.

☆ Hints and tips
Indian head massage and any other form of massage such as aromatherapy can ease the symptoms of the disease as part of palliative care for patients with advanced incurable cancer but should not be considered where the patient is undergoing treatment for the disease.

Necessary actions

The therapist should be aware of the possible actions to take if the client presents with a contraindication:

- encourage the client to seek medical advice
- explain why the treatment cannot be carried out
- modify the treatment.

Treatment objectives

The objectives of the treatment should be discussed during the consultation to ensure the satisfaction of the client. If they want to feel relaxed by the treatment it is imperative to make this the focus of the treatment, although other benefits through adaptations of the treatment can be achieved by the therapist. Possible treatment objectives are:

- feelings of relaxation/sedation
- a sense of well-being
- an uplifting/invigorating feeling

- improvement of hair and scalp condition
- feelings of stimulation.

Suitable adaptations to the IHM treatment for these individual objectives are given below under the heading 'Planning treatment'.

Assessing lifestyle patterns

The increasing popularity of IHM as a treatment may be because of an increase in stress levels caused by our lifestyles. When questioning your client you should consider their:

- occupation
- diet
- exercise levels
- alcohol consumption
- smoking
- stress levels.

Visual assessment

Your visual assessment during consultation should include notes on the following physical characteristics.

Posture

By viewing the client's posture much can be learnt about their physical and mental state. Someone who is feeling depressed or is in pain will hold themselves very differently to someone who is not. Pain can also show itself in facial expression resulting in a frown and/or a downward turn to the mouth. Postural faults such as round shoulders and a forward head tilt can cause neck pain and headaches.

Skin condition

Skin type and condition such as normal, dry, oily, combination, sensitive and dehydrated will help you to choose a suitable massage oil if one is being used and can also be an indicator of the general health of the client. It is important to note differences in the skin related to age, such as thinness of skin or poor elasticity, as this will affect the depth of your massage movements. The distinction between non-medical treatable skin conditions and those which should be referred to a doctor should be noted on the client's record card. Some treatable skin conditions such as psoriasis are improved by Indian head massage and the application of therapeutic massage oils.

Hair condition

The density, texture and length of the hair can give an indication of health of the scalp and the client generally. The effects of cosmetic procedures such as colouring can leave the hair dry and cause breakage. Healthy hair will be shiny, silky and smooth to the touch.

Scalp condition

The colour of the scalp is an indicator of the blood supply to the hair follicles and the health of the hair. A pale scalp can mean a lack of nutrients and oxygen getting to the hair and results in poor growth. Note the degree of sebum present or flakes of skin or dandruff, which may indicate disease or disorder. Note also the tightness of the scalp to the bony structure underneath; a healthy scalp will appear slightly pink, be free of debris and be able to move freely over the bones of the skull.

Manual

Often, manual techniques are used to confirm aspects of the client's condition that have been determined by the other consultation techniques. However, occasionally the manual assessment can contradict the other techniques and further questioning of the client may be necessary.

Muscle tone

Determining the degree of muscle tone is subjective but a comparison between muscles of the same client can give an indication of where there is a high degree of tension in the muscles, which could be an indicator of poor posture, stress, overworked muscles and/or a build-up of waste products within the muscle itself.

More information on all these aspects of body analysis can be found in Chapter 7 Skin and body analysis.

Referral to client records

By referring to the client's record card the therapist can remind themselves of the details of the client's previous treatment and the short-term effects. This can then be followed up by questioning the client on the long-term effects of the previous treatment. This information will inform the therapist of adaptations to the products or techniques to bring about beneficial effects.

A skilful therapist will be able to practise these techniques to perform an effective consultation that is probing and determines the client's requirements. The consultation will inform decisions surrounding the products and techniques to use that will best suit the client's skin type and condition and their treatment objectives. This will ensure the best result is achieved with the aim of achieving client satisfaction and their return of business.

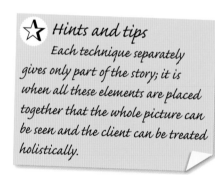

Hints and tips
Each technique separately gives only part of the story; it is when all these elements are placed together that the whole picture can be seen and the client can be treated holistically.

Planning treatment

Treatment planning involves collating the information gleaned from the consultation and using it to decide on the:

- proposed treatment including the length and cost
- frequency of treatment, i.e. whether weekly or fortnightly
- massage medium, including type of oils to use if appropriate

- movements/manipulation and techniques to use
- adaptations to the routine to suit the client's needs and treatment objectives
- time of day for the treatment.

The proposed treatment plan should be discussed with the client and their approval sought in the form of a signature on the client record. Although this will not protect a therapist from prosecution if the client were to start litigation, it is required as part of the industry's code of practice and membership of a relevant professional body and will influence the outcome of an insurance claim.

Treatment time for Indian head massage

A time of 45 minutes for Indian head massage has been determined by the industry as a standard commercial timing and should be used during the practical assessment.

Contra-actions

It is important to explain the treatment and the possible contra-actions at the time of the consultation to gain the client's trust and to ensure their satisfaction with the treatment. The client can then ask questions to clarify and can make an informed decision as to whether to continue with the treatment. Adaptations to the treatment can be put in place if necessary. The contra-actions to Indian head massage treatment are:

- allergies
- depression
- insomnia
- hallucination
- respiratory reactions
- headache
- nausea
- muscle aches
- skin irritations
- increased secretions
- lethargy
- heightened emotions.

These conditions may be brought about by some of the effects of the treatment, as indicated in Table 12.4.

> ⭐ *Hints and tips*
> *As it is intended that there should be an improvement in the client's condition, the treatment plan should be reviewed periodically as improvements are made.*

▽ Table 12.4 Contra-actions to IHM

Contra-action	Cause and action to take
Allergies Skin irritations	Action of the massage oil on the skin. Perform the IHM without oil through clothing or perform a sensitivity test with another oil.
Headache Nausea	Action of the massage movements releasing toxins held in the tissues into the blood circulation. Advise the client to rest and drink plenty of water to flush out the toxins via the kidneys.
Increased secretions	Action of the hands over the skin stimulates the sebaceous and sweat glands to increase activity with the resulting increased sebum and sweat. If these are undesirable the massage could be performed through clothing.
Respiratory reactions	Cold-like symptoms can develop as the sinuses are emptied and stimulated to produce more cleansing mucous. Rest and clear airways as necessary until the symptoms pass.
Depression Insomnia Hallucination Heightened emotions	Often known as the 'healing crisis', these contra-actions are the result of the psychological effects of the treatment and although they can be traumatic at the time, once over, a great release of tension is experienced and a sense of well-being replaces the anxiety. The client is more able to cope with the stresses they are experiencing in their lives.
Muscle aches	The action of the movements release toxins and local nerve fibres are stimulated, resulting in muscle ache. Rest will give time for the tissues to heal and return to normal. These symptoms are a sign that the treatment has worked and will pass in a short period of time. If concerned, inform the therapist at the next treatment.
Lethargy	Caused by the release of toxins into the blood stream, affecting the muscles and nerve tissues in the brain. Rest and allow the body to return to normal.

Prepare for treatment

The trolley should be prepared with the chosen massage medium and disinfectant hand wipes for the removal of oils from the hands if required. A small bowl containing dry pads of cotton wool and a bottle of eau de cologne may be required to remove excess oil after the treatment.

Environmental conditions

- Warmth: as Indian head massage can be performed through or without upper outer clothing the temperature, of the room should be adjusted accordingly.

- Ventilation: adequate ventilation to allow a steady exchange of air to prevent fatigue should be provided but this should not cause a drop in temperature, which could ruin the client's enjoyment of the treatment.

- Lighting: subdued lighting is required to encourage the relaxation of the client but not so dark as to be sedating. Avoid bright artificial lighting as this is not conducive to the treatment.

- Privacy: when performed through the clothing the treatment area need not be so private, but a quiet area for the promotion of relaxation is required.

- Volume and type of music/sounds: the correct music and its volume can also induce relaxation. Music with lyrics can be detrimental to the treatment as the client may recite them internally instead of emptying the mind to allow the energy channels to open and flow.

- Pleasant aroma: the use of essential oils burnt within the treatment area can promote relaxation as certain oils have an effect on the limbic system when inhaled. A clean fresh aroma can be obtained through oils such as peppermint and/or tea tree.

Avoid the use of floral smells such as lavender when treating male clients.

Preparation of the therapist

The therapist should prepare themselves mentally before the performance of an Indian head massage. A calm and relaxed approach is needed by the therapist if they are to avoid passing on their own stresses from everyday life and self-protection techniques should be practised if they are not to get involved with the client's problems.

Preparation of the client

Before the treatment begins the client should receive a thorough consultation to determine safety to treat and their treatment objectives; they should be prepared physically and mentally for the treatment. Where there are concerns surrounding a possible allergic reaction, a sensitivity test or patch test should be undertaken at least 24 hours before treatment by cleaning an area of skin either behind the ear or in the crease of the elbow and placing a little of the intended product onto the area. The client should be informed of the signs to watch out for, such as irritation, redness, itching or swelling and that if any of these occur to inform you immediately as the treatment cannot go ahead. If after 24 hours there are no such signs the treatment can go ahead as planned.

Removal of accessories

The client should be asked to remove appropriate outer clothing as necessary and to put on a wrap-around gown or a towel under the arms to leave the upper back and shoulders exposed. This stage can be omitted if the treatment is to take place without oil and through the clothing or if the client is male when a gown may not be necessary. A towel can be placed around the shoulders if there are concerns surrounding the temperature of the room. The client's clothing should be folded neatly and placed away from the immediate treatment area to prevent spoiling through accidental spillage of massage oil.

⭐ *Hints and tips*
     Tea tree essential oil has anti-viral properties and when burnt in the treatment room can protect the therapist and clients from air-borne viruses that cause colds and flu.

Activity ✿

Practise these exercises before and after an Indian head massage treatment:

1   Deep breathing: place your hands with fingers loosely interlocked over your abdomen; breathe in deeply through the nose pushing the abdomen outwards so the fingers move apart; breathe out through the mouth, allowing the fingers to return to their original position.

2   Close your eyes with your arms loosely down by your sides. Imagine all the negative feelings and tension in your body coming up from your feet, through your legs and body and down into your arms and out of your fingers. Flick your hands and your fingers so that the negative energy is 'flicked away' into the room.

3   Have regular Indian head massage treatments, concentrating on the rebalancing of the chakras.

The client should also be asked to remove any jewellery in the area being treated such as bracelets, watches, necklaces, earrings and other piercings such as those found in the eyebrow.

Removal of the shoes and the placing of the feet on the floor, covered with disposable paper, is thought to 'ground' the client and enable the energy channels to flow more effectively. Mentally the client should be prepared with deep breathing exercises as the therapist places their hands lightly on the client's shoulders to emulate the breathing pattern. In this way the therapist can calm the breathing pattern if needed through deep breathing exercises.

Perform Indian head massage

Effects and benefits of Indian head massage

The effects and benefits of Indian head massage are not only accredited to the treatment area of the shoulders, arms, neck, scalp, ears and face but to the whole body. The holistic nature of the treatment ensures that the whole body is treated through the spiritual as well as physical application of the Indian head massage techniques.

The benefits and uses of Indian head massage are to:

- aid relaxation and stress relief
- improve blood and lymph circulation
- improve skin and hair texture
- improve scalp condition
- improve muscle tone
- improve memory
- reduce tension headaches
- improve concentration
- improve sleep patterns
- improve sinus problems
- reduce tinnitus.

The effects of Indian head massage can be divided into physical, physiological and psychological.

Physical

Shoulder, neck, face and scalp muscles are relaxed by the action of the massage techniques and the increase in heat to the area caused by the increase in blood circulation. This relieves muscle tension and improves joint mobility, increasing flexibility and improving posture, and this can result in the alleviation of headaches. In the case of the facial muscles around the eyes in particular, the relaxation relieves tired eyes and eye strain. The stimulated lymphatic system also reduces any inflammation in the tissues, which is often associated with muscular pain and tension. Consequently muscle pain is relieved and the stress on joints and muscles released.

Health and safety

In rare cases it is possible for a client to have an extreme reaction in the form of an anaphylactic shock involving the swelling of the tissues in the mouth and respiratory system. If this occurs the situation is an emergency and an ambulance should be called. If the client is a known sufferer of such a condition they may carry an antihistamine pen (Epipen) which should be administered by the client as soon as symptoms arise.

Physiological

Massage increases the blood circulation, resulting in an increase in nutrients and oxygen within the area being treated. The increase in nutrients to the upper body can be seen in the improvement in the growth and health of the hair and scalp and benefits to the face can be seen in the health and glow of the skin. An increase in nourishment also promotes healing, which is important for scarring caused by acne and an increase in oxygen to the brain relieves mental fatigue, improving concentration and promoting clearer thinking.

The waste removal system of the body, the lymphatic system, is also stimulated by massage, improving lymphatic circulation and the stimulation of the lymph nodes. Being part of the immune system, this improves the body's immunity, promotes health and improves the fight against disease. It also aids in the removal of toxins and by doing so eliminates accumulations in the skin, lymph nodes and scalp and reduces swelling by releasing the accumulation of lymph that could lead to oedema.

The autonomic nervous system is also affected by Indian head massage, having great beneficial effects, both long and short term. The sympathetic nervous system when stimulated by the massage techniques will slow the pulse and breathing rate, lowering blood pressure, reducing anxiety and symptoms of stress. Activating the parasympathetic nervous system promotes sleep and relaxation. The brain is stimulated, which releases the 'feel good' hormones called endorphins. These elevate the mood, lifting depression, relieving physical and mental pain and releases emotions and repressed feelings.

Psychological

The massage encourages the release of stagnant energy within the body through chakra balancing and restores the natural energy flow of the body. This promotes whole body healing and creates a feeling of balance and calm.

Massage mediums

The traditional massage mediums used in India for thousands of years were vegetable oils obtained from locally grown plants and therefore relied on whether the plant was in season. Sesame, mustard, almond, coconut and olive oil derived from the plant material were extracted using simple methods such as distillation or pressing not only to nourish and improve the condition of hair, skin and scalp, but because they are absorbed into the blood stream, where they have positive health benefits and improve the functioning of the body's systems.

Massage oils

- Coconut oil: this has a beautiful aroma and helps to keep the head cool, so is popular for use in the hot summer months. It is a medium to light oil that is highly moisturising to the skin and scalp and can help the hair, scalp and skin become more vibrant and alive. The oil is extracted by pressing the macerated white kernel flesh.

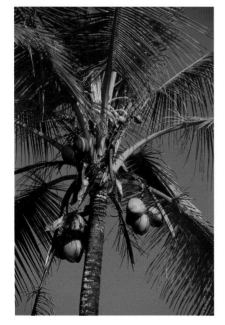

△ Palm tree and coconut

- Olive oil: this is classed as a 'winter' oil. It has a strong smell and highly moisturising properties so is used for excessively dry hair and scalps. It is a safe oil so suitable for use with children. It is extracted by grinding the ripe olives into a paste, which is then pressed to extract the oil.

- Sesame oil: one of the most popular choices among Indian families. It helps to relieve swellings and muscular pains and strengthens and moisturises the hair and skin. It is known as a 'summer' oil, due to its availability at that time of year. It has a light texture that is non-clinging and absorbs quickly and easily. The oil is extracted by hot or cold pressing of the ripe seeds; the differences in the colour of the oil are obtained by roasting the seeds before extraction.

- Mustard oil: this is a very warming oil, popular for use in the winter months. It opens the pores and has a strengthening and moisturising effect on the skin. It increases body heat within the tissues being massaged and relieves pain, reduces swellings and relaxes stiff muscles, making it useful in the treatment of arthritis. Mustard oil is extracted from black mustard seeds which have been macerated in warm water by steam or water distillation.

- Grapeseed oil: the seed of the grapes are cold pressed to release the oil but the oil is also a by-product of the wine-making industry, making it cheap to buy. The resulting oil has regenerative and restructuring qualities and can reduce the appearance of scar tissue; it is also highly moisturising.

- Almond oil has a strong smell and is used for excessively dry hair and scalp due to its great properties as an emollient. It is a 'winter' oil and is suitable for use on children. The almond kernels are pressed to extract the oil.

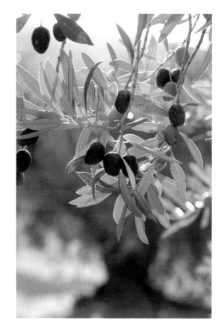

△ Olive tree and olive fruit

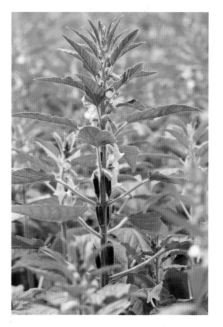

△ A sesame plant and seed

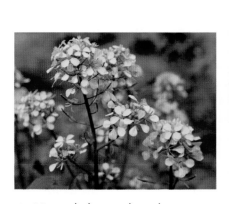

△ Mustard plant and seed

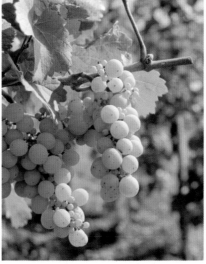

△ Grape vine and seed

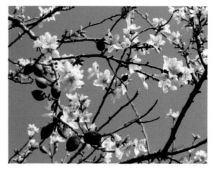

△ Almond tree and nut

Powder/talc

Powder or talc can be used successfully to perform Indian head massage as it provides 'slip' but facilitates effective massage movements and manipulations. In the hair it can also absorb excess sebum leaving the hair and scalp less greasy when brushed out after treatment.

Talc is a mineral mined from the Earth which is very soft and can be cut easily. Its softness allows it to be ground down into a fine powder. Usually a slight perfume is added to talc.

Indian head massage techniques

The massage movements employed within an IHM treatment are those classified by other massage treatments in the Western world. These massage movements are called effleurage, petrissage, tapotement and frictions. Additionally, there is the inclusion of cleansing and/or breathing techniques to bring about deep relaxation and the spiritual side of the treatment of the Marma points and chakras.

Effleurage

Effleurage is a stroking movement performed with the whole palmar surface of the hand on large areas of the body or with part of the hand such as the pad of the thumb for small areas like the face. In Swedish massage it is traditionally performed towards the heart, encouraging venous blood flow and lymphatic drainage, but in complementary therapies this is not always the case and 'reverse effleurage' is often used. The movement is used at the beginning of a massage routine in a particular area to prepare the area and the client for the deeper massage movements to come. The first touch should begin light, with more depth and speed added with consecutive strokes. It is also used to link movements together or return to the starting point of a series of other movements (reverse effleurage) and between deeper movements such as petrissage to remove toxins that may have accumulated.

The massage routine in a particular area should be completed by a series of effleurage movements in an appropriate direction, with the pressure starting firmly and quickly and becoming more superficial and slower as the last stroke is performed to signal to the client the completion of the routine in that area.

Effleurage prepares the area and client for further massage techniques while spreading the massage medium and the introduction of touch has an immediate relaxation on the client. It desquamates and warms the skin tissues through the friction of the hands on the area and increases blood circulation (arterial flow) with the result of an erythema and venous flow with the removal of waste products from the area being massaged. The arterial flow brings fresh nutrients and oxygen to the tissues, both superficially and deeper, as the stroke is applied more deeply. This increases the temperature of the deeper tissues, creating relaxation in muscle tissues and the release of fibrous adhesions.

Petrissage

Petrissage is a kneading or rubbing movement performed in a circular motion with the whole hand or part of the hand, such as fingers, thumb, heel of the palm, knuckles, thumb pad. These movements are performed on the soft tissues, muscle and adipose tissue once they have warmed and relaxed by effleurage and are often performed following or across the fibres to manipulate the soft tissues against more rigid structures such as the bones. The pressure should be firm but take into account the amount of soft tissue being massaged. Areas of bony or delicate tissue should be avoided completely when performing petrissage massage movements. The firm kneading and manipulation of muscle tissue causes the blood capillaries within to dilate, bringing valuable nutrients and oxygen to the cells. The increase in nutrients and oxygen enables the muscle tissue to perform at its optimum and removes accumulated waste products, including lactic acid which returns to its natural form, glycogen, found in all muscle tissue. Fibrous adhesions that are associated with muscle stiffness and discomfort are reduced and muscle tissue is stretched, bringing about muscle relaxation and the relief of stress and tension.

Tapotement

Tapotement are tapping movements of a light, brisk, springy nature applied with the outside of both hands (hacking) and the finger tips (tapping). They are performed on areas of tissue bulk but bony protuberances should be avoided. The effect of tapotement is to stimulate nerve endings in the skin and tissues, creating an increase in local blood circulation and the formation of an erythema. The muscle fibres are temporarily toned through stimulation and the action brings about a 'brightening' to the skin and the psyche.

Friction

Frictions are a deeper, more penetrating massage movement that should only be performed after more superficial movements have been performed in preparation. They are performed with the flat palm, thumbs or fingertips for specific benefits. These intense movements are applied with considerable pressure to fibrous adhesions to encourage their dissipation or on areas of stiffness or tension within the muscle tissue. They generate local heat through the rubbing action of the tissues against each other, dilating the capillaries and increasing blood circulation, breaking down and freeing adhered tissue. Frictions also promote lymphatic drainage and stimulate the local nerves, relieving pain.

Marma points

The term 'Marma points' applies to the pressure points on the body that stimulate life force, similar to those used in acupressure massage. They are thought to be the energy control points and are linked to the chakras (but not in a positional sense) **and** can be thought of as the access points in the physical body to the world of energy. There are 37 Marma points that can be treated, controlled, directed or manipulated in various ways during IHM. The idea is that massaging the Marma points will cleanse blocked energy flow, using the finger tips to either stimulate or calm the Marma point and thereby promoting physical, emotional and spiritual balance.

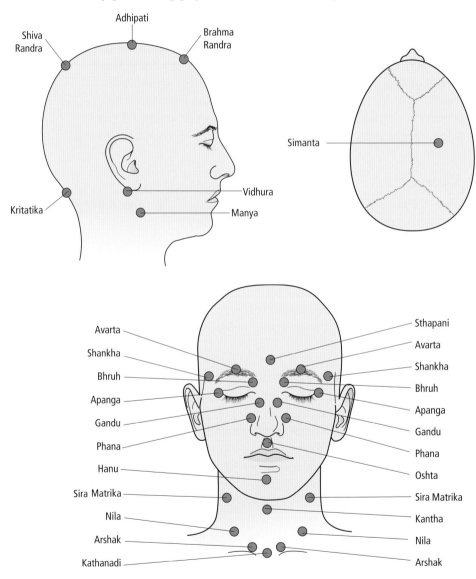

△ Marma points of the head, face and neck

The word 'Marma' can also be associated with tenderness (pain), secretion or vital places. The head has the greatest concentration of Marma points in the human body, with special points governing the eyes, ears, nostrils, mouth and brain. The essential oils penetrate easily at Marma points and influence the entire physical body by affecting the energy bodies. The link between the Marma points and the chakras can easily be seen here and an IHM should incorporate movements that work these energy release points in order to bring about the full beneficial effects of the treatment.

Working the Marma points can unblock the body's energy channels, treat a dosha imbalance or a specific system or organ of the body. The methods used are to locate the Marma point, usually a sensitive, hard or tender place within the tissues. Apply pressure with the finger tips, increasing the pressure as deep breaths are exhaled. Alternatively, a circular motion can be employed with the fingertips on the Marma point: a clockwise movement to stimulate or energise an organ; anti-clockwise to unblock or release a stagnant energy channel. The Marma points can also be treated with heat and essential oils to bring about specific effects.

Indian head massage routine

An Indian head massage treats the following areas of the body:

- face
- head
- chest and shoulders
- arms and hands
- back
- chakras.

A suggested routine is described below. You may be taught a routine that varies slightly from this; each routine will have its own merits. The routine described is broken down into the areas of the body being treated for ease of learning but when performing the treatment it should be continuous.

Upper back and shoulder massage

1 Standing behind the client, place hands lightly on the client's shoulders and together perform three deep breaths in through the nose and out through the mouth.

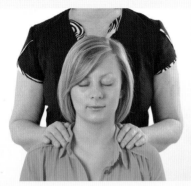

△ Starting position

2 Hover the hands close to but not touching the client's head and hold for one minute to centre and focus both the therapist and client to the treatment.

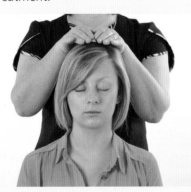

△ Centring for the treatment

3 With right hand resting on the client's right shoulder, use the left hand to perform effleurage movements that begin just below the medial border of the scapula, up the centre of the back and out over to the left shoulder and return to the starting point. Repeat three times on the left and then three on the right.

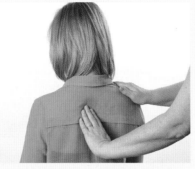

△ Effleurage to the left shoulder

4 With the fingers of both hands resting lightly on the top of the shoulders, reach down with the thumbs and with pressure bring the thumbs up to meet the fingers. Repeat the movement, fanning outwards in three sections. Repeat the whole movement three times.

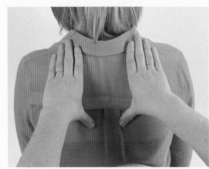

△ Thumb sweeps

5 With right hand resting on the client's right shoulder, perform frictions with the heel of the hand by moving the hand briskly back and forth. Start at the point of the shoulder, along the top edge of the scapula, down the medial border and along the bottom edge to form a reverse C shape and repeat three times. Repeat three times on the right side.

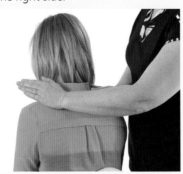

△ Heel frictions

6 Repeat the above movement but using the fingertips. Keep the fingers together and straight and point them away from the spine.

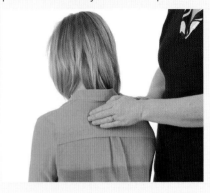

△ Fingertip frictions

7 Repeat effleurage movement as point 3.

8 With one hand resting on the client's shoulder, perform knuckle pressures down the spine using the middle joint of the fore and third fingers of the other hand. Apply the pressure as the client breathes out, release the pressure and slide down the spine. Repeat, dropping about one inch at a time until you reach the lowest point of the scapula. Repeat three times.

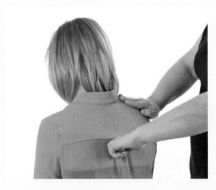

△ Knuckle pressures

9 Place both hands on the caps of the client's shoulders with your thumbs extending medially along the top edge of the scapula on the trapezius muscle. Push the thumbs away over the shoulders towards the chest, release and move medially towards the spine. Repeat until whole of the upper fibres of the trapezius has been treated in this way.

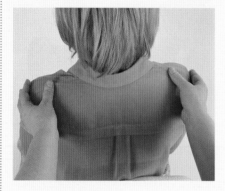

△ Thumb pushes

10 Place the thumbs both sides of the spine close to the upper and medial borders of the scapula and place the fingers over the shoulders to the front of the client's body. Keeping the thumbs still lift the upper fibres of the trapezius by pulling the fingers back towards the thumbs. Repeat along the top of the shoulders, working outwards toward the cap of the shoulders.

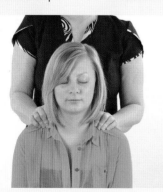

△ Trapezius squeezes

11 Repeat the movement above but use the heel of the hands instead of thumbs to lift the upper fibres of the trapezius and then push the heel forward, allowing the muscle to roll and release from your hands. Repeat along the top of the shoulders working outwards toward the cap of the shoulders.

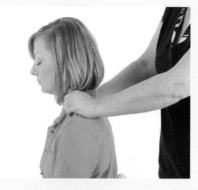

△ Heel pushes

12 Place the inside of your forearms on top of the shoulders close to the neck. Apply downward pressure and slide outwards, rotating the forearms as you go to finish with the inner arm upwards. Repeat three times.

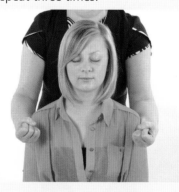

△ Forearm rolls

13 With the knees bent, place the hands flat on the upper back of the client and with a brisk sliding movement bring the fingers together to pinch the tissues between them and then release. Repeat over the entire upper back.

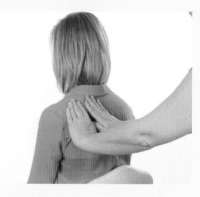

△ Chopping on the upper back

14 Perform double-handed hacking, with the hands held loosely in a prayer position, over the left and right sides of the upper back avoiding the spine. This movement comes from the wrist which should be relaxed and loose.

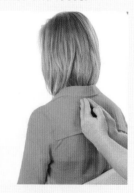

△ Double-handed hacking

Upper arm massage

1 With both hands on the left upper arm, fingers to the front and thumbs to the back, pick up and squeeze the deltoid muscle of the shoulder.

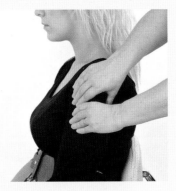

△ Deltoid squeeze

2 Standing to the side of the client, place one hand on the biceps and one on the triceps with fingers pointing towards the floor. Squeeze the hands together and release, starting near the shoulder and working down the upper arm to the elbow. Gently slide to return to the starting position and repeat three times.

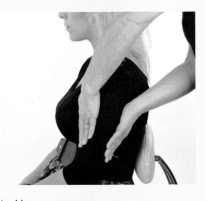

△ Upper arm squeezes

3 Stand behind the client again and grasp the deltoids, one in each hand, fingers to the front and heels of the hand behind. Roll the hands forward to move the deltoid and allow the muscle to release from the grasp. Repeat three times and then move down the upper arm to work on the triceps muscle until you reach above the elbow, each time repeating three times.

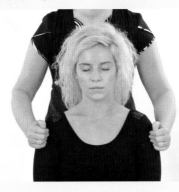

△ Heel rolls to the upper arm

4 With the fingers pointing downwards and towards the back of the arm and the thumbs at the front, lift and roll the triceps and biceps, starting from the shoulder and working down towards the elbow. Slide to the starting position and repeat three times.

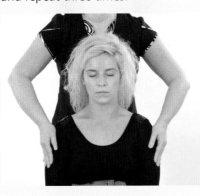

△ Upper arm rolls

5 Standing to the side of the client with one hand on the shoulder and the other lifting and supporting the elbow, circle the shoulder joint three times in one direction and three in the other, taking the joint through its complete range of movement. Repeat on the other side.

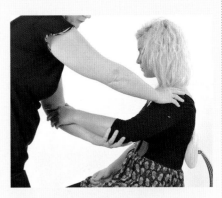

△ Shoulder circumduction

6 Support the client's forearm along the length of your arm and using the free hand squeeze the muscles of the forearm and release, starting at the elbow and working towards the wrist. Repeat three times.

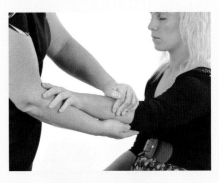

△ Forearm squeezes

7 Support the client's forearm and perform circle pressures, using the thumb into the metacarpal spaces of the hand.

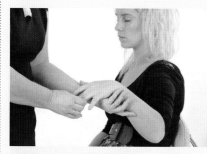

△ Thumb circles to metacarpal spaces

8 Turn the hand upwards and perform thumb pressures in circles into the palm of the hand.

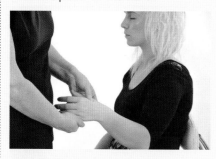

△ Thumb circles to the palm

9 Take each digit between the fingers and thumb and squeeze and release, working from the knuckle to the fingertips.

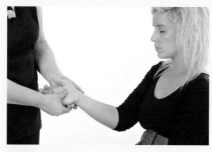

△ Digit squeezes

10 Stand behind the client and perform shoulder drops by lifting the arms with the elbows bent and then allowing them to drop. Repeat three times.

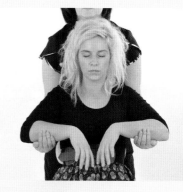

△ Shoulder drops

11 Perform forearm rolls to complete, as in point 12 of the upper back massage.

427

Head massage

1 Standing to the side of the client with one hand at the occipital and the other on the forehead above the eyebrows, gently rock the head forwards and backwards. Repeat three times.

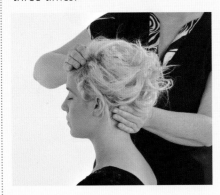

△ Head rocking

2 Keeping the hand on the forehead, squeeze and release the trapezius using the inner borders of the fore finger and the thumb, starting at the occipital and working downwards towards the base of the neck.

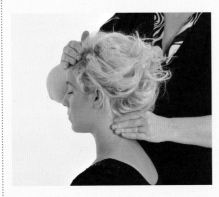

△ Trapezius squeezes

3 Still with the hand on the forehead, allow the client's head to drop slightly to one side so that it is supported along the forearm and the trapezius muscle is slightly stretched. Using the tips of the fingers, perform finger frictions in a zigzag motion to the trapezius border, starting at the occipital and finishing at the shoulder. Repeat three times and then three on the opposite side.

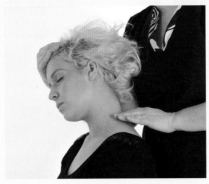

△ Frictions to the border of the trapezius

4 Perform thumb pushes along the border of the trapezius while supporting the head as before. Place the fingers to the front and push with the thumb, covering the area from the top to the shoulder as before. Repeat to the other side.

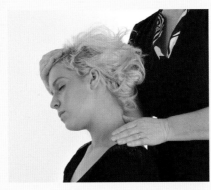

△ Thumb pushes to the border of the trapezius

5 Still supporting the head as before, squeeze the border of the trapezius using the inner border of the forefinger and the thumb, starting at the base of the neck upwards towards the ear.

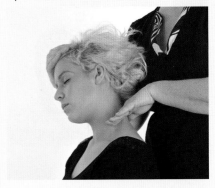

△ Squeezes to the border of the trapezius

6 Support the forehead with one hand while the other performs finger frictions along the base of the skull at the occipital bone.

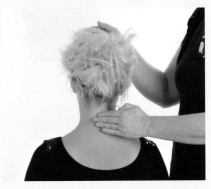

△ Finger frictions along the base of the skull

Chapter 13
MASSAGE USING PRE-BLENDED AROMATHERAPY OILS

This chapter covers the following units:

NVQ unit B24 Carry out massage using pre-blended aromatherapy oils

City & Guilds VRQ unit 309 Provide massage using pre-blended aromatherapy oils

VTCT VRQ unit UV30425 Provide massage using pre-blended aromatherapy oils

LEARNING OBJECTIVES

This chapter is about the skills involved in preparing clients for and the delivery of massage using pre-blended aromatherapy oils. It is essential that you are able to adapt and modify the use of pre-blended oils and massage techniques to suit individual client needs.

The learning outcomes for NVQ unit B24 are:

  Be able to maintain safe and effective methods of working when carrying out massage using pre-blended aromatherapy oils

  Be able to consult, plan and prepare for treatments with clients

  Be able to massage the body using pre-blended aromatherapy oils

  Understand organisational and legal requirements for carrying out massage using pre blended aromatherapy oils.

  Understand how to work safely and effectively when carrying out massage using pre-blended aromatherapy oils

  Understand how to consult with clients

  Be able to prepare to carry out massages using pre-blended aromatherapy oils

  Understand anatomy and physiology related to massage treatments

  Understand contraindications and aromatherapy oils

  Understand how to use pre-blended aromatherapy oils

  Understand the principles behind massage techniques using pre-blended aromatherapy oils

  Understand how to provide aftercare advice

You will need to be successful in all of these outcomes to be competent in massage using pre-blended aromatherapy oils, to qualify for insurance and be able to perform the treatment on members of the public.

NVQ evidence requirements

For the NVQ your assessor will need to observe you perform this treatment successfully on at least four occasions involving different clients. Two of these must be full-body massage treatments including the face. You must practically:

1 Use the consultation techniques of:
- questioning
- visual
- manual
- reference to record cards.

2 Check these physical characteristics:
- weight
- height
- posture
- muscle tone
- age
- health
- skin condition.

3 Be able to take the necessary actions of:
- encouraging the client to seek medical advice
- explaining why the treatment cannot be carried out
- modification of the treatment.

4 Have different treatment objectives that are:
- relaxation
- sense of wellbeing
- uplifting
- anti-cellulite
- stimulating.

5 Massage techniques to be used are:
- effleurage
- petrissage
- tapotement
- pressure point.

6 Treatment areas to include are:
- face
- head
- chest and shoulders
- arms and hands
- abdomen
- back
- gluteals
- legs and feet.

7 Aftercare advice that covers:
- avoidance of activities which may cause contra-actions
- future treatment needs
- modifications to lifestyle patterns
- healthy eating and exercise advice
- suitable homecare products and their uses.

VRQ practical evidence requirements

There are different evidence requirements for the VRQ qualifications, depending on the awarding body.

City & Guilds unit 309 Provide massage using pre-blended aromatherapy oils

The final summative observation should be undertaken when the candidates have completed a minimum of three formative massage treatments using pre-blended aromatherapy oils to meet three of the following objectives:

- relaxation
- uplifting
- sense of wellbeing
- stimulation.

Each observation should be accompanied by a treatment plan which should include the following information:

- client's history, lifestyle factors that may influence the treatments and client expectations
- pre-blended aromatherapy oils selected to suit client's skin type and condition
- massage techniques that were selected and adapted to suit the area of the body being treated
- contra-actions that may occur during and following treatment and how to respond.

For the final observation the candidate will be assessed carrying out one massage treatment using pre-blended aromatherapy oils.

VTCT unit UV30425 Provide massage using pre-blended aromatherapy oils

Four observations to include the following range:
Used all consultation techniques:

- questioning
- visual
- manual
- reference to client records

Dealt with all physical characteristics of clients:

- weight
- height
- posture
- muscle tone
- age
- health
- skin condition

Dealt with a minimum of one of the necessary actions:

- encouraging the client to seek medical advice
- explaining why the treatment cannot be carried out
- modification of treatment

Met all treatment objectives:

- relaxation
- sense of wellbeing
- uplifting
- anti-cellulite
- stimulating

Covered all treatment areas:

- face
- head
- chest and shoulders
- arms and hands
- abdomen
- back
- legs and feet

Used all massage techniques:

- effleurage
- petrissage
- tapotement
- vibration
- friction

Given all types of advice:

- avoidance of activities which may cause contra-actions
- future treatment needs
- modifications to lifestyle patterns
- healthy eating and exercise advice
- suitable home care products and their use

In all cases simulation is NOT allowed.

VRQ knowledge requirements

City & Guilds unit 309 Provide massage using pre-blended aromatherapy oils	VTCT unit UV30425 Provide massage using pre-blended aromatherapy oils	Page no.
Learning outcome 1: Be able to prepare for massage using pre-blended aromatherapy oils		
Practical skills/observations		
Prepare themselves, client and work area for body treatment using pre-blended aromatherapy oils		460–1
Use suitable consultation techniques to identify treatment objectives		203–6
Advise the client on how to prepare for the treatment		461

Introduction

Aromatherapy is the use of essential oils to bring about a healing process to the recipient as well as encouraging good health and increasing well-being. It can aid in balancing the mind, body and spirit. As a natural treatment, aromatherapy has always been popular with clients because the aromatic qualities and properties of the essential oils are supported by the manual approach of massage.

Aromatherapy is often used as an alternative or complement to conventional medicine and drugs. When used as an alternative treatment aromatherapy is used in place of conventional treatments while as a complementary treatment aromatherapy is managed together with a conventional treatment to provide support. Aromatherapy can assist in treating many different conditions, including headaches, muscular tension, anxiety and high blood pressure.

The history of the use of plants for therapeutic effect goes back thousands of years. Primitive man found the leaves, berries and roots gathered for food could make them unwell or heal the sick. The different woods they burned gave off aromas that caused them to feel calm or excited. Egyptians collected botanical plants to grow which produced herbs, woods and resins to be used in cosmetics, medicines and for embalming. During the fourteenth century sachets of lavender were worn around the neck during the Black Death (plague) and pomanders of orange and lavender were also used.

The aim of aromatherapy massage is to ensure penetration of the oils through the skin and into the bloodstream via massage. Combining the senses of touch and smell make the recipient feel physically and mentally relaxed and emotionally nourished and cared for. Aromatherapy aids immunity by boosting the immune system, lymphatic and blood circulations. It also acts on the nervous system to stimulate, revive or relax, depending on the oils used. The treatment can help to relieve specific ailments and balance the body's energy levels through a holistic approach.

> **Key term**
>
> **Pomander** – a mixture of aromatic substances enclosed in a ball-shaped bag or box and used to scent clothes and linens; formerly carried to guard against infection.

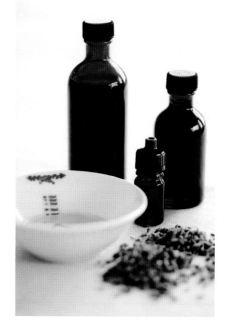

△ Essential oils

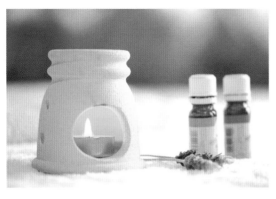

△ Oil burner

The benefits of aromatherapy can be gained directly through massage, used in a bath or used in candles, infusers and burners.

Essential oils and their properties

Essential oils are highly aromatic substances that come from different parts of plants including the leaf, stem, petals, peel and bark. During the initial stage they are known as 'essences'; these are the 'life force' of the plant, becoming an oil only after extraction. Three elements make up essential oils: carbon, hydrogen and oxygen. Essential oils are blended together with a carrier oil to make the pre-blended oils that are used during aromatherapy massage. Depending on the client's individual treatment objectives, the blend of essential oils used will vary and could be for relaxation, a sense of well-being, uplifting, anti-cellulite or stimulating.

Different essential oils possess different therapeutic effects and can act on an emotional and/or physical level. However, once extracted, all essential oils have the same basic properties:

- volatility

- light and non-greasy

- aroma

- highly concentrated

- mix with vegetable oil, mineral oil and alcohol

- do not mix with water.

Different essential oils have differing volatility rates (i.e. speed of evaporation). Every essential oil will fall into one of the classifications shown in Table 13.1, based on their volatility and referred to as 'notes'.

▽ Table 13.1 Classification of notes based on volatility of essential oils

	Top	**Middle**	**Base**
Volatility	Highly volatile	Moderately volatile	Low volatility
Effect	Uplifting	Balancing	Sedating and relaxing
Aroma	Sharp	Warm, soft and mellow	Deep, heavy and intense
Speed	Fast acting, penetrates the skin quickly	Moderate, penetrating the skin at a reasonable speed	Slow penetration of the skin
Lasting effects	Less than 24 hours	1–2 days	5–7 days
Examples	Clary sage Eucalyptus Lemon Tea tree	Camomile Geranium Lavender Rosemary	Rose Sandalwood Ylang-ylang

Methods of entry into the body

There are four basic entry routes into the body for essential oils, as shown in Table 13.2 below.

▽ Table 13.2 Essential oil entry routes into the body

Location	Method of entry	
Skin	The essential oils enter the body when massage is performed via the pores and hair follicles of the skin. Essential oils are small in molecular structure which enables them to penetrate the epidermis. They are then passed between the cells via the glue that holds the cells together into the upper layer of the dermis, where they enter the blood stream via the blood capillaries. From here the oils are distributed around the body.	△ Application of massage with essential oils
Lungs	Through inhalation the essential oils penetrate the lining of the lungs and pass into the bloodstream via the blood capillaries surrounding the alveoli. From here the oils are distributed around the body.	△ Inhalation via the nose into the lungs

Location	Method of entry
Olfactory system	Via inhalation the essential oils penetrate high up inside the nasal cavity to the olfactory mucous membrane which then stimulates a nerve impulse. This impulse is transmitted along the small nerve fibre to one of the main olfactory nerves in the olfactory lobe and finally along the olfactory tract to the brain. Inside the brain instinctive behaviour or memory is triggered: ● The primary olfactory cortex and higher olfactory areas are responsible for recognising what we have smelt and associating it with other information, e.g. a perfume may remind you of somebody who wears it. ● The limbic system, which activates instinctual behaviour and emotion, e.g. the smell of food can make you salivate. The oils can also have an effect on the nerve pathways themselves, resulting in sedative or stimulated effects.
Digestive system	Essential oils enter the digestive system when they are taken orally. This is not a practice used by a therapist due to the high risk of toxicity and irritation of the delicate membrane lining the digestive system. Clients should be warned against this method. △ Ingestion via the mouth is not recommended

Excretion of essential oils

Essential oils are excreted through urine, faeces, perspiration and exhalation. Excretion generally takes 3–6 hours in a normal healthy body but can take up to 14 hours in an obese or unhealthy body. The method of excretion differs from oil to oil. For example, sandalwood can be detected by its aroma in urine; garlic, even when applied to the skin, will be passed out through exhalation, while geranium is detected in perspiration.

Extraction methods of essential oils

Essential oils are extracted from plants in a variety of ways. Different methods are used to ensure that the extracted oil is of the highest natural quality. Extracting oils from plants can be a very expensive process, so many manufacturers now produce synthetic oils, which although they smell similar, do not have the same therapeutic properties. There are five extraction methods:

1 Distillation

2 Enfleurage

3 Maceration

4 Expression

5 Solvent extraction.

Distillation

This is the oldest, cheapest and most frequently used method of extraction. The plant material is placed into a still with water or steam or both, and is heated. The heat produces steam, which cause the walls of the specialised plant cells that hold the essence to break down and release it in the form of a vapour. The vapour is channelled into a condenser where the vapour is left to condense. The resulting liquid is separated into the essential oil and water. Being lighter, the oil floats on top of water (with the exception of clove, which is heavier). This process can take up to 18 hours and the stills can vary in size. The first distillation is usually the best quality with the most therapeutic properties; subsequent distillations are inferior and therefore cheaper. The distilled water can also be of use and is often sold as flower water.

Enfleurage

Enfleurage works on the principle that fat will absorb essential oils. This method is used to extract the finest quality essences from delicate flowers such as rose and jasmine that cannot be heated. The essential oils obtained from this method are expensive to purchase as it can take many millions of flower petals to produce just 1 kilo of essential oil. Because of this it is rarely used today as a method of extraction.

Sheets of glass are smeared thinly with fat and the freshly picked flowers are sprinkled on top. The glass sheets are then stacked in tiers in wooden frames and left for up to 70 days. Occasionally the dead petals are removed and replaced with new ones until the fat can absorb no more oil. Once the fat is saturated with the oils it is collected and cleaned of any debris and is known at this stage as a pomade. This is diluted in alcohol, mechanically agitated and the essential oils are transferred to the alcohol. This mixture is called an 'absolute', which is a very high quality essential oil. The resultant liquid is heated gently so that the alcohol evaporates, leaving the pure essential oil.

> ### Key terms
>
> **Absolute** – a very high quality essential oil.
>
> **Pomade** – a fat substance saturated with essential oil, before the oil has been separated out.

Maceration

This is a method whereby the plant material is soaked in a base oil or dipped into hot fat and kept warm for 2–3 weeks. As the petals and leaves turn brown they are replaced with fresh material until the base oil has absorbed the plant's perfume and therapeutic properties. The process is used on flowers that do not go on generating oils after harvesting, but is now an out-dated method of extraction.

Expression

Expression is used most commonly for the citrus family, for example, lemon, bergamot, orange and grapefruit. The peel is pressed either by machine or by hand, releasing the essential oil and some fruit juice, which are absorbed by sponges. The sponges are squeezed to release the mixture, which is left to stand so the essential oil floats on the top.

Solvent extraction

This process involves the use of solvent, which is allowed to slowly flow over racks of plants and dissolves the plant oils as it does so. The solvent is then returned for reuse, leaving the semi-solid perfume material known as a 'concrete'. This is the aromatic plant material together with natural plant waxes. Like the pomade, the concrete is agitated with alcohol to remove the plant waxes, leaving an 'absolute'.

Essential oils index

Table 13.3 shows a breakdown of the benefits and effects of essential oils.

▽ Table 13.3 Benefits and effects of essential oils

Essential oil		
Camomile: **Roman Chamomile** *(Chamaemelumnobile)* **German** **Chamomile** *(Matricariarecutita)* △ Chamomile	**Appearance**	A small, yellow and white flower which looks like a daisy. The flowers are used for extraction
	Country of origin	Europe and Egypt
	Benefits and effects	Both Roman and German chamomile have excellent calming properties; Roman chamomile has a sweeter fragrance and is more effective for irritation. It is good at treating menstrual and menopausal problems. German chamomile is excellent on the skin to soothe, calm and regenerate. It is dark blue in colour and has a very strong aroma
	Note	Middle

Clary sage *(Salivias clarea)* △ Clary sage	**Appearance**	Green herb with purple flowers. The flowers and the leaves are used for extraction
	Country of origin	France and Bulgaria
	Benefits and effects	Clary sage is an antidepressant and good for the regulation of the menstrual cycle. It promotes a sense of well-being and is very relaxing. It should not be used in pregnancy or if drinking alcohol
	Note	Top
Eucalyptus *(Eucalyptus globulus)* △ Eucalyptus	**Appearance**	A tall tree (300 feet high), with white bark and long pointed leaves. The leaves are used for extraction
	Country of origin	Australia
	Benefits and effects	Eucalyptus is a stimulant that has an antiseptic, anti-bacterial and germicidal effect. It is an expectorant so is useful in treating colds, mucus and catarrh
	Note	Top
Geranium *(Pelargonium odorantissimum)* *(Pelargonium robertianum)* △ Geranium	**Appearance**	Can be various; usually a plant with pink or red flowers and serrated pointed leaves. The leaves are used for extraction
	Country of origin	North Africa, Southern France, Spain and Kenya
	Benefits and effects	Geranium is a balancer and has sedating effects; it is good for irregular menstruation and regulating menopause symptoms. It works well on the digestive system, assisting with irritable bowel syndrome and constipation. It has antiseptic properties and is used in many skincare products
	Note	Middle
Lavender *(Lavandulaofficinalis)* △ Lavender plant	**Appearance**	Lavender blue flowers which are used for extraction
	Country of origin	Southern Europe, North West Africa and many other parts of the world
	Benefits and effects	Lavender is a very commonly used essential oil and can treat just about everything. It has many benefits and effects and is one of very few essential oils that can be used neat on the skin. It has antiseptic properties and can be used on bites, boils and acne. It is a diuretic and therefore good for cellulite. It can help to treat headache, migraines and depression and has a balancing effect
	Note	Middle

Essential oil		
Lemon (*Citrus limon*) △ Lemon	**Appearance**	A yellow fruit; small dark green tree. It is the skin of the fruit that is used for extraction
	Country of origin	North India, Europe, California, Australia, South Africa
	Benefits and effects	Lemon is very stimulating and invigorating. It has antiseptic and diuretic properties and is good for cellulite and insect bites and stings. It is also good for oily skin; can cause mild photosensitivity
	Note	Top
Lemongrass (*Cymbopogon citratus*) △ Lemongrass	**Appearance**	Long thin grass that has a lemon aroma; the grass is used for extraction
	Country of origin	West Indies, Sri Lanka
	Benefits and effects	Lemongrass is a stimulant that increases the circulation and is energising. It is good for oily skins and in treating cellulite
	Note	Top
Marjoram (*Origanum majorana*) △ Marjoram	**Appearance**	A green herb where the leaves are used for extraction
	Country of origin	Mediterranean, Yugoslavia, Hungary
	Benefits and effects	Marjoram has sedating, analgesic and comforting properties. It is good for respiratory problems, high blood pressure and rheumatism and arthritis. It may cause drowsiness so care must be taken
	Note	Middle
Neroli (*Citrus aurantium*) △ Neroli	**Appearance**	Neroli is extracted from the yellow and white flowers from the bitter orange tree
	Country of origin	France and Tunisia
	Benefits and effects	This oil is used in many skincare products as it is excellent at calming stressed, dry, sensitive skins. It has sedative properties and is used for depression, anxiety and insomnia. It is also good at treating stress-related digestive problems
	Note	Base

Rose (Damask) *(Rosa damascena)* △ Rose	**Appearance**	White to red petals, the rose is a well-known flower. The petals are used for extraction
	Country of origin	Bulgaria, Turkey and Morocco
	Benefits and effects	Rose has antiseptic and aphrodisiac properties. It is sedating and calming. Rose is a good female oil as it is used to treat painful and irregular periods and the menopause. It is used in many skincare products for dry skin
	Note	Base
Rosemary *(Rosemarinus officinalis)* △ Rosemary	**Appearance**	Shrubs with rigid branches which have scaly bark, needle-like leaves and pale blue flowers. It is the herb and root that are used for extraction
	Country of origin	Southern Europe, North Africa, South West Asia, Mediterranean
	Benefits and effects	Rosemary is a stimulant and is good for low blood pressure; it also has diuretic properties. It is good for the treatment of cellulite and increases circulation. It should not be used in pregnancy or with a client who has high blood pressure
	Note	Middle
Sandalwood *(Santalum album)* △ Sandalwood	**Appearance**	Small evergreen tree; the wood is used for extraction
	Country of origin	East and West India and Australia
	Benefits and effects	Sandalwood is calming and sedating. It has an expectorant effect, which makes it useful for treating coughs, catarrh and bronchitis. It has a suitable masculine aroma and is used widely in skincare; also has an aphrodisiac effect
	Note	Base
Tea tree *(Melaleuca alternifolia)* △ Tea tree	**Appearance**	Small tree; the leaves are used for extraction
	Country of origin	Australia
	Benefits and effects	Tea tree is antiseptic and has anti-fungal, anti-viral and anti-bacterial properties. It is one of very few essential oils that can be used neat on the skin
	Note	Top

Ylang-ylang (*Cananga odorata*)	Appearance	A tree that produces yellow flowers; the flowers are used for extraction
	Country of origin	Seychelles, Mauritius, Philippines
	Benefits and effects	Ylang-ylang has deeply calming and sedative effects on the body. It reduces high blood pressure and slows the heart rate down. It also has aphrodisiac properties. It should not be used on someone who suffers with low blood pressure
△ Ylang-ylang	Note	Base

Essential oils that relate to treatment objectives

Table 13.4 shows a list of essential oils that relate directly to the assessment range set by HABIA. You should use this list to plan your treatments to meet all of the treatment objectives required.

▽ Table 13.4 Required treatment objectives with related essential oils

Relaxation	Sense of well-being	Uplifting	Anti-cellulite	Stimulating
Chamomile Clary sage Geranium Lavender Marjoram Neroli Rose Ylang-ylang	Chamomile Clary sage Geranium Lavender Neroli Rose Ylang-ylang	Eucalyptus Lemon Lemongrass Rosemary Tea tree	Lavender Lemon Lemongrass Rosemary	Geranium Lemon Rosemary

Carrier oils

Carriers are the substances used to 'carry' the essential oils into the body. In aromatherapy massage the most likely carrier to use is vegetable oils as they have properties of their own that can assist the client and their condition and they also contain nutrients. Unlike essential oils, vegetable oils are greasy so they facilitate the massage movements. They do not evaporate, that is to say they are 'fixed', and they will leave an oily mark on absorbent paper. A mineral oil should not be used because their large molecular structure means they cannot be absorbed through the skin.

The properties of a good carrier oil are:

- little or no aroma
- not soluble in water or alcohol
- low volatility
- medium viscosity
- does not alter the therapeutic effect of the essential oils.

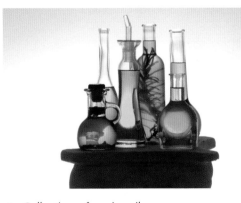

△ Collection of carrier oils

Some commonly used carrier oils are described below.

- Apricot kernel (*Prunus armeniaca*): pale yellow in colour, this oil contains Vitamin A. It penetrates well and is nourishing to dry skin.

- Avocado oil (*Persea americana*): avocado oil is a fruit-based oil that has a rich, thick texture. It contains essential fatty acids, proteins, minerals and vitamins A, B, D and E. Very nourishing and moisturising, it aids dermal regeneration so is suitable for skins in need of restorative treatment such as dry and dehydrated skins, ageing skins, eczema or those with sun damage. Best used in conjunction with a lighter-textured oil such as sweet almond or grapeseed.

- Calendula oil (*Calendula officinalis*): an infusion of the lipid-soluble active properties of the marigold flower, calendula is a light carrier oil. It has tissue regenerating properties so promotes the healing of wounds, scars, burns and other injuries. It can be used on all skin types but is best mixed with another carrier oil for general use.

- Evening primrose (*Oenothera biennis*): a golden yellow, fine-textured seed-based oil. It is rich in vitamins and minerals, particularly gamma-linolenic acid (GLA). It is often used as a nutritional supplement; the oil is useful in the treatment of eczema, psoriasis, pre-menstrual tension, menopausal problems and nappy rash. The oil is a good moisturiser so is indicated for dry, chapped or ageing skins. It has natural healing properties and so can accelerate wound healing.

- Grapeseed oil (*Vitus vinifera*): seed-based oil with a fine, light texture and greenish in colour. It is quickly and deeply absorbed into the skin but is best blended with more nutritious oils as it contains low levels of vitamins, minerals and proteins.

- Hazelnut oil (*Corylus avellana*): beneficial for oily or combination skin types and effective for acne; this oil is stimulating to the circulation and has astringent properties.

- Jojoba oil (*Simmondsia chinesis*): this golden coloured 'oil' is actually a liquid wax with high penetrating properties. It closely resembles the skin's natural oil, sebum, with excellent softening and moisturising qualities. It contains proteins, minerals and an anti-inflammatory agent. Suitable for all skin types including oily and spotty skins as it helps to unclog the pores. Also good for inflamed, irritated skin conditions and dandruff or dry scalps.

- Macadamia oil (*Macadamia ternifolia*): a nut-based oil so not to be used with those clients with nut allergies. Medium in texture and useful for all skin types in dilution with other carrier oils. It is highly emollient and nourishing to dry and mature skins as it has anti-ageing properties.

- Olive oil (*Olea europaea*): a good emollient, but it is thick in texture and is more suitable when diluted with another oil; soothing to inflamed skin and good for bruises.

> ## Key terms
>
> **Viscosity** – the quality that describes a fluid's resistance to flow.
>
> **Volatility** – how fast a substance evaporates.

- Peach kernel oil (*Prunus persica*): fruit-based oil, pale gold in colour. It contains minerals and vitamins, particularly vitamin E. It is easily absorbed and is recommended for use on ageing, dry and sensitive skins and those with broken capillaries.

- Safflower oil (*Carthamus tinctorius*): light in texture and beneficial for bruising; safflower oil is highly moisturising with an exceptionally high amount of oleic acids.

- Sunflower seed (*Helianthus annuus*): light-textured, non-greasy oil which contains Vitamins A, B, C, D and E. It has a healing effect on the skin and is beneficial to skin ulcers, bruising and skin diseases.

- Sweet almond oil (*Prunus amygdalus*): a pale yellow nut oil, rich in vitamins, minerals and protein. Light and easily absorbed, it is an excellent lubricant with revitalising and nourishing qualities. Sweet almond is useful for dry, sensitive and irritated skin conditions. Care must be taken with clients with nut allergies.

- Wheat germ oil (*Triticum vulgare*): a seed-based oil, heavy and rich in texture and a dark reddish-orange colour. It has a strong wheat/earthy odour but is rich in vitamins, particularly vitamin E, proteins and minerals. It stimulates tissue regeneration so is useful for treating ageing skins prone to lines and wrinkles, scars and stretch marks, especially as a preventative measure and also sun damaged skins. The oil may cause sensitivity in those prone but it can be added to other oils to preserve them as it has good antioxidant properties.

Key terms

Gamma-linolenic acid – an omega 6 fatty acid.

Oleic acid – an unsaturated fatty acid that is important for cell structure.

Health and safety

Remember that clients with nut allergies must not be treated with a nut-based carrier oil.

Pre-blended aromatherapy oils

There are many benefits to using pre-blended aromatherapy oils instead of blending the oils yourself. Many professional product companies now make their own pre-blended aromatherapy oils and a reputable, well-known brand name will be instantly recognisable to clients. Many of these large companies market their products worldwide and offer a wide range of choice and retail products. They are likely to provide promotional marketing material as well as blending, bottling and packaging their products. Do be aware however, that the blend is not personal to the client, and there may be an essential oil within the pre-blended product that is not suitable for an individual.

Maintain safe and effective methods of working when providing massage using pre-blended aromatherapy oils

Aromatherapy can offer a perfectly safe and natural approach to overall well-being but there are some precautions that a therapist must follow. For general health and safety please refer back to Chapter 1 Monitoring health and safety.

Sensitivity to aromatherapy oils

Ensure that you carry out a sensitivity test to establish your client's response and suitability to treatment. This should be conducted at least 24 hours prior to treatment and the results thoroughly recorded on the client's record card.

Certain groups of people will be more vulnerable to possible dangers from the use of essential oils, for example, pregnant women, epileptics and clients with high blood pressure. Oils that should be avoided all together on these clients are shown below.

- Pregnant women: aniseed, basil, cinnamon, camphor, carrot seed, cedarwood, clary sage, clove, cypress, fennel, hyssop, jasmine, juniper berry, marjoram, nutmeg, origanum, parsley, peppermint, rosemary, sage, savoury, thyme.

- Epileptics: fennel, hyssop, rosemary, sage, thyme.

- High blood pressure: hyssop, rosemary, sage, thyme.

A much diluted blend of oils should be used on these groups, as well as on babies, young children and older people treatment should be less frequent.

In some cases the use of essential oils can cause problems of dermal sensitivity, photosensitisation or toxicity to the client and/or the therapist.

Dermal sensitivity

This is caused by the application of an irritant, such as an essential oil, to the skin. The degree of sensitivity varies and irritation is defined as a simple reaction following contact with an irritant substance. In some cases even diluted essential oils can cause dermal sensitivity and repeated applications increase the chance of a skin reaction. The reaction takes the form of erythema, itching and blotchy skin.

Photosensitisation

Some oils enhance the effects of ultra-violet light on the skin and therefore should not be used before exposure to sunlight, sun beds or other sources of ultra-violet light. These essential oils are angelica, bergamot, lemon, lime and orange.

Toxicity

The majority of essential oils are non-toxic and perfectly safe when used in accordance with the correct blending and application guidelines. Some, however, are highly toxic even in low concentrations and others can give rise to toxicity if used over a long period of time.

Using any oil repeatedly over a long period of time is unwise as residues may build up in the body and give rise to toxic effects. In addition the body may stop responding to them if used continually.

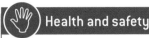
Banned oils

Below is a list of essential oils that have been banned because of their potential dangers and should not be used at all.

- almond (Bitter)
- boldo leaf
- calamus
- horseradish
- jaborandi leaf
- mugwort
- mustard
- pennyroyal
- rue

- sassafras
- savin
- southernwood
- tansy
- thuja
- wintergreen
- wormseed
- wormwood

Storage of pre-blended aromatherapy oils

Essential oils evaporate more quickly than fixed oils and consequently can be spoiled if stored incorrectly, leading to a loss of therapeutic effect and fragrance. They should be stored:

- in a cool dark place
- in an airtight container
- in a dark glass bottle
- away from sunlight and heat.

An unopened bottle of essential oil should last 2–4 years, depending on the type of oil. Citrus oils such as lemon and grapefruit have a shorter shelf life of approximately six months. Old and new blends of essential oils should not be mixed together. Plastic containers are not good for the storage of essential oils, as the oils tend to permeate the plastic.

Hints and tips
Not every client will like the same fragrance – another reason to ensure adequate room ventilation.

Ventilation

Always ensure your treatment room has appropriate ventilation as some essential oils can be very potent in smell. Good ventilation will reduce the negative effects that the aroma of essential oils can have on you and other clients during the course of the day.

Consult, plan and prepare for treatments with clients

It is essential that a therapist has a clear understanding the theory of the structure of the skin and systems of the body when performing massage using pre-blended aromatherapy oils. Details of relevant anatomy and physiology relating to this chapter can be found in Chapter 4. For consultation, planning and preparing for treatments with clients see Chapter 6 Professional practices.

Treatment timings

Table 13.5 shows the different aromatherapy massage treatments and their associated timings.

▽ Table 13.5 Treatment timings for aromatherapy massage treatments

Treatment area	Timing
Back, neck and shoulder pre-blended aromatherapy massage	30 minutes
Full body pre-blended aromatherapy massage	60 minutes
Full body pre-blended aromatherapy massage including face and head	75 minutes

Contraindications to massage using pre-blended aromatherapy oils

The specific contraindications to massage using pre-blended aromatherapy oils are divided into two groups – those that prevent treatment and those that restrict treatment. These are shown in Table 13.6.

▽ Table 13.6 Contraindications to massage using pre-blended aromatherapy oils

Conditions that prevent treatment	Conditions that restrict treatment
Fungal, bacterial and viral infections Infestations Severe eczema and psoriasis Severe skin conditions Eye infections Deep vein thrombosis During chemotherapy and radiotherapy treatment	Broken bones Recent scar tissue Hyper-keratosis Skin allergies Cuts and abrasions Epilepsy Diabetes Heart disease/conditions High and low blood pressure Skin disorders Recent fractures and sprains Undiagnosed lumps and swellings Product allergies Respiratory and circulatory conditions Dysfunctions of the muscular and nervous systems Phlebitis Pregnancy

Contra-actions to massage using pre-blended aromatherapy oils

A contra-action can be identified as a condition which may arise during the treatment which would indicate that the treatment must stop. It may also be something that arises on completion of the treatment. After a massage using pre-blended aromatherapy a client may feel particularly relaxed if oils were chosen for this effect. Always discuss possible contra-actions with your client after treatment. Contra-actions from massage using pre-blended aromatherapy oils include:

- an allergic reaction to the products used
- possible insomnia or difficulty sleeping
- low mood or feelings of melancholy
- hallucinations

- excessive redness or skin irritation from the essential oils
- respiratory reactions
- feeling faint (caused by an alteration of blood pressure levels)
- headaches (caused by dehydration and the release of toxins around the body)
- nausea
- muscles aches
- increased secretions and urination
- lethargy
- heightened emotions.

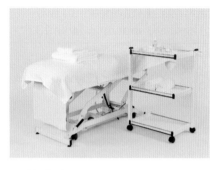

△ Typical set up

Setting up for massage using pre-blended aromatherapy oils

Your set-up for massage using pre-blended aromatherapy oils should reflect high standards. It is important to instil confidence in your client and you must ensure your appearance is appropriate. A client will expect you to be professional both in appearance and manner, with a washed and ironed uniform, hair tied up neatly and securely off your face and short clean nails free from polish.

Back to basics

Equipment checklist

Your trolley should be equipped with:

- Sterilising agent for the client's feet.
- Cleanser in case make up needs to be removed.
- Cotton pads and tissues.
- Bolsters for additional support.
- A lined bowl for client's jewellery.
- A choice of pre-blended aromatherapy oils.
- Consultation form, client record card and pen.

The massage couch should be equipped with:

- Towels to cover the client and the couch.
- Couch roll, to cover the couch and dispose of on completion of treatment.
- A covered waste bin.

The treatment environment

One of the most important requirements for massage using pre-blended aromatherapy is the room environment. You must ensure that the client is warm, comfortable and provides privacy when changing. Your treatment room should always be well ventilated with suitable lighting and music.

The couch should be covered over with clean towels and new couch roll. Your trolley should be set up accordingly with your chosen pre-blended aromatherapy oil on your trolley.

Preparation of the client before treatment

Once your consultation is complete, you need to give the client directions on how to prepare for the treatment. Sufficient privacy, space and time should be allocated to this so the client does not feel rushed. Instruct the client to remove their clothing to their underwear and to place their clothes in a suitable place. A female client may be more comfortable removing her bra for treatment so reassure her that her modesty will be maintained and she will be covered over with towels at all times. Remind the client to remove all jewellery and put in a safe place. Ask the client to lie under the towels in either a supine or prone position (depending on your routine and areas to be treated) and to wait for your return to the treatment room.

Wash your hands for hygiene, ensure the client is covered sufficiently and place any pillow or bolster support for comfort as required. You may need to cleanse the client's face of make up before you commence your treatment. Always clean the client's feet and then rewash your hands. Verbally check that the client is warm and comfortable and inform them that you are about to begin.

Perform massage using pre-blended aromatherapy oils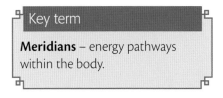

Now both you and your client are prepared and ready for the treatment to begin. You will continue to use the massage movements that you learned in Chapter 11 Body massage treatments. The massage movements used are effleurage, petrissage, tapotement, pressure point, vibrations, frictions, neuromuscular and lymphatic drainage. You will need to adapt and use a variety of these movements in varying depth, rhythm and pressure to suit the individual needs of your client and meet the treatment objectives.

> **Key term**
>
> **Meridians** – energy pathways within the body.

▽ Table 13.7 Specialist techniques for pre-blended aromatherapy massage

Specialist techniques for pre-blended aromatherapy massage	
Pressure point	Techniques for pressure point massage relate to energy pathways in the body. Adapted from Shiatsu massage techniques, the movements follow meridians or energy pathways to increase or decrease energy levels. Points across the body should be pressed in light to moderate pressure and last for 3–7 seconds, on the client's exhaled breath
Neuromuscular	The pressure for neuromuscular massage is much firmer than that used in Swedish techniques and the movements are intended to affect and stimulate the nerves. The direction of massage is to follow the sensory nerve roots

☆ *Hints and tips*
When massaging the back of your client's body it is a lovely gesture to place an ornate bowl of warm water with a few drops of the same pre-blended oil in on the floor under the face hole so your client can inhale the aroma.

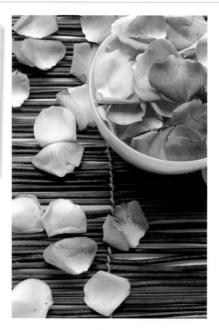

△ Bowl containing oils and petals

The treatment will begin with the client lying face up (supine) and the sequence is as follows:

- Front of right leg and foot
- Front of left leg and foot
- Abdomen
- Left arm and hand
- Right arm and hand
- Chest and shoulders
- Face and head

  Turn client over, so they are lying prone.
- Back of right leg and gluteals
- Back of left leg and gluteals
- Back

Treatment technique: massage routine

A suggested massage routine is shown below.

Front of leg:

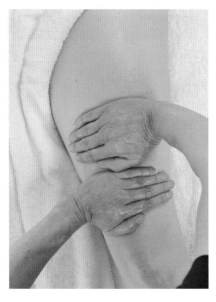

1 Double-handed effleurage, from toes to top of leg × 6.

2 Double-handed effleurage, from toes to knee × 3.

3 Alternate hand effleurage, from toes to knee × 3.

4 Alternate deep hand petrissage on outer then inside of leg from ankle to knee.

5 Light circles around the knee and over the top of the patella.

6 Double-handed effleurage from knee to thigh × 3.

7 Double-handed lifting of upper leg.

8 Kneading to the upper leg.

9 Light lymphatic drainage movement from knee to inguinal node.

10 Double-handed effleurage, from toes to top of leg × 6.

11 Finish with pressure at foot and cover over leg with towel.

7 Still with the forehead supported, perform heel frictions along the base of the skull at the occipital bone.

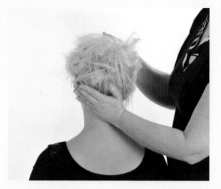

△ Heel frictions along the base of the skull

8 Effleurage the base of the skull using the flat of the hand, still with the forehead supported.

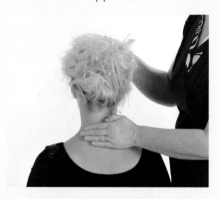

△ Effleurage the base of the skull

9 Turning the hand to point the fingers downwards, apply finger pressure points to the centre at the occipital, then either side of the trapezius where it attaches to the skull. Each time gently rock the head back into the pressure, hold and then release by rocking the head slightly forwards. Repeat three times.

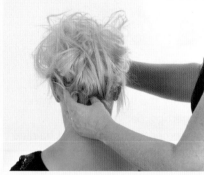

△ Finger pressure points to the occipital

10 Standing behind the client, support the head in the forearm as before as the client takes their head to one side. Using the free arm, place the inner forearm at the base of the neck and apply pressure. Gently hold before sliding the arm out towards the cap of the shoulder, turning it as you do so. Repeat three times and then on the other side.

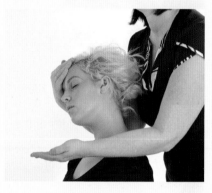

△ Forearm pressures

11 Effleurage the base of the skull as in point 8.

Scalp massage

1 Supporting the head with one hand, perform heel frictions to the sides of the head, front above and behind the ears. Repeat on the other side.

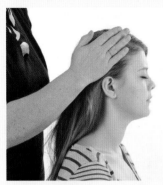

△ Heel frictions to the sides of the head

2 Repeat using finger frictions.

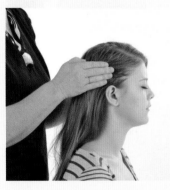

△ Finger frictions to the sides of the head

3 Rub the entire scalp using the fleshy part of one hand then the other.

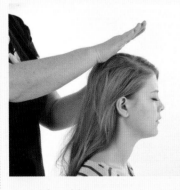

△ Scalp rubbing

4 Perform whole hand frictions to the entire scalp using one hand and then the other.

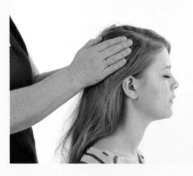

△ Whole hand frictions

5 Claw the hands and using the fingertips, perform zigzag movements from the front hairline to the nape to ruffle the hair.

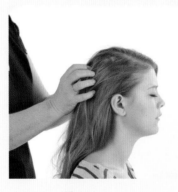

△ Hair ruffling

6 Taking large sections of the hair, perform hair tugging.

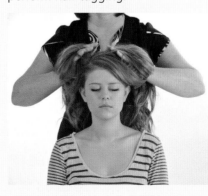

△ Hair tugging

7 Using the hands alternately, effleurage the scalp using the fingertips from front hairline through to the nape.

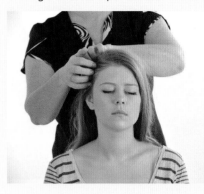

△ Effleurage of the scalp using fingertips

8 Hover the hands over the head closely and perform finger tapotement movements by drumming with straight fingers. Cover the entire scalp.

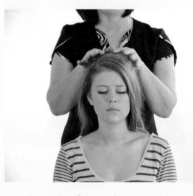

△ Fingertip drumming

9 Stretch the fingers and starting at the front hairline, perform finger pressure points over the scalp, pressing and holding for a second before releasing, then move back about an inch and repeat. Cover the entire scalp in this way.

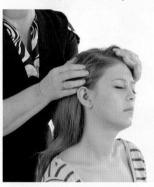

△ Finger pressure points over the scalp

10 Using the inner borders of the forefinger and thumb, squeeze and lift the scalp, working over the entire surface of the scalp.

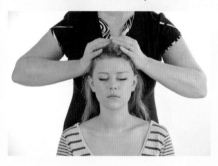

△ Scalp squeeze

11 Using both hands at the same time on either side of the head, perform heel frictions by turning at the wrist so fingers start facing forward and finish pointing upwards. Work from in front of the ear, above and then behind.

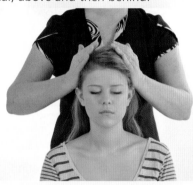

△ Circular heel frictions to the sides of the head

12 Standing at the side of the client, place one hand at the front hairline and the other at the back and gently squeeze the head between the palms of the hands. Repeat three times.

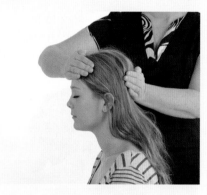

△ Head compressions

13 Repeat effleurage to the scalp as in point 7.

Face massage

1 Support the client's head into your body; place the hands along the jawline, fingertips at the chin, and gently draw the fingers back towards the ears. Replace one hand at a time but higher to repeat the movement across the cheeks and then the forehead. Repeat three times.

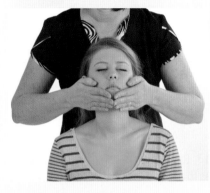

△ Effleurage to the face

2 Using the forefinger and third finger, perform pressure points on the forehead in three sections: in the centre, above the right eyebrow and then the left. Begin at the eyebrow and work towards the hairline, press and hold for a second before releasing then slide up.

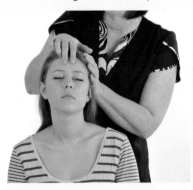

△ Pressure point massage to the forehead

3 Starting at the bridge of the nose and using the fingertip of the forefinger, perform pressure points around the entire border of the eye socket.

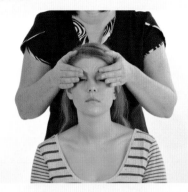

△ Pressure point massage around the eye socket

4 Starting at the nostrils, perform pressure points out along but under the cheekbones to finish at the hairline.

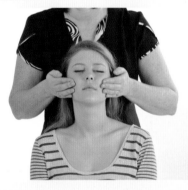

△ Pressure point massage along the cheekbones

5 With the forefinger and third finger, perform circular frictions at the temple.

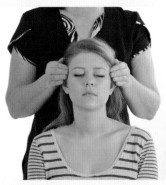

△ Circular frictions to the temple

6 Pinch the ear lobe and circle with the thumb and inner border of the forefinger. Work up and around the edge of the ear.

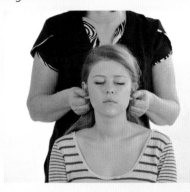

△ Massage of the ear

7 Cup the jawline in the hands and apply gentle pressure and hold for a couple of seconds before moving up the face, cup the cheekbones and then the forehead.

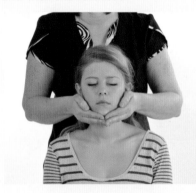

△ Cupping of the face

Chakra balancing

1 Place one hand over the top of the client's head (the crown chakra) and the other over the throat chakra but without touching the client. Keep fingers together and keeping still ask the client to take three deep breaths, in through the nose and out through the mouth.

2 Keeping the hand over the crown chakra move the other up to cover the brow chakra and repeat the breathing.

3 Move both hands up to cover the crown chakra and repeat the breathing.

4 Place the hands gently on the client's shoulders and pause before taking a big step backwards out of the client's aura and gently shake the hands to release the energy.

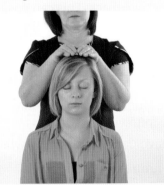

△ Crown chakra

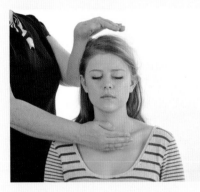

△ Crown and throat chakras

Adaptation to suit client requirements

- Relaxation/sedation: for a relaxing treatment, use a warm, private, quiet treatment area, with subdued lighting, suitable music and relaxing oils burning such as lavender to give a pleasant aroma. The routine should be adapted to contain more of the stroking, rubbing and effleurage movements.

- Sense of well-being: the emphasis should be placed on the mental state of the client and concentrate on the neck and shoulder areas to relieve stress and tension and the chakra balancing to promote well-being and self-healing.

- Uplifting/invigorating: the treatment area can be brighter with livelier music playing and refreshing oils burning. Any movement that is performed is done so briskly; rubbing and frictions should be performed for longer to invigorate. Minimise the relaxing movements that can sedate a client.

- Improvement of hair and scalp condition: concentrate the massage on the scalp, performing more of the movements and using beneficial oils that will nourish the hair and feed the scalp.

- Stimulation: prepare the treatment area as for the uplifting massage and perform all the movements with more speed and pressure to stimulate the tissues.

Completing the treatment

It is important the client is satisfied and the therapist should allow time for the client to feed back and ask questions to improve the service provided. This will not only ensure their repeat business but they may recommend you to a friend or relative for treatment.

It is important that the client's records are completed accurately with the details of the treatment, including the results of tests and the client feedback. This can ensure continuity of treatment should the therapist be absent for their next visit and can assist in the event of becoming involved in legal proceedings.

Aftercare advice for Indian head massage

The aftercare advice for massage treatment can be considered under the following headings:

- avoidance of activities which may cause contra-actions
- future treatment needs
- modification of lifestyle patterns
- healthy eating and exercise advice
- suitable homecare products and their use.

Avoidance of activities which may cause contra-actions

For 12–24 hours following treatment the client should be advised to:

- rest, to give the tissues time to recover/heal
- drink plenty of water to rid the body of toxins that have been released into the blood stream
- avoid physical exercise as the muscles need to rest to recover
- ensure light food intake; indigestion is likely if a heavy meal is eaten as the blood supply has been diverted to the muscles, etc.
- avoid alcohol as this will add more toxins to the body
- take extra care when driving as the senses may be dull and fatigue may mean reactions are slower
- leave the oils on for up to eight hours as they will be absorbed through the skin and will provide beneficial effects.

Future treatment needs

The client should be advised to:

- return for further Indian head massage treatment about once per week if needed
- consider the use of regular treatments to control their stress levels

Remember...

As a reminder, the contra-actions to Indian head massage are:

- allergies
- depression
- insomnia
- hallucination
- respiratory reactions
- lethargy
- headache
- muscle ache
- nausea
- skin irritations
- increases secretions
- heightened emotions.

- consider further complementary therapies such as aromatherapy to help with specific conditions
- consider seeing a counsellor/lifestyle coach/alternative therapist as appropriate.

Modification of lifestyle patterns

The client should be advised to:

- perform relaxation techniques such as deep breathing exercises
- allocate time for self and take up a hobby or interest that is absorbing
- monitor sleep patterns, avoid alcohol in the evening and go to bed at a reasonable time if sleeping is a problem
- promote sleep by the use of essential oils on the pillow
- have a relaxing bath before bedtime to induce sleep
- avoid stimulants such as cola drinks, tea, coffee and alcohol after 6pm
- give up smoking or at least cut down on the number of cigarettes smoked in a day
- eat regularly and healthily
- be aware of posture and make changes to facilitate better posture such as changing the height of a work chair, for example.

Healthy eating and exercise advice

The client should be advised to:

- perform postural exercises to help relieve aches and pains
- perform stretching exercises for those muscles that have shortened and toning exercises for those that have lengthened
- walk briskly for 30 minutes a day
- eat light meals frequently
- eat five portions of fruit and vegetables per day
- reduce sugar intake as this gives a 'sugar high' followed by an extreme low and can lead to low metabolism and diabetes
- reduce alcohol levels and have at least three days per week that are alcohol free
- drink plenty of water and fruit juice
- reduce the intake of coffee and other high caffeine drinks
- avoid low-calorie diets as they lower the metabolism.

Suitable homecare products and their use

The client should be advised to use aromatherapy oils at home in the bath, to burn or to place on the pillow to aid sleep.

Methods of evaluating

It is professional practice to reflect on the Indian head massage treatment in order to review, describe, analyse and evaluate the experience and therefore inform practice. During this process it is also helpful to discuss and review the outcomes of the treatment and its effectiveness with clients. Encourage clients to offer their opinions, and where continued treatment is considered advisable, agree revised goals and further treatment. Encourage clients to think how they might promote their own health and well-being.

Reflection may take place during the treatment in the form of decisions made to change the original treatment plan as it progresses and to adapt the treatment to suit circumstances that arise and develop during the treatment. The advantage of reflection on performance to clientele is an ever-improving service and increased benefits of the treatment. Adaptation to techniques during the treatment as matters arise also maintains safety and maximum gain for the client.

The benefits of stringent reflective practice to a complementary therapy business will be evident from the increase in client satisfaction and their return of custom. It will also result in an improved reputation, leading to an increase in clients and business profitability and ultimately ensures the success of the business.

 Want to know more?

The following professional bodies offer membership, information on changes in practices including health and safety, insurance and continued professional development.
www.babtac.com
www.itecworld.co.uk
www.fht.org.uk
www.beautyguild.com
See also the industry lead body Habia: www.habia.org and the Health and Safety Executive: www.hse.gov.uk

NVQ assessment checklist

To complete this unit you must have the following theoretical and practical skills. Check against the list below and refer back to the relevant section for information on anything you are unsure about.

1. **Be able to maintain safe and effective methods of working when providing Indian head Massage**

❏ **1.1** set up and maintain the treatment area to meet legal, hygiene and service requirements

❏ **1.2** maintain personal hygiene, protection and appearance that meets accepted industry and organisational requirements

❏ **1.3** clean all tools and equipment using the correct methods

❏ **1.4** position equipment and massage medium for safety and ease of use

❏ **1.5** position the client and themselves to minimise fatigue and risk of injury and in a way suitable for the treatment

❏ **1.6** use accepted industry hygiene and safety practices throughout the treatment to minimise cross-infection

❏ **1.7** adopt a positive, polite and reassuring manner towards the client at all times

❏ **1.8** maintain the client's modesty, privacy and comfort at all times

❏ **1.9** complete the treatment within a commercially viable time

❏ **1.10** keep records up to date, accurate, complete, legible and signed by the client and practitioner

❏ **1.11** leave the treatment area in a condition suitable for future treatments

2. **Be able to consult, plan and prepare for treatments with clients**

❏ **2.1** use consultation techniques to determine the client's treatment needs

❏ **2.2** obtain signed, written and informed consent prior to carrying out the treatment from the client or parent/guardian if the client is a minor

❏ **2.3** explain to the client what the treatment entails in a way they can understand

❏ **2.4** identify the client's medical history, physical characteristics and lifestyle pattern by asking questions

❏ **2.5** consult effectively with the client to identify any contraindications to massage treatments, recording the client's responses and take any necessary action

❏ **2.6** provide client advice without reference to a specific medical condition and without causing undue alarm or concern

❏ **2.7** explain and agree the projected cost, duration and frequency of treatment needed

❏ **2.8** agree in writing the client's needs expectations and treatment objectives ensuring they are realistic and achievable

❏ **2.9** adapt client preparation procedures to suit the environment in which the massage is to be undertaken

❏ **2.10** protect clothing, hair and accessories prior to beginning massage

❏ **2.11** select suitable resources and massage medium to meet the treatment objectives

3. **Be able to perform Indian head massage**

❏ **3.1** provide suitable support and cushioning, as necessary, to specific areas of the body during the treatment

❏ **3.2** adapt massage techniques, sequence and use of massage medium to meet the client's physical characteristics and treatment area(s)

❏ **3.3** vary the depth, rhythm and pressure of massage movements to meet treatment objectives, treatment area(s) and client's physical characteristics and preferences

❏ **3.4** co-ordinate breathing techniques with that of the client

❏ **3.5** apply massage medium to ensure minimal waste

❏ **3.6** take prompt remedial action if contra-actions or discomfort occur during the course of treatment

❏ **3.7** allow the client sufficient post-treatment recovery time

❏ **3.8** check that the finished result is to the client's satisfaction and meets the agreed treatment objectives

❏ **3.9** provide aftercare advice specific to the client's individual needs

4. **Understand organisational and legal requirements for providing Indian head massage**

❏ **4.1** explain own responsibilities under current health and safety legislation, standards and guidance

❏ **4.2** explain own responsibilities under local authority licensing regulations for themselves and their premises

❏ **4.3** explain the importance of not discriminating against clients with illnesses and disabilities and why

❏ **4.4** state the age at which an individual is classed as a minor and how this differs nationally

❏ **4.5** explain why minors should not be given treatments without informed and signed parental or guardian consent

❏ **4.6** explain why it is important, when treating minors under the age of 16, to have a parent present

❏ **4.7** explain the legal significance of gaining signed, informed consent to treatment

❏ **4.8** explain manufacturer's and organisational requirements for waste disposal

❏ **4.9** explain the importance of the correct storage of client records in relation to the Data Protection Act

❏ **4.10** explain how to complete client records and the reasons for keeping records of treatments and gaining client signatures

❏ **4.11** explain own responsibilities and reasons for maintaining personal hygiene, protection and appearance according to accepted industry and organisation requirements

❏ **4.12** explain the organisation's requirements for client preparation

❏ **4.13** explain the organisation's service times for Indian head Massage and the importance of completing the service in a commercially viable time

❏ **4.14** explain the organisation's requirements for treatment area maintenance

5. Understand how to work safely and effectively when providing Indian Head Massage

❏ **5.1** explain how to set up the work area for Indian head massage

❏ **5.2** explain the necessary environmental conditions for Indian head massage (including lighting, heating, ventilation, sound and general comfort) and why these are important

❏ **5.3** explain the importance of and reasons for disinfecting hands and how to do this effectively

❏ **5.4** explain how to position themselves and the client for Indian head massage taking into account individual physical characteristics

❏ **5.5** explain what repetitive strain injury (RSI) is, how it is caused and how to avoid developing it when delivering massage treatments

❏ **5.6** explain the importance of adopting the correct posture throughout the treatment and the impact this may have on themselves and the outcome of the treatment

❏ **5.7** explain the reasons for maintaining client modesty, privacy and comfort during the treatment

❏ **5.8** explain why it is important to maintain standards of hygiene and the principles of avoiding cross-infection

❏ **5.9** explain how to minimise and dispose of waste treatments

6. Understand how to consult with clients

❏ **6.1** explain how to use consultation techniques when communicating with clients from different cultural and religious backgrounds, ages, disabilities and genders for this treatment

❏ **6.2** explain why it is important to encourage and allow time for clients to ask questions

❏ **6.3** explain the importance of questioning clients to establish any contraindications to Indian head massage

❏ **6.4** explain why it is important to record client responses to questioning

❏ **6.5** explain the legal significance of client questioning and recording the client's responses

❏ **6.6** explain how to give effective advice and recommendations to clients

❏ **6.7** explain how to visually assess the physical characteristics

❏ **6.8** explain how to assess posture and skeletal conditions that may be present and how to adapt and change the massage routine

❏ **6.9** explain how to recognise different skin types and conditions

❏ **6.10** explain how to recognise different scalp conditions and hair types

❏ **6.11** explain the reasons why it is important to encourage clients with contraindications to seek medical advice

❏ **6.12** explain the importance of and reasons for not naming specific contraindications when encouraging clients to seek medical advice

❏ **6.13** explain why it is important to maintain client's modesty, privacy and comfort

❏ **6.14** explain the relationship between lifestyle patterns and effectiveness of treatment

❏ **6.15** explain the beneficial effects which can result to the client's lifestyle pattern

7. Understand how to prepare for providing Indian head massages

❏ **7.1** explain the importance of giving clients clear instructions on the removal of relevant clothing, accessories and general preparation for the treatment

❏ **7.2** explain why it is important to reassure clients during the preparation process whilst also maintaining the client's modesty and privacy

❏ **7.3** explain how to select the appropriate massage oil suitable for skin, scalp and hair type and condition

❏ **7.4** explain how and when to adapt client preparation for working in different environments

❏ **7.5** explain how to practically and mentally prepare themselves for carrying out the treatment

8. Understand anatomy and physiology related to Indian head massages

❏ **8.1** explain the structure and function of muscles, including the types of muscles within the treatment areas

❏ **8.2** explain the positions and actions of the main muscle groups within the treatment areas

❏ **8.3** explain the position and action of the primary bones and joints of the skeletal system within the treatment areas

❏ **8.4** explain how to recognise postural faults and conditions within the treatment areas

❏ **8.5** explain the structure, function and location of blood vessels and the principles of circulation, blood pressure and pulse within the treatment areas

❏ **8.6** explain the interaction of lymph and blood within the circulatory system

❏ **8.7** explain the structure and function of the lymphatic system

❏ **8.8** explain the position and function of the sinuses

❏ **8.9** explain the basic principles of the central nervous system and autonomic system

❏ **8.10** explain the basic principles of the endocrine and respiratory systems

❏ **8.11** explain the structure and function of skin

❏ **8.12** compare the skin characteristics and skin types of different ethnic client groups

❏ **8.13** explain the effects of Indian head massage on the individual systems of the body

❏ **8.14** summarise the physical and psychological effects of Indian head massage

9. Understand contraindications and contra-actions that affect or restrict body massage treatments

❏ **9.1** explain the contraindications that prevent treatment and why

❏ **9.2** explain the contraindications which may restrict treatment or where caution should be taken, in specific areas and why

❏ **9.3** explain the possible contra-actions which may occur during and post treatment and how to deal with them

10. Understand different Indian head massage mediums

❏ **10.1** explain how to store and maintain Indian head massage mediums in a safe and hygienic manner and why this is important

❏ **10.2** explain how to use Indian head massage mediums safely and effectively

❏ **10.3** explain the types of Indian head massage oils available and their beneficial properties e.g. mustard, coconut, olive and sesame

11. Understand the principles of Indian head massage

❏ **11.1** explain the key aspects of the origins and traditions of Indian head massage

❏ **11.2** summarise the basic principles of Ayurveda

❏ **11.3** explain the principles of body, mind and spiritual wellness

❏ **11.4** explain the principles and practices of marma (pressure) points application (of which 37 are in the treatment area) and their purpose

❏ **11.5** explain the principles and practices of the 7 primary chakras and their importance in relation to the Indian head massage treatment

❏ **11.6** explain the importance of getting the client to remove their shoes before treatment

❏ **11.7** explain why it is important to maintain correct posture during Indian head massage and to complete stretching exercises to prevent repetitive strain injury

❏ **11.8** explain the correct use and application of Indian head massage techniques to meet a variety of treatment objectives

❏ **11.9** explain how to adapt the Indian head massage sequence, depth and pressure to suit different client physical characteristics, areas of the body and preferences

❏ **11.10** explain why effective client breathing is necessary prior to starting the treatment

❏ **11.11** explain how own breathing techniques can enhance the effectiveness of the treatment process

❏ **11.12** evaluate the advantages of Indian head massage

❏ **11.13** explain how and why support and cushioning would be used during the treatment

❏ **11.14** explain the importance of evaluating the effectiveness of Indian head massage treatments

12. Understand how to provide aftercare advice

❏ **12.1** explain why it is important to give post-treatment advice

❏ **12.2** explain the benefits of a course of treatment

❏ **12.3** explain the lifestyle factors and changes that may be required to improve the effectiveness of the treatment

❏ **12.4** explain post-treatment restrictions and future treatment needs

❏ **12.5** explain products for home use that will benefit the client and those to avoid and why

Test yourself

1. What are the 'Chakras' used in Indian head massage treatments?

2. The solar plexus chakra can be found in the

   a) chest

   b) stomach

   c) throat

   d) pelvis.

3. Which of the following best describes an imbalance in the brow chakra?

    a) Poor sleep pattern
    b) Difficulty in expression
    c) Poor concentration
    d) Sinus problems

4. Which one of the following conditions would prevent Indian head massage?

    a) Pregnancy
    b) Severe psoriasis
    c) Whiplash
    d) Nervous dysfunctions

5. What is the most important reason for gaining client agreement prior to treatment?

    a) To prevent the client from changing their mind
    b) To fix the cost of the treatment
    c) To meet health and safety legislation
    d) To ensure the client understands treatment procedure

6. What is the commercially acceptable treatment time for an Indian head massage treatment?

7. Why should you remove the client's jewellery prior to treatment?

8. Give four benefits of an Indian head massage.

9. Name six contra-actions to Indian head massage treatment.

10. Which of the following is the best description of the term 'petrissage'?

    a) A tapping movement
    b) A stroking movement
    c) A kneading movement
    d) A trembling movement

11. State four vegetable oils that were popularly used in India to perform Indian head massage.

12. What are 'marma points'?

13. How many marma points are there in the head and neck?

14. Which of the following is a property of mustard oil?

    a) Cooling
    b) Warming
    c) Soothing
    d) Moisturising

15. What is the aftercare advice for Indian head massage?

Foot:

1 Effleurage all over foot × 6.

2 Deep effleurage over foot × 3.

3 Finger circles around the tarsals.

4 Deep circles to the Achilles tendon.

5 Massage over the heel of the foot.

6 Deep effleurage across the whole underneath of foot.

7 Knuckle across the whole underneath of foot.

8 Thumb crosses over the whole underneath of foot.

9 Massage the top of the foot.

10 Massage down between each metatarsal.

11 Light lymphatic drainage between each metatarsal.

12 Massage each toe, finish with a gentle tug.

13 Effleurage the whole foot, starting deeper and getting lighter × 6.

14 Finish with a pressure to the foot and cover over with towel.

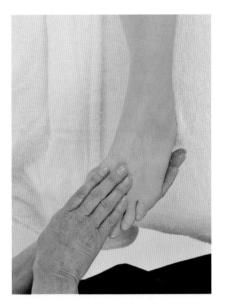

Abdomen:

1 Effleurage in clockwise movement to apply oil.

2 Thumb stroking on solar plexus.

3 Prayer movement from solar plexus, both hands out under ribcage and pull in at waist.

4 Circles with reinforced hands in clockwise direction.

5 Side lifting – effleurage, on one side then the other, gentle pressure in centre.

6 Cover over with towel.

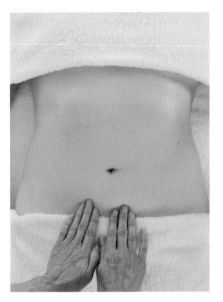

Arm and hand:

1 Alternate-hand effleurage from hands to shoulder.

2 Double-handed effleurage from hands to shoulder.

3 Single-handed deeper effleurage to top of arm

4 Bend elbow and support on the chest – palmer stroking from elbow to shoulder, deep to light.

5 Circles around the shoulder.

6 Linking effleurage to elbow.

7 Circles around the elbow.

8 Deep effleurage to front and back of forearm.

9 Massage around the carpals.

10 Deep massage to palm of hand.

11 Light massage over top of hand.

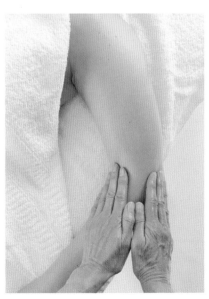

12 Massage between each metacarpal.

13 Light drainage between each metacarpal.

14 Massage each phalange and finish with a slight tug.

15 Pressure to finish, cover over with a towel.

Chest and shoulders:

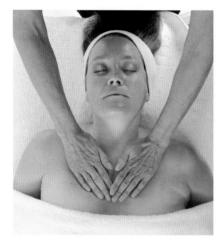

1 Effleurage down from front of neck, over chest and around shoulders to the back of the neck.

2 Draining movement – press on chest. Retain pressure as hands move out towards axillae area. Turn hands and push down on shoulders.

3 Move thumbs to apply pressure under clavicle towards axillae and light drainage with thumbs.

4 Move head from side to side, supporting with both hands.

5 Effleurage over décolleté, around to shoulders and massage trapezius with thumbs and knuckles.

6 Light effleurage over whole chest area; finish with pressure in occipital hollow.

Face:

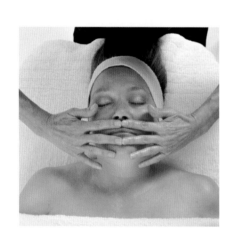

1 Full face lift effleurage × 3.

2 Reinforced thumb pressure, from between eyebrows, up centre of forehead to top of crown.

3 Thumb stroking in centre of forehead × 4.

4 Thumb pressure up the forehead × 3.

5 Thumb stroking on forehead × 4.

6 Thumb pressure across the forehead × 3.

7 Draining from centre of forehead out to temples.

8 Forefinger pressure from notch at upper inside corner of eye socket and work along eyebrow and around eye socket (gently).

9 Lifting and pinching eyebrow with thumb and index finger.

10 Rotary movements on the temples – 2 fingers.

11 Thumbs on the forehead, finger pressures on the cheeks and under cheekbones (3 rows).

12 Draining on the cheeks with finger tips (3 rows) along same pathways.

13 Finger rotation on the masseter muscles.

14 Turn face round to one slide.

15 Gently massage ear lobe, working around ear.

16 Place hands over ears (not touching) and hold for 6–10 seconds.

17 Turn head over and repeat steps 15 and 16 on other ear.

18 Effleurage down from chin, over chest and shoulders, finish with a pressure at shoulders.

Head:

1 Thumb pressures from centre of head right down, working a step out each time.

2 Shampoo massage movements on the scalp slowly, covering all areas.

3 Gentle hair tugging.

4 Palm strokes from top of scalp down.

5 If you are able to, create a ponytail and tug gently, if not, pressure at the crown chakra and release.

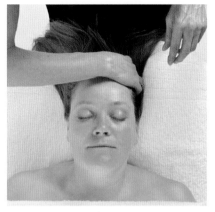

Back of legs:

1 Effleurage from foot to thigh × 6.

2 Deep effleurage from foot to inside knee × 3.

3 Raise lower leg and massage using the heal of hand down centre of calf muscles.

4 With leg still raised, gentle lymphatic drainage to the popliteal lymph nodes.

5 Return leg flat, deep effleurage to top of thigh.

6 Knead top of thigh.

7 Palmar stroke top of thigh.

8 Light lymphatic drainage into inguinal node.

9 Effleurage from foot to thigh ×6.

10 Finish with pressure at ankle, cover over.

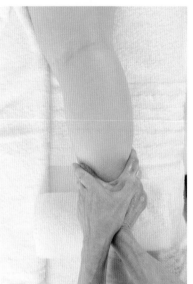

Back:

1 Spinal stretch applying oil.

2 From top of couch, reverse effleurage down either side of spine, sweep out over buttocks and pull in at waist. Return up either side of spine and heel of hands to neck. Press both hands out across shoulders to deltoid and sweep around scapular and return to neck with heel of hands again.

3 Return to side of couch, figure of eight with both hands, crossing over spine.

4 Reinforced hand, effleurage up each side of spine and circle shoulders, middle and lower back.

5 Thumb pressures down the side of the spine between the vertebrae to the hips.

6 Thumb pressure and slide down sides of spine to hips.

7 Place hands on top of each other and push firmly up side of spine with both hands, going right around shoulder blades and down to waist, push up and around scapula and down to hips. Push up and over waist and gluteals and finish at base of spine.

8 Thoracic drain, effleurage to the top of the shoulders and hold, to the armpit at the axillary nodes and lastly to the waist and drain out to both sides.

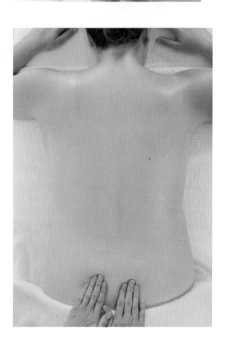

9 Pleating with gentle scissor movement.

10 Fingertip draining from spine outwards, across back.

11 Two-fingered pressure down either side of the spine, working from neck down to coccyx.

12 Thumb kneading on the sacrum and out over the gluteals × 3 rows.

13 Full back effleurage × 6.

14 Cover over with towel, finish with spinal stretch.

LO12 Provide aftercare advice

Aftercare and homecare advice should always been given to the client following massage using pre-blended aromatherapy oils.

Avoidance of activities which may cause contra-actions

For 12–24 hours following treatment the client should be advised to:

- rest, to give the tissues time to recover/heal

- drink plenty of water to rid the body of toxins that have been released into the blood stream

- avoid physical exercise as the muscles need to rest to recover

- ensure light food intake; indigestion is likely if a heavy meal is eaten as the blood supply has been diverted to the muscles, etc.

- avoid alcohol as this will add more toxins to the body

- take extra care when driving as the senses may be dull and fatigue may mean reactions are slower

- leave the oils on for up to eight hours as they will be absorbed through the skin and will provide beneficial effects.

Future treatment needs

The client should be advised:

- to return for further aromatherapy massage treatments. These can be carried out to suit the client's needs, but every 2–3 weeks is often recommended

- about retail products that encourage the client to use essential oils safely at home. These can include essential oil bathing products, candles, infusers and oil burners and pre-blended essential oil skin products

- to consider lifestyle changes such as taking exercise, maintaining a healthy diet, regular fluid intake and methods of relaxation

- of the need for postural awareness.

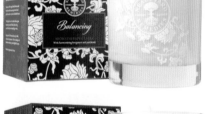
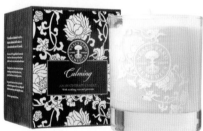
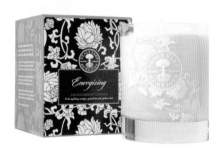

△ Retail aromatherapy candles

Want to know more?

A French chemist, Rene-Maurice Gattefosse, wrote the first modern book on the benefits of essential oils in 1937 and coined the phrase 'aromatherapy'. After burning his hand in his laboratory he used the essential oil of lavender to soothe his skin and was surprised at how quickly his burn healed and with very little scarring. This began a fascination with essential oils and Gattefosse went on to write several books on the subject.

You may find it interesting to research farms whose plants are used for extraction of essential oils. Many of these farms have times when they are open to visitors. Lavender is grown nationwide and is in season between the months of June and July where you will see a beautiful abundance of purple fields. Lavender is generally harvested from July through to September.

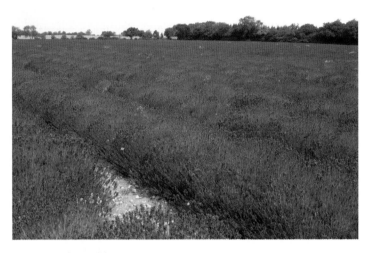

△ Lavender fields

For more on aromatherapy oils refer to the HABIA website: www.habia.org.uk.

NVQ assessment checklist

To complete this unit you must have the following theoretical and practical skills. Check against the list below and refer back to the relevant section for information on anything you are unsure about.

1. Be able to maintain safe and effective methods of working when carrying out massage using pre-blended aromatherapy oils

❏ **1.1** set up and maintain the treatment area to meet organisation and manufacturers' instructions

❏ **1.2** maintain personal hygiene, protection and appearance meets accepted industry and organisational requirements

❏ **1.3** clean all equipment using the correct methods

❏ **1.4** position equipment and pre-blended oils for safety and ease of use

❏ **1.5** position the client and themselves to minimise fatigue and risk of injury and in a way suitable for treatment

❏ **1.6** use accepted industry hygiene and safety practices throughout the treatment to minimise the risk of cross-infection

❏ **1.7** adopt a positive, polite and reassuring manner towards the client at all times

❏ **1.8** maintain the client's modesty, privacy and comfort at all times

❏ **1.9** complete the treatment within a commercially viable time

❏ **1.10** keep records up to date, accurate, easy to read and signed by the client and practitioner

❏ **1.11** leave the treatment area and equipment in a suitable condition for future treatments

2. Be able to consult, plan and prepare for treatments with clients

❏ **2.1** use effective consultation techniques to determine the client's treatment needs

❏ **2.2** obtain signed, written, informed consent prior to carrying out the treatment from the client or parent/ guardian if the client is a minor

❏ **2.3** explain to the client the treatment procedure in a way they can understand

❏ **2.4** question the client to identify the client's medical history, physical characteristics and lifestyle pattern

❏ **2.5** consult with the client to identify any contraindications to aromatherapy treatments, recording the clients responses, and take any necessary action

❏ **2.6** encourage clients to ask questions and clarify any points

❏ **2.7** carry out a sensitivity test to establish response and suitability for treatment

❏ **2.8** provide client advice without reference to a specific medical condition and without causing undue alarm or concern

❏ **2.9** explain and agree the projected cost, likely duration, frequency and types of treatment needed

❏ **2.10** agree in writing the client's needs, expectations and treatment objectives, ensuring they are realistic and achievable

❏ **2.11** protect client's clothing, hair and accessories

❏ **2.12** select suitable pre-blended aromatherapy oils which meet the treatment objectives which are fit for purpose

3. Be able to massage the body using pre-blended aromatherapy oils

❏ **3.1** provide suitable support and cushioning to specific areas of the body during the treatment if necessary

❏ **3.2** adapt massage techniques, sequence and use of pre-blended oil to meet the client's physical characteristics and treatment area(s)

❏ **3.3** vary the depth, rhythm and pressure of massage movements to meet treatment objectives, treatment area(s) and client's physical characteristics and preferences

❏ **3.4** apply and use pre-blended oil to minimise waste

❏ **3.5** take prompt remedial action if contra-actions or discomfort occur during the course of treatment

❏ **3.6** give the client sufficient post-treatment recovery time

❏ **3.7** check that the finished result is to the client's satisfaction and meets the agreed treatment objectives

❏ **3.8** provide aftercare advice

4. Understand organisational and legal requirements for carrying out massage using pre blended aromatherapy oils

❏ **4.1** explain own responsibilities under current health and safety legislation, standards and guidance

❏ **4.2** explain own responsibilities under local authority licensing regulations for themselves and the premises

❏ **4.3** explain the importance of not discriminating against clients with illnesses and disabilities and why

❏ **4.4** explain the age at which an individual is classed as a minor and how this differs nationally

❏ **4.5** explain why it is important, when treating minors under 16 years of age, to have a parent or guardian present

❏ **4.6** explain why minors should not be given treatments without informed and signed parental or guardian consent

❏ **4.7** explain the legal significance of gaining signed, informed consent to treatment

❏ **4.8** explain own responsibilities and reasons for maintaining personal hygiene, protection and appearance according to accepted industry and organisational requirements

❏ **4.9** explain the manufacturers' and organisational requirements for waste disposal

❏ **4.10** explain the importance of the correct storage of client records in relation to the Data Protection Act

❏ **4.11** explain how to complete client records, the importance of and reasons for keeping records of treatments and gaining client signatures

❏ **4.12** explain the organisation's requirements for client preparation

❏ **4.13** explain the organisation's service times for massage treatments and the importance of completing the service in a commercially viable time

❏ **4.14** explain the organisation's and manufacturers' requirements for the treatment area, maintenance and cleaning of equipment

5. Understand how to work safely and effectively when carrying out massage using pre-blended aromatherapy oils

❏ **5.1** explain how to set up the work area for massage treatments

❏ **5.2** explain the necessary environmental conditions for body massage treatments (including lighting, heating, ventilation, sound and general comfort) and why these are important

❏ **5.3** explain the importance and reasons for disinfecting hands and how to do this effectively

❏ **5.4** explain how to position themselves and the client for massage treatments taking into account individual physical characteristics

❏ **5.5** explain what repetitive strain injury (RSI) is, its cause and how to avoid developing it when delivering massage treatments

❏ **5.6** explain the importance of adopting the correct posture throughout the treatment an the impact this may have on themselves and the outcome of the treatment

❏ **5.7** explain the reasons for maintaining client modesty, privacy and comfort during the treatment

❏ **5.8** explain why it is important to maintain high standards of hygiene and the principles of avoiding cross-infection

❏ **5.9** explain how to minimise and dispose of waste treatments

6. Understand how to consult with clients

❏ **6.1** explain how to use effective consultation techniques when communicating with clients from different cultural and religious, backgrounds, ages, disabilities and genders for this treatment

❏ **6.2** explain why it is important to encourage and allow time for clients to ask questions

❏ **6.3** explain the importance of questioning clients to establish any contraindications to head and body massage treatments

❏ **6.4** explain why it is important to record client responses to questioning

❏ **6.5** explain the legal significance of client questioning and the recording of client responses

❏ **6.6** explain how to give effective advice and recommendations to clients

❏ **6.7** explain how to visually assess the clients' physical characteristics

❏ **6.8** explain how to asses posture and skeletal conditions that may be present and how to adapt and change the massage routine

❏ **6.9** explain how to recognise different skin types and conditions

❏ **6.10** explain how to effectively carry out a skin sensitivity test for allergies to pre-blended aromatherapy oils

❏ **6.11** explain the types of reactions that can occur as a result of using pre-blended aromatherapy oils and how to recognise them

❏ **6.12** explain the reasons why it is important to encourage clients with contraindications to seek medical advice

❏ **6.13** explain the importance of and reasons for not naming specific contraindications when encouraging clients to seek medical advice

❏ **6.14** explain why it is important to maintain client's modesty and privacy

❏ **6.15** explain the relationship between lifestyle patterns and effectiveness of treatment

❏ **6.16** summarise the beneficial effects which can result from changes to the client's lifestyle pattern

7. Be able to prepare to carry out massages using pre-blended aromatherapy oils

❏ **7.1** explain the importance of giving clients clear instructions on the removal of relevant clothing, accessories and general preparation for the treatment

❏ **7.2** explain why it is important to reassure clients during the preparation process whilst also maintain the client's modesty and privacy

❏ **7.3** explain how to select the appropriate pre-blended aromatherapy oil suitable for skin type, condition and treatment objectives

❏ **7.4** explain how to cleanse different areas of the body in preparation for treatment e.g. face and feet

8. Understand anatomy and physiology related to massage treatments

❏ **8.1** explain the structure and function of cells and tissues

❏ **8.2** explain the structure and function of muscles, including the types of muscle

❏ **8.3** explain the positions and actions of the main muscle groups within the treatment areas of the body

❏ **8.4** explain the position and function of the primary bones and joints of the skeleton

❏ **8.5** explain how to recognise postural faults and conditions

❏ **8.6** explain the structure, function and location of blood vessels and the principles of circulation, blood pressure and pulse

❏ **8.7** explain the interaction of lymph and blood within the circulatory system

❏ **8.8** explain the structure and function of the lymphatic system

❏ **8.9** explain the basic principles of the central and autonomic nervous system

❏ **8.10** explain the basic principles of the endocrine, respiratory, digestive and excretory system

❏ **8.11** explain the structure and function of the skin

❏ **8.12** explain the skin characteristics and skin types of different ethnic client groups

❏ **8.13** explain the structure and location of the adipose tissue

❏ **8.14** summarise the effects of massage using pre-blended aromatherapy oils on the individual systems of the body

❏ **8.15** summarise the physical and psychological effects of massage using pre-blended aromatherapy oils

❏ **8.16** explain how to recognise erythema and its causes

9. Understand contra-indications and aromatherapy oils

❏ **9.1** explain the contraindications that prevent treatment and why

❏ **9.2** explain the contraindications which may restrict treatment or where caution should aromatherapy oils be taken, in specific areas and why

❏ **9.3** explain possible contra-actions which may occur during and post treatment, why and how to deal with them

10. Understand how to use pre-blended aromatherapy oils

❏ **10.1** explain how to store and maintain pre-blended aromatherapy oils in a safe and hygienic manner

❏ **10.2** explain how to use pre-blended aromatherapy oils safely and effectively, including the effects of volatility

❏ **10.3** summarise the types of pre-blended aromatherapy massage oils available, their purpose

❏ **10.4** explain how to adapt their choice of pre-blended aromatherapy oils to meet specific clients' physical and emotional needs

11. Understand the principles behind massage techniques using pre-blended aromatherapy oils

❏ **11.1** explain why it is important to maintain correct posture during massage and complete their own stretching exercises to prevent repetitive strain injury

❏ **11.2** explain the correct use and application of massage techniques to meet a variety of treatment objectives

❏ **11.3** explain how to adapt the massage sequence, depth and pressure to suit different client physical characteristics, areas of the body and preferences

❏ **11.4** explain how to adapt massage treatments for male and female clients

❏ **11.5** explain the areas of the body and body characteristics needing particular care when undertaking massage using pre-blended aromatherapy oils

❏ **11.6** explain the advantages of massage using pre-blended aromatherapy oils

❏ **11.7** explain how and why support and cushioning would be used during the treatment

❏ **11.8** explain the limitations of using pre-blended aromatherapy oils and when and why to refer clients onto a clinical aromatherapist

❏ **11.9** explain the importance of evaluating the effectiveness of massage using pre-blended aromatherapy oils

12. Understand how to provide aftercare advice

❏ **12.1** evaluate the lifestyle factors and changes that may be required to improve the effectiveness of the treatment

❏ **12.2** explain post-treatment restrictions and future treatment needs

❏ **12.3** explain products for home use that will benefit and protect the client and those to avoid and why

❏ **12.4** explain how eating and exercise habits can affect the effectiveness of treatment

Test yourself

1. Which of the following contraindications restricts aromatherapy treatment?
   a) Deep vein thrombosis
   b) High/low blood pressure
   c) Severe skin conditions
   d) Eye infections

2. Why is a patch test for pre-blended aromatherapy treatment given to clients?
   a) To see if the client likes the smell
   b) To see if the client likes the feel of the oil on their skin
   c) To check the client is suitable for treatment and does not have an allergic reaction
   d) Because you have to do one

3. Which of the following is a property of an essential oil?
   a) They mix with water
   b) They do not have an aroma
   c) They do not evaporate
   d) They evaporate

4. Which of the following is a 'top note' oil?
   a) Tea tree
   b) Lavender
   c) Ylang-ylang
   d) Rose

5. Which of the following is a 'middle note' oil?

   a) Tea tree

   b) Lavender

   c) Ylang-ylang

   d) Rose

6. Which of the following is a 'base note' oil?

   a) Neroli

   b) Rose

   c) Chamomile

   d) Lemon

7. Which essential oil from the following list can be used neat on the skin?

   a) Rose

   b) Lavender

   c) Rosemary

   d) Lemongrass

8. Which of the following essential oils is stimulating in its effect?

   a) Lavender

   b) Rose

   c) Rosemary

   d) Chamomile

Chapter 14
STONE THERAPY MASSAGE

This chapter covers the following units:

NVQ unit B28 Provide stone therapy treatments

City & Guilds VRQ unit 322 Apply stone therapy massage

VTCT VRQ unit UV30475 Apply stone therapy massage

LEARNING OBJECTIVES

This chapter is about the skills involved in providing hot and cold stone therapy treatments. It looks at the massage, placing of stones and the selection of different types of stones. It is essential that you are able to adapt and modify stone therapy treatments to suit individual client needs.

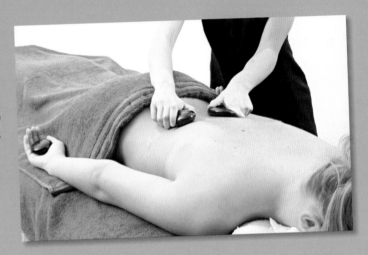

The learning outcomes for NVQ unit B20 are:

- Be able to maintain safe and effective methods of working when providing stone therapy treatments
- Be able to consult, plan and prepare for treatments with clients
- Be able to perform stone therapy treatments
- Understand organisational and legal requirements
- Understand how to work safely and effectively when providing stone therapy
- Understand how to consult with clients
- Understand how to prepare to provide stone therapy treatments
- Understand anatomy and physiology related to stone therapy treatments
- Understand contraindications and contra-actions that affect or restrict stone therapy treatments
- Understand how to use stone therapy equipment
- Understand the principles behind stone therapy techniques and how to use them
- Understand how to provide aftercare advice

You will need to be successful in all of these outcomes to be competent in stone therapy treatments, to qualify for insurance and be able to perform the treatment on members of the public.

NVQ evidence requirements

For the NVQ your assessor will need to observe you perform this treatment successfully on at least four occasions involving different clients. Two of these must be full-body stone therapy treatments including the face. You must practically cover:

1   Using the following equipment:
    professional stone heater
    stones
    accessories
    cooling systems.

2   Use the consultation techniques of:
    questioning
    visual
    manual
    reference to record cards.

3   Check these physical characteristics:
    weight
    height
    posture
    muscle tone
    age
    health
    skin condition.

4   Be able to take the necessary actions of:
    encouraging the client to seek medical advice
    explaining why the treatment cannot be carried out
    modification of the treatment.

5   Have different treatment objectives that are:
    relaxing
    balancing
    uplifting
    create a sense of wellbeing
    perform local decongestion
    give relief from muscular tension.

6   Use different types of stones that are:

    basalt
    marine
    marble
    semi-precious.

7   Use stone techniques that include:
    rotatio\rature management.

8   Treatment areas to include are:
    face
    head
    neck, chest and shoulders
    arms and hands
    abdomen
    back
    legs and feet.

9   Treatment techniques to be used are:
    effleurage
    petrissage
    friction
    tapping
    tucking
    placement
    trigger point.

10 Aftercare advice that covers:
    avoidance of activities which may cause contra-
        actions
    future treatment needs
    modifications to lifestyle patterns
    suitable homecare products and their uses.

VRQ practical evidence requirements

There are different evidence requirements for the VRQ qualifications depending on the awarding body.

City & Guilds unit 322 Apply stone therapy massage

The final observation should be undertaken when the candidates have completed a minimum of three formative stone therapy massage treatments.

Each observation should include:

client's history, lifestyle, factors that may influence the treatment and client expectations

findings of the body analysis and relevant tests

stones selected for the treatment and the reasons why

how the treatment was selected and adapted to suit the treatment need

contra-actions that may occur during and following treatment and how to respond.

For the final summative observation the candidate will be assessed carrying out one stone therapy massage treatment to include hot and cold stones.

VTCT unit UV30475 Apply stone therapy massage

Four observations to include the following range:

Used all consultation techniques:

questioning

visual

manual

reference to client records

Dealt with a minimum of one necessary action:

encourage the client to seek medical advice

explain why treatment cannot be carried out

modify the treatment

Used all types of equipment:

professional stone heater

stones

accessories

cooling systems

Dealt with all client physical characteristics:

weight

height

posture

muscle tone

age

health

skin condition

Met all treatment objectives:

relaxing

balancing

uplifting

sense of well-being

local decongestion

relief from muscular tension

Used a minimum of three out of four types of stones:

basalt

marine

marble

semi-precious stones

Used all stone therapy techniques:

rotation of stones

alternation of hot and cold stones

use of hot stones only

use of cold stones only

combination of stone types and sizes

temperature management

Covered all treatment areas:

face

head

neck, chest and shoulders

arms and hands

abdomen

back

legs and feet

Used all treatment techniques:

effleurage

petrissage

frictions

tapping

tucking

placement

trigger point

Given all types of advice:

avoidance of activities which may cause contra-actions

future treatment needs

modifications to lifestyle patterns

suitable home care products and their use

In all cases simulation is *not* allowed.

VRQ knowledge requirements

City & Guilds unit 322 Apply stone therapy massage	VTCT unit UV30475 Apply stone therapy massage	Page no.
Learning outcome 1: Be able to prepare for stone therapy massage		
Practical skills/observations		
Prepare themselves, client and work area for stone therapy massage		481–4
Use suitable consultation techniques to identify treatment objectives		203–6
Carry out body analysis and relevant tests		481
Provide clear recommendations to the client		470
Select products, tools and equipment to suit client treatment needs		483
Underpinning knowledge		
Describe salon requirements for preparing themselves, the client and work area		481–4
Describe the environmental conditions suitable for stone therapy massage		483
Describe the different consultation techniques used to identify treatment objectives		203–6
Explain the importance of carrying out a detailed body analysis and relevant tests		481
Describe how to select products, tools and equipment to suit client treatment needs		482
Explain the contraindications that prevent or restrict stone therapy massage		481
Describe the types of stones, their properties and uses		476–80
Describe the historical and cultural background for stone therapy massage		476
Describe how stones should be stored		480
Learning outcome 2: Be able to carry out stone therapy massage		
Practical skills/observations		
Communicate and behave in a professional manner		183–4
Follow health and safety working practices		482–90
Position themselves and client correctly throughout the treatment		484
Use products, tools, equipment and techniques to suit client treatment needs		483
Complete the treatment to the satisfaction of the client		484–90
Evaluate the results of the treatment		490
Provide suitable aftercare advice		490
Underpinning knowledge		
Explain how to communicate and behave in a professional manner		183–4
Describe health and safety working practices		482–90
Explain the importance of positioning themselves and the client correctly throughout the treatment		484
Explain the importance of using products, tools, equipment and techniques to suit client treatment needs		483
Describe how treatments can be adapted to suit client treatment needs		483
State the contra-actions that may occur during and following treatments and how to respond		482

Introduction

Stone therapy is the use of hot and cold stones to bring about a balance within the body. Stone therapy is an ancient healing therapy that was practised in Native America, Egypt and China and was used for many different ailments and as a natural source of hot and cold.

Stone therapy is a popular treatment offered by many salons and spas worldwide. It has become a favourite with clients who enjoy traditional massage and it includes a combination of temperatures and a holistic approach that treats the mind, body and spirit. It is popular treatment among therapists as it enables them to use deeper pressure with the added benefits of hot and cold, without causing injury to themselves.

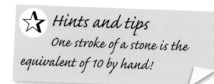

☆ *Hints and tips*
One stroke of a stone is the equivalent of 10 by hand!

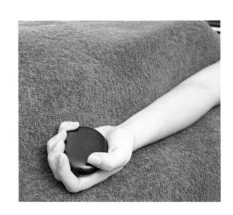

△ Hot stones in the hand

Benefits of stones

Stone therapy affects the body both physically and psychologically. Physically, the stones assist the therapist to work to deeper levels, providing advanced relaxation and relief to muscular tension while protecting the therapist against injury such as repetitive strain injury (RSI). The effects vary depending on the temperature of the stones. Heated stones increase the body's temperature and stimulate blood and lymphatic circulation. They give warmth on cooler days and to cold areas such as hands and feet during treatment. The skin will redden and hyperaemia is produced as the blood vessels dilate. The treatment can also be performed with just cold stones or a combination of stone temperatures. Cold stones will decrease blood circulation and the client's body temperature will drop. The skin will become lighter in colour and a numbing affect will occur on the superficial nerve endings. Cold stones can feel very therapeutic when used for drainage on the face, especially if a client suffers with congestion such as sinusitis and

☆ *Hints and tips*
Always complete a thorough consultation and check with your client their likes and dislikes relating to the temperature of the stones. A client who feels the cold will not appreciate the unexpected shock of cold stones if they are hoping to gain warmth and deep relaxation from their treatment.

puffiness in this area. Generally, cold stones will provide an invigorating, toning and stimulating effect. A combination of hot and cold stones can be used to treat sluggish circulation and even cellulite, especially if the massage is of a firm pressure and in the direction of the lymphatic nodes. Cold stones can also be used to avoid overheating the body during treatment or cooling on a hot day. All areas of the body, face and head benefit from the stones, as do the chakras.

Psychologically, the effects can be deeply calming, soothing, comforting, grounding and sedating. The purpose of using stones can range from grounding the client, dispersing deep-seated tension and clearing and balancing the chakras.

Types of stones

Basalt

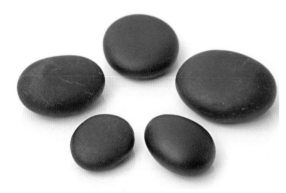

△ Basalt stones for massage

Black basalt stones are the most common to be used during this treatment. They are volcanic in origin and are widespread throughout the world. They are often found on riverbeds and range from grey to black in appearance and are smooth to the touch. The inside of a basalt stone is like honeycomb and the small pockets within the stone help to retain heat. Basalt stones range in size, from tiny toe stones which are placed in between the toes, medium stones which fit nicely in the palm of the therapist's hand and are used on the arms and lower legs, large stones for placement or massaging bigger areas such as the back, and contour stones which are oval in shape and can be used on specific areas to release tension.

Marine

Ranging from green to grey in colour, stones of marine origin are excellent for using cold. They are smooth and dense and come from sedimentary rock. Again, different sizes are recommended so they can be used on different areas of the body, for example small stones for the removal and drainage of congestion in the face.

Marble

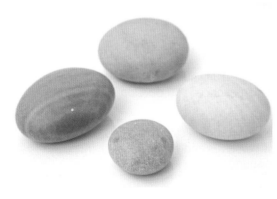

△ Marine stones for massage

Marble stones are used for cool massage treatments and are specifically shaped for size and smoothness for this treatment. They are ideally used at room temperature as they feel slightly cooler than body temperature; sometimes no additional cooling treatment is needed. Marble stones are often used for facial, neck and palm massage and are particularly good at reducing puffiness around the eye area.

Semi-precious stones

Semi-precious stones are most often placed on the corresponding chakras during stone therapy treatment. However, a stone could equally be placed in the client's hand or next to them on the couch. Semi-precious stones, or crystals, come from one unified source, the Earth. They are created from the magma or Earth's inner core

477

and have gone through a geological process of heating, cooling and displacement on their way to their present form. Semi-precious stones will either be in their natural form and just washed to remove the dirt that has accumulated on them over thousands of years, or they may be cut into a particular shape and polished smooth.

Ancient civilisations used semi-precious stones for healing; each stone is said to emit an energy signature or frequency. The stone's colour also plays a dynamic role in its healing energy and can stimulate or calm, purify or heal and balance the mind, body and spirit.

A client can either choose their own stone, simply by identifying the crystal they are most drawn to, or the therapist can choose on the client's behalf after conducting a detailed consultation and identifying the client's objectives and physical and emotional health.

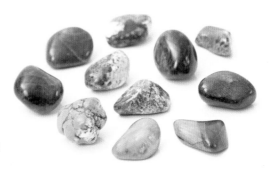

Chakras

△ A range of semi-precious stones

A chakra is a spinning wheel of energy that receives and transmits energy. There are seven main chakras in the body and all have a corresponding colour, crystals and physical and psychological associations (see Table 14.1). They run in one straight vertical line through the centre of the body, starting above the head and finishing at the base of the trunk. If any one of these chakras has a blockage the energy cannot pass through; if a blockage occurs it is believed that physical and/or emotional changes can occur at the place of the blocked chakra. For the body to work in complete harmony all chakras need to have energy flowing freely and this is the main focus of the stone therapy treatment.

> **Key term**
>
> **Geology** – the scientific study of the Earth and the processes by which it evolves.

▽ Table 14.1 The seven chakras and their associations

Chakra number	Chakra	Colour	Corresponding crystals	Association
7	Crown	Clear or violet	Clear Quartz, Diamond	Represents intuition and knowingness and signifies will, thought and spirituality. Its element is spirit
6	Third eye	Purple	Amethyst	Provides us with clarity and clear sight. We gain wisdom through our experiences and develop intellect. The element is light
5	Throat	Blue	Turquoise	This is used for communication and tells how honestly we express ourselves and where we seek truth. The element is sound
4	Heart	Pink or green	Pink quartz, Jade	Represents your love centre, with both personal and emotional empowerment, compassion and trust. Its element is air
3	Solar plexus	Yellow	Citrine, Tiger's Eye	Defines self-esteem and gut instinct; it is used to gain personal power and calm. Its element is fire
2	Sacral	Orange	Amber	This is concerned with physical strength, vitality and procreation. It is linked to relationships. Its element is water
1	Root/ base	Red	Blood Stone, Red Jasper	This gives animation to the physical body and is linked to the material world and our success. It represents being grounded. Its element is earth

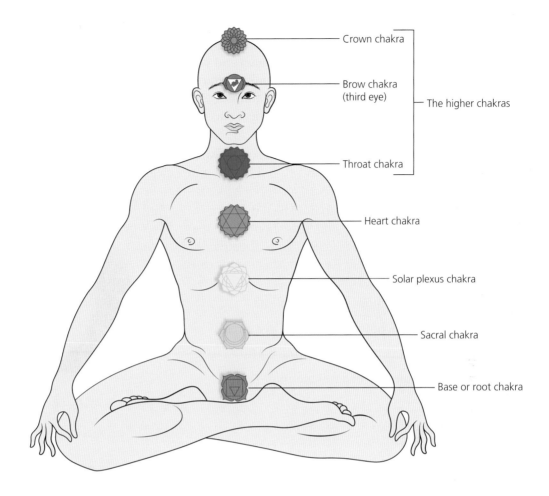

△ The seven chakras of the body

   Maintain safe and effective methods of working when providing stone therapy treatments

For health and safety that relates to this unit, refer back to Chapter 1 Monitoring health and safety. The following pieces of health and safety legislation relate specifically to providing stone therapy treatments:

- Health and Safety at Work Act 1974

- Electricity at Work Regulations 1989

- Provisions and Use of Work Equipment Regulations 1998

- Data Protection Act 1998.

Looking after your stones

A set of good quality stones can be quite expensive, so looking after them properly will ensure they last for many years and will also mean they work effectively. If stones are not looked after they can become sticky with the residue of massage mediums, become a health and safety concern and not retain their heat successfully during treatment.

Stones should be washed thoroughly in warm soapy water after each treatment, wiped with a disinfectant and stored together in a clean, dry place.

As stones begin to lose their ability to hold heat during a treatment they will need re-energising. This should be done on a regular basis to guarantee each client gets a treatment where the stones work effectively. Re-energising stones can be done in a number of different ways:

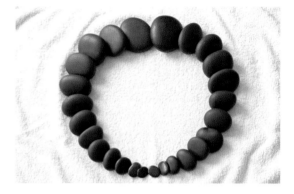

- storing stones in a container with natural salt

- placing the stones touching one another in a circle

- placing the stones outside on the natural earth

- placing the stones outside in a full moon or in the sunlight.

△ Stones in a circle re-energising

Hot stone heaters

There are many types of professional hot stone heaters available which vary in size and capacity. You should always use a heater that has been designed specifically for the beauty industry and heating stones; do not attempt to use a heater intended for domestic use as you may find you are in breach of your insurance policy. Always follow the manufacturer's instructions for your heater. Professional heaters are thermostatically controlled with a safe section for water to maintain the stones at a constant working temperature. Lay the stones flat and evenly in the heater and allow enough time for all the stones to heat up evenly. The usual temperature is 50–55°C but remember to check your manufacturer's instructions as each heater is different. Always have a thermometer in the water so you can check the temperature at any point during the treatment and adjust the heater accordingly.

Health and safety

Do not forget to have your hot stone heater checked as part of your annual Portable Appliance Test (PAT).

Consult, plan and prepare for treatments with clients

It is essential that a therapist has a clear understanding relating to the theory of the structure of the skin and systems of the body when performing stone therapy massage. Details of relevant anatomy and physiology relating to this chapter can be found in Chapter 4 Anatomy and physiology. For consultation, planning and preparing for treatments with clients please refer back to Chapter 6 Professional practices.

The therapist must undertake a tactile sensation and heat sensitivity test with each client to accurately determine the client's skin response to hot and cold temperatures. They must also be able to make a brief yet precise assessment of the client's skin in order to select the correct massage medium to choose, whether oil or cream. A therapist must use a good quality massage medium otherwise the stones will stick and not slip and glide easily. This will cause discomfort to the client and interrupt the flow of the massage. Plain carrier oils can be used or a pre-blended oil containing essential oils may be preferable to enhance the treatment's relaxing or invigorating outcome. If using a medium containing essential oils, the therapist should ensure that the client has had a skin test and is not contraindicated to the product.

> ☆ **Hints and tips**
> If your client has never had a stone therapy treatment before you can introduce them to it slowly by using stones in other treatments, for example, when performing hand and arm massage in a manicure.

Treatment time for stone therapy massage

A time of 90 minutes for full body stone therapy massage including head and face has been determined by the industry as a standard commercial timing and should be used during the practical assessment. The price for this treatment is likely to be about £90; however, this is an example and a luxury spa retreat or cruise liner will probably charge more than a salon with local competition. Pricing of a treatment is determined by many things but you should always consider any competition from other businesses and your overheads.

Contraindications to stone therapy treatment

The specific contraindications to stone therapy massage treatment are divided into two groups – those that *prevent* treatment and those that *restrict* treatment. These are shown in Table 14.2.

▽ Table 14.2 Contraindications to stone therapy massage

Conditions that prevent treatment	Conditions that restrict treatment
Fungal, bacterial and viral infections	Broken bones
Infestations	Recent scar tissue
Severe eczema and psoriasis	Cuts and abrasions
Severe skin conditions	Varicose veins
Dysfunctions of the muscular and nervous systems	Epilepsy
	Diabetes
Deep vein thrombosis	High and low blood pressure
During chemotherapy and radiotherapy treatment	Recent fractures and sprains
	Respiratory and circulatory conditions
	Pregnancy

Contra-actions to stone therapy treatment

A contra-action can be identified as a condition which may arise during the treatment which would indicate that the treatment must stop. It may also be something that arises on completion of the treatment. During treatment the therapist must be alert at all times to changes happening which result in an unwanted reaction. Contra-actions to stone therapy massage include:

- an allergic reaction to the massage medium used
- excessive redness or skin irritation from the temperature of the stones
- bruising caused by incorrect use of the stones
- burning from inappropriate temperature of the hot stones
- feeling faint (caused by an alteration of blood pressure levels)
- headaches (caused by dehydration and the release of toxins around the body).

The following actions should be taken if a client shows any sign of a contra-action, either during or after their treatment.

- Remove any product straight away and apply a cold compress if a skin reaction is present.
- Ensure the client is lying down if they feel faint.
- If the skin is burned, run under cold water and apply a non-sticky sterile dressing. Ensure that the client seeks medical advice.
- Advise the client to seek medical advice should any reaction continue or occur after treatment.

Setting up for stone therapy

Your set-up for stone therapy massage should reflect high standards. It is important to instil confidence in your client and you must ensure your appearance is appropriate. A client will expect you to be professional both in appearance and manner, with a washed and ironed uniform, hair tied up neatly and securely off your face and short, clean nails free from polish.

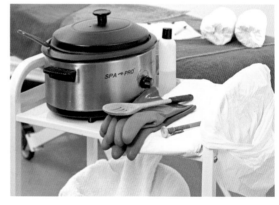

△ Setting up for hot stone treatment

 Hints and tips
Always give your client enough time to get up off the couch slowly after the treatment and to get changed. Offer your client a glass of water and discuss aftercare and homecare advice while they are sitting down. This will help to eliminate some possible contra-actions.

Health and safety
You must ensure hot stones are a suitable temperature to use on your client's skin. If in doubt wait a little longer until they have cooled sufficiently.

Remember . . .
It is imperative that you record any contra-actions on the client's record card. Include details of the date, time and as much detail of the reaction as you can.

Back to basics

Equipment checklist

Your trolley should be equipped with:

- Sterilising agent for the client's feet.
- Cleanser if make-up needs to be removed.
- Cotton pads and tissues.
- Bolsters for additional support.
- A lined bowl for client's jewellery.
- Professional hot stone heater, with towel under to catch drips.
- Selection of stones.
- Heat-resistant gloves for taking stones out of the heater.
- Thermometer to constantly check the temperature of the stone healer.
- Ice for cooling the marine or marble stones.
- A large bowl with a towel in which to place used stones.
- Massage medium.
- Consultation form, client record card and pen.

The massage couch should be equipped with:

- Towels and linen to cover the client, couch and tuck the stones under.
- Couch roll, to cover the couch and dispose of on completion of treatment.
- A covered waste bin.

The treatment environment

One of the most important requirements for stone therapy massage is the environment of the treatment room. You must ensure that the client is warm, comfortable and has privacy when changing. Your treatment room should always be well ventilated with a pleasant aroma and suitable lighting and music.

The couch should be covered over with clean towels and new couch roll. Your trolley should be set up accordingly and should be placed near the plug socket with no trailing wires. You will not be able to move your trolley around during this treatment as it will be very heavy and will need to stay near the electricity source, so everything should be placed within easy reach. A small towel should be placed next to the heater so you are able to place stones to dry and cool sufficiently before use.

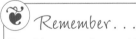 Remember . . .

Provide your client with bolster support under their knees and ankles as required.

483

Preparation of the client before treatment

Once your consultation is complete, you need to give the client directions on how to prepare for the treatment. Make sure you allocate sufficient privacy, space and time for this so the client does not feel rushed. Instruct the client to remove their clothing to their underwear and place their clothes in a suitable place. A female client may be more comfortable removing her bra for treatment so reassure her that her modesty will be maintained and she will be covered over with towels at all times. Remind the client to remove all their jewellery and put in a safe place. Ask the client to lie under the towels in either a supine or prone position (depending on your routine and areas to be treated) and to wait for your return to the treatment room.

Wash your hands for hygiene and ensure the client is covered over sufficiently, placing any pillow or bolster support for comfort as required. You may need to cleanse the client's face of make-up before you begin your treatment. Always ensure you clean their feet and then re-wash your hands. Verbally check that the client is warm and comfortable and inform them that you are about to begin.

Modifications and adaptations to treatment

There will be times when you need to adapt or modify your treatment to suit individual client needs. A professional therapist should always be willing to accommodate the client's needs and they should be identified at the point of consultation. Adaptations to stone therapy massage can include:

- changing the size of the stones and pressure used to suit individual preferences and client size

- taking care over bony areas, avoiding them completely if possible

- remembering the client's desired outcome and using the most suitable stone temperature and massage medium

- working around any areas that are restricted to treatment.

> **Remember . . .**
> Always adjust the couch at the beginning of the treatment so it is at a comfortable working height throughout the treatment.

Perform stone therapy massage treatment LO3 LO7 LO10 LO11

Now both you and your client are prepared and ready for the treatment to begin. You will continue to use the massage movements that you learned in Chapter 11 Body massage treatments.

Beginning treatment

Slowly introduce the stones to the client's skin, after the massage medium has been dispersed onto the chosen area. One stone should be familiarised first, followed by the other, and each stone should have been rolled in the therapist's hand already to cover the stone lightly in oil for slip and glide and to avoid the risk of them overheating. The massage movements used are effleurage,

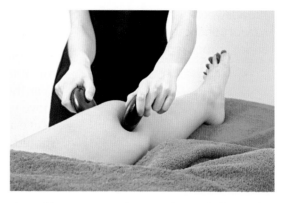

△ Holding stone and massaging with the oval side for deeper work

petrissage, frictions and tapping. Tapotement is not used in stone therapy massage as you will bruise your client if performing these movements with stones. When using effleurage and petrissage, you should hold the stones so the flat sides are used. For frictions you can use the oval sides of the stones to create deeper pressure and work on dispersing fibrous adhesions.

The specialist stone techniques are referred to as 'tucking' and 'placement'.

- Tucking: this is the placement of stones around the body for warmth and in readiness to be used. The stones can be tucked under a towel to keep them warm until they are needed; once used they can be tucked under an area of skin.

- Placement: relates to the direct placing of stones on an area of the body. This could be a semi-precious stone on a chakra or a basalt stone in the palm of the hand, for example.

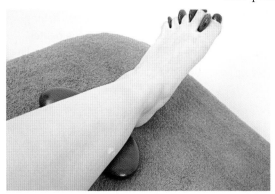

△ Stone tucked under area of skin

The treatment will begin with the client lying face up (supine) and the sequence consists of:

- Client lying supine underneath a spinal layout, with chakra stones in place as required
- Front of right leg and foot
- Front of left leg and foot
- Abdomen
- Left arm
- Right arm
- Chest and neck
- Face and head
- Turn client over, lying prone with chakra and back stones in place as required
- Back of right leg
- Back of left leg
- Back.

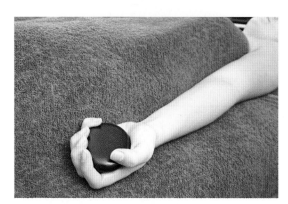

△ Stone placement in hand

Treatment technique: placement of stones

Before you begin the stone therapy massage you will place stones on the front of the body and a spinal layout underneath your client's back for the stones to warm, relax the muscles and ground the client while you are treating the front of their body.

For the spinal layout you need to:

1. Remove six or eight stones (depending on the length of the client's back) of similar sizes from the stone heater and lay them on the towel to dry and cool slightly.

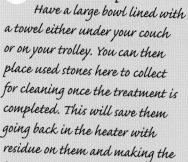

☆ *Hints and tips*

Have a large bowl lined with a towel either under your couch or on your trolley. You can then place used stones here to collect for cleaning once the treatment is completed. This will save them going back in the heater with residue on them and making the heater more difficult to clean.

2 Help the client to sit up so you are able to place the spinal layout stones.

3 Visually assess the client's back and place the stones in pairs on the couch, on either side of the spine, from the lower arch in the lumbar section of the back, right up to the top of the trapezius muscle.

4 Cover the stones over with a towel to protect against burning.

5 Help to lower your client slowly back onto the stones and move around any that feel uncomfortable.

Initially, the spinal layout may feel slightly strange to a client who has never had a stone therapy massage before, but as long as the stones are placed in an even and comfortable position they will soon forget they are there.

For the front of the body you need to:

1 Take up to three medium-sized stones out of the heater and blot dry.

2 With the client's exhale of breath, place the stones over the towel on the sacrum, solar plexus and heart chakra areas.

3 A cold stone can be placed over the third eye chakra if desired.

4 Take a further two medium-sized stones out of the heater and blot dry.

5 Place these in the palm of the client's hand.

6 Remove from the heater the small toe stones in their net and blot dry.

7 Place four toe stones in between the toes on each foot.

Once the front of the body has been massaged you will need to remove each stone from the couch and client, including the toe stones. Sit your client up to remove the spinal layout and help to turn the client over onto the front of their body. Now you need to place stones for the back of the body.

For the back of the body you need to:

1 Remove three to four large stones from the heater and blot dry.

2 Cover the client's back with a hand towel. On the client's exhale breath, place the stones along the client's spine.

3 Cover the stones over with another hand towel to retain their heat.

4 Take a further two medium stones out of the heater and blot dry.

5 Place a stone each in the palm of the client's hand.

Once you have finished your massage remove all the stones, turn your client over and sit them up slowly. Offer them a glass of water and allow them plenty of time to get changed. You will then be able to give aftercare advice. Remember to check the treatment was to the client's satisfaction and met the agreed treatment objectives.

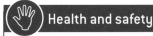

Health and safety

Do not forget to cover the spinal layout stones with a towel; having just come out of the stone heater they will be too hot for a client to lie back on them without protection.

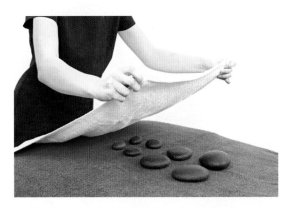

△ Spinal layout of stones on the couch with the client sat up

Hints and tips

You can rest any corresponding semi-precious chakra stone onto the front of the client's body in their correct place, give the client the crystal to hold or lay it next to them on the couch for chakra balancing.

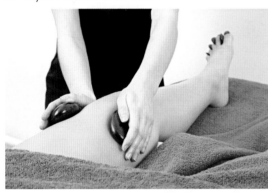

△ Layout of stones for foot

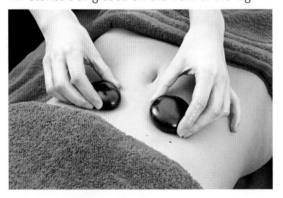

△ Stones being used on the front of the leg

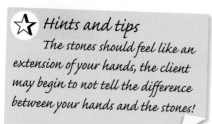

△ Stones being used on the abdomen

Treatment technique: massage routine

Front of leg and foot:

1 Select four medium-sized stones from the heater and blot dry.

2 Tuck two stones under the towel by the client's thigh area.

3 Place two stones on the couch roll by the ankle.

4 Place a ten-pence size of oil in the palm of your hands and begin to effleurage from ankle to thigh.

5 Take the stones from the ankle area and roll them in the palm of your hands to coat with oil, to check the temperature and to disperse some of the heat.

6 Perform more effleurage movements using your warmed hands.

7 Introduce the stones to the legs (one at a time if necessary) using effleurage.

8 Perform a simple leg massage routine.

9 As those stones begin to cool, tuck them under the client's leg and pick up your two new stones that were placed earlier by the thigh.

10 Continue with your leg massage routine.

11 Cover the leg over with a towel and use the current two stones to perform a simple foot massage.

12 Tuck the stones once cooled and cover the foot over to keep warm.

13 Repeat on the other leg and foot.

Abdomen:

1 Remove the chakra stones from the client's abdomen.

2 Take two medium-sized stones out of the heater and blot dry.

3 Place a small amount of oil in the palm of your hands and distribute around the client's abdomen.

4 Roll the two stones in the palm of your hands to coat with oil, to check the temperature and to disperse some of the heat.

5 Introduce the warm stones to the abdomen area slowly and perform a simple massage, remembering to follow the direction of the colon.

6 Once the stones are cooled place them under the client's waist, cover the abdomen with a towel and replace the chakra stones.

Arm:

1 Take two medium-sized stones out of the heater and blot dry.

2 Place the stones next to the arms on the couch roll.

3 Place a small amount of oil in the palm of your hands and distribute along the length of the client's arm.

4 Roll the two stones in the palm of your hands to coat with oil, to check the temperature and to disperse some of the heat.

5 Introduce the warm stones to the arm area slowly and perform a simple arm and hand massage.

6 Leave a warm stone in the palm of the client's hand and cover with a towel.

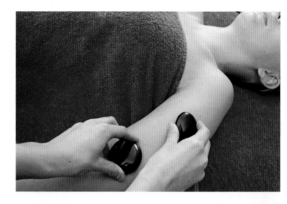

△ Stones being used on the arm

Chest and neck:

1 Take two small stones out of the heater and blot dry.

2 Place the stones next to the shoulders on the couch roll.

3 Remove the cold stone from the third eye chakra, if placed there earlier.

4 Place a small amount of oil in the palm of your hands and distribute along the décolleté.

5 Perform a manual massage in this area.

6 Roll the two stones in the palm of your hands to coat with oil, to check the temperature and to disperse some of the heat.

7 Introduce the warm stones to the arm area slowly and use the stones to gently massage over the décolleté and use them at an angle on any fibrous adhesions on the trapezius.

8 Turn the client's head to one side and use one stone to massage the neck, repeat on the other side.

9 Leave the warm stones tucked under the trapezius muscle.

Face and head:

1 Take two small stones out of the heater and blot dry (you could use cold stones here).

2 Place the stones next to the shoulders on the couch roll.

3 Place a small amount of facial oil in the palm of your hands and distribute over the face.

4 Perform a manual massage in this area.

5 Roll the two stones in the palm of your hands to coat with oil, to check the temperature and to disperse some of the heat.

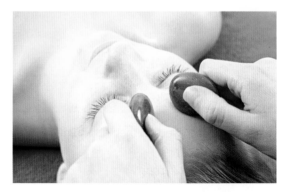

△ Stones being used on the face and head

6 Introduce the warm stones to the arm area slowly and use the stones to gently massage over the jaw line, cheek bone, forehead and finish at the temples.

7 Leave a stone on the third eye chakra.

8 Perform a simple scalp massage.

Back of leg:

1 Select four medium-sized stones from the heater and blot dry.

2 Tuck two stones under the towel by the client's thigh area.

3 Place two stones on the couch roll by the ankle.

4 Place a ten pence size of oil in the palm of your hands and begin to effleurage from ankle to thigh.

5 Take the stones from the ankle area and roll them in the palm of your hands to coat with oil, to check the temperature and to disperse some of the heat.

6 Perform more effleurage movements using your warmed hands.

7 Introduce the stones to the legs (one at a time if necessary) using effleurage.

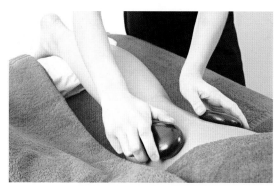

△ Stones being used on the back of the leg

8 Perform a simple leg massage routine.

9 As those stones begin to cool, tuck them under the client's leg and pick up your two new stones that were placed earlier by the thigh.

10 Continue with your leg massage routine.

11 Cover the leg over with a towel and use one of the stones to perform a massage on the sole of the foot.

12 Leave this stone resting on the sole of the foot; cover the foot over to keep warm.

13 Repeat on the other leg and foot.

Back:

1 Select two large stones and two medium-sized stones from the heater and blot dry.

2 Tuck the two large stones under the towel by the client's lower back.

3 Tuck the two medium stones under the couch by the client's shoulders.

4 Remove the stones from the client's back.

5 Place a large amount of oil in the palm of your hands and begin to effleurage over the back.

6 Take the two large stones from under the towel by the lower back and roll them in the palm of your hands to coat with oil, to check the temperature and to disperse some of the heat.

7 Perform more effleurage movements using your warmed hands.

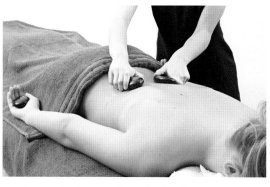

△ Stones being used on the back

8 Introduce the stones to the lower back (one at a time if necessary) using effleurage.

9 Perform a simple back massage routine.

10 As those stones begin to cool, tuck them under the client's waist and pick up your two new stones that were placed under the towel by the client's shoulders.

11 Continue with your back massage routine.

12 When you come to the end of your routine place those two stones under the client's shoulders.

13 Cover the back with a towel.

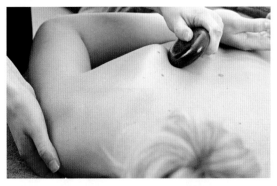

△ Using stones around the scapula

Provide aftercare advice

Aftercare and homecare advice should always been given to the client following stone therapy massage.

Avoidance of activities which may cause contra-actions

For 12–24 hours following treatment the client should be advised to:

- rest, as they may feel deeply relaxed
- drink plenty of water to avoid dehydration
- avoid physical exercise
- ensure light food intake
- avoid alcohol and caffeine.

Future treatment needs

The client should be advised:

- to return for further stone therapy massage treatments. These can be carried out to suit the client's needs, but every 2–3 weeks is often recommended
- about retail products that will enhance the appearance and quality of their skin
- to consider lifestyle changes such as taking exercise, maintaining a healthy diet, regular fluid intake and methods of relaxation
- of the need for postural awareness.

> ☆ *Hints and tips*
> *You can alternate between hot and cold stones during treatment or use hot or cold stones only.*

> ☆ *Hints and tips*
> *It is good practice to use a combination of stone sizes, to suit your hands and the different areas of the client's body.*

Key term

Geothermal therapy – the use of alternate hot and cold temperatures on the body.

> **Want to know more?**
>
> Mary Nelson of Arizona, USA, developed and introduced the La Stone Therapy service. She is a pioneer in research and development of 'Geothermal therapy' which is a technique that uses alternate hot and cold stones on the body. More information can be found on the website by visiting www.lastonetherapy.com
>
> You can also refer to the HABIA website: www.habia.org.

NVQ assessment checklist

To complete this unit you must have the following theoretical and practical skills. Check against the list below and refer back to the relevant section for information on anything you are unsure about.

1. **Be able to maintain safe and effective methods of working when providing stone therapy treatments**

❏ **1.1** set up and maintain the treatment area to meet legal, hygiene and service requirements

❏ **1.2** maintain personal hygiene, protection and appearance that meets accepted industry and organisational requirements

❏ **1.3** remove and handle stones in a way which avoids injury to themselves and the client

❏ **1.4** clean all tools and equipment using the correct methods

❏ **1.5** disinfect stones after each treatment

❏ **1.6** heat, cool and store stones according to manufacturers instructions and in a way which effectively energises them

❏ **1.7** position equipment and treatment products for safety and ease of use

❏ **1.8** use suitable materials to protect the client's skin against extremes of temperature during stone replacement

❏ **1.9** use accepted industry hygiene and safety practices throughout the treatment

❏ **1.10** adopt a positive, polite and reassuring manner towards the client throughout the treatment

❏ **1.11** maintain the client's modesty, privacy and comfort at all times

❏ **1.12** use treatment products to minimise waste

❏ **1.13** dispose of waste materials safely and correctly

❏ **1.14** carry out the treatment within a commercially viable time

❏ **1.15** keep records up to date, accurate, easy to read and signed by the client and practitioner

❏ **1.16** leave the treatment area and equipment in a suitable condition for future treatments

2. **Be able to consult, plan and prepare for treatments with clients**

❏ **2.1** use consultation techniques to determine the client's treatment needs

❏ **2.2** obtain signed, written and informed consent prior to any service from the client or parent/guardian if the client is a minor

❏ **2.3** explain to the client what the treatment entails in a way they can understand

❏ **2.4** consult with the client to identify their medical history, physical characteristics and lifestyle pattern, recording their responses

❏ **2.5** consult with the client to identify if they have any contraindications to stone therapy treatments, recording their responses and taking any necessary action

❏ **2.6** actively encourage clients to ask questions and clarify points

❏ **2.7** position themselves and the client to minimise the risk of fatigue and injury to themselves and the client

❏ **2.8** carry out a test patch to determine the client's skin response to hot and cold temperature

❏ **2.9** provide client advice without reference to a specific to a specific medical condition and without causing undue alarm and concern

❏ **2.10** explain and agree the projected cost, likely duration, frequency and types of treatment needed

❏ **2.11** agree in writing the client's needs, expectations and treatment objectives, ensuring they are realistic and achievable

❏ **2.12** clean and prepare the client's skin to suit the areas to be treated

❏ **2.13** protect the client's clothing, hair and accessories

❏ **2.14** select types of stone suitable to meet the treatment objectives

3. **Be able to perform stone therapy treatments**

❏ **3.1** explain to the client the sensation created by the stones

❏ **3.2** explain the treatment procedure to the client in a clear and simple way at each stage in the process

❏ **3.3** provide suitable support and cushioning to specific areas of the body during the treatment if necessary

❏ **3.4** use suitable material to protect the client's skin against extremes of temperature during front and back placement

❏ **3.5** place suitable types of stone on the chakra points, when required, to meet the agreed treatment objectives

❏ **3.6** place suitable types of stone under the body, when required, ensuring client comfort

❏ **3.7** lubricate the skin to allow the smooth, continuous movement of the stones over the skin to avoid risk of overheating

❏ **3.8** use stone therapy techniques in a way which avoids alarm to the client, is suitable for their physical characteristics, the treatment area(s) and treatment objectives

❏ **3.9** adapt the treatment techniques and sequence to meet the client's physical characteristics and treatment area(s)

❏ **3.10** vary the depth, rhythm and pressure of treatment techniques to meet treatment objectives, treatment area(s) and client's physical characteristics and preferences

❏ **3.11** check the client's well-being throughout the stone therapy treatment

❏ **3.12** handle stones to avoid excessive noise and disturbance to the client throughout the treatment

❏ **3.13** assist to reposition the client in a controlled manner to minimise disturbance of the treatment process

❏ **3.14** take prompt remedial action if contra-actions or discomfort occur during the course of treatment

❏ **3.15** allow the client sufficient post-treatment recovery time

❏ **3.16** check that the finished result is to the client's satisfaction and meets the agreed treatment objectives

❏ **3.17** give the client aftercare advice

4. Understand organisational and legal requirements

❏ **4.1** explain own responsibilities under relevant health and safety legislation, standards and guidance

❏ **4.2** explain own responsibilities under local authority licensing regulations for themselves and their premises

❏ **4.3** explain the importance of checking current insurance guidelines for the delivery of stone therapy treatment

❏ **4.4** explain the importance of not discriminating against clients with illnesses and disabilities and why

❏ **4.5** explain the age at which an individual is classed as a minor and how this differs nationally

❏ **4.6** explain why it is important, when treating minors under 16 years of age, to have a parent present

❏ **4.7** explain why minors should not be given treatments without informed and signed parental or guardian consent

❏ **4.8** explain the legal significance of gaining signed, informed consent to treatment

❏ **4.9** explain own responsibilities and reasons for maintaining their own personal hygiene, protection and appearance according to accepted industry and organisational requirements

❏ **4.10** explain the manufacturers' and organisational requirements for waste disposal

❏ **4.11** explain the importance of the correct storage of client records in relation to the Data Protection Act

❏ **4.12** explain how to complete client records and the reasons for keeping records of treatments and containing client signatures

❏ **4.13** explain the organisation's requirements for client preparation

❏ **4.14** explain the organisation's service times for stone therapy treatments and the importance of completing the service in a commercially viable time

❏ **4.15** explain own responsibilities and reasons for keeping their nails short, clean, well-manicured and free of polish for massage treatments

❏ **4.16** explain the organisation's and manufacturers' requirements for treatment area, equipment maintenance and equipment cleaning regimes

5. Understand how to work safely and effectively when providing stone therapy

❏ **5.1** explain how to set up the work area for stone therapy treatments effectively when providing stone therapy treatments

❏ **5.2** explain the necessary environmental conditions for stone therapy treatments (including lighting, heating, ventilation, sound and general comfort) and why these are important

❏ **5.3** explain the importance and reasons for disinfecting hands and how to do this effectively

❏ **5.4** explain what contact dermatitis is, how to avoid developing it when carrying out stone therapy treatments

❏ **5.5** explain the importance of disinfecting stones after each treatment and how to do this effectively

❏ **5.6** explain how to position themselves and the client for stone therapy treatments taking into account individual physical characteristics

❏ **5.7** explain repetitive strain injury (RSI), how it is caused and how to avoid it when carrying out stone therapy treatments

❏ **5.8** evaluate the advantages to the therapist of using stone therapy as a means of avoiding RSI

❏ **5.9** explain the importance of using the correct sized stones for the therapist's own hands and the client's physical characteristics

❏ **5.10** explain the importance of adopting the correct posture throughout the treatment and the impact this may have on themselves and the outcome of the treatment

❏ **5.11** explain the reasons for maintaining client modesty, privacy and comfort during the treatment

❏ **5.12** explain why it is important to maintain standards of hygiene and the principles of avoiding cross-infection

❏ **5.13** explain how to minimise and dispose of waste treatments

❏ **5.14** explain why it is important to check the client's well-being at regular intervals during stone therapy treatments

6. Understand how to consult with clients

❏ **6.1** explain how to use effective consultation techniques when communicating with clients from different cultural and religious backgrounds, age, disabilities and gender, for this treatment

❏ **6.2** explain why it is important to encourage and allow time for clients to ask questions

❏ **6.3** explain the importance of questioning clients to establish any contraindications to head and stone therapy treatments

❏ **6.4** explain why it is important to record client responses to questioning

❏ **6.5** explain the legal significance of client questioning and the recording of client responses

❏ **6.6** explain how to give effective advice and recommendations to clients

❏ **6.7** explain how to visually asses the clients physical characteristics

❏ **6.8** explain how to carry out and interpret thermal tests

❏ **6.9** explain how to assess posture and skeletal conditions that may be present and how to adapt and change the stone therapy treatment routine

❏ **6.10** summarise how to recognise different skin types and conditions

❏ **6.11** explain the reasons why it is important to encourage clients with contraindications to seek medical advice

❏ **6.12** explain the importance of and reasons for not naming specific contraindications when encouraging clients to seek medical advice

❏ **6.13** explain why it is important to maintain client's modesty and privacy

❏ **6.14** evaluate the relationship between lifestyle patterns and effectiveness of treatment

❏ **6.15** evaluate the beneficial effects which can result from changes to the client's lifestyle pattern

❏ **7.** **Understand how to prepare to provide stone therapy treatments**

❏ **7.1** explain the importance of giving clients clear instructions on the removal of relevant clothing, accessories and general preparation for the treatment

❏ **7.2** explain why it is important to reassure clients during the preparation for the treatment

❏ **7.3** explain how to select the appropriate oil suitable for stone therapy treatment

❏ **7.4** explain how to cleanse different areas of the body in preparation for treatment

❏ **8.** **Understand anatomy and physiology related to stone therapy treatments**

❏ **8.1** explain the structure and function of cells and tissues

❏ **8.2** explain the structure and function of muscles, including the types of muscle i.e. voluntary and involuntary

❏ **8.3** explain the positions and actions of the main muscle groups within the treatment areas

❏ **8.4** explain the position and function of the primary bones and joints of the skeleton

❏ **8.5** explain the position and function of the sinuses

❏ **8.6** explain how to recognise postural faults and conditions

❏ **8.7** explain the structural, function and location of blood vessels and the principles of circulation, blood pressure and pulse

❏ **8.8** explain the interaction of lymph and blood within the circulatory system

❏ **8.9** explain the structure and function of the lymphatic system

❏ **8.10** explain the basic principles of the central nervous system and autonomic system

❏ **8.11** explain the basic principles of the endocrine, respiratory, digestive and excretory systems

❏ **8.12** explain the structure and function of skin

❏ **8.13** explain the skin characteristics and skin types of different ethnic client groups

❏ **8.14** explain the structure and location of the adipose tissue

❏ **8.15** summarise the effects of hot and cold stone therapy on the individual systems of the body

❏ **8.16** evaluate the psychological effects of hot and cold stone therapy treatment

❏ **9.** **Understand contraindications and contra-actions that affect or restrict stone therapy treatments**

❏ **9.1** explain the contraindications that prevent treatment and why

❏ **9.2** explain the contraindications which may restrict treatment or where caution should be taken, in specific areas and why

❏ **9.3** explain possible contra-actions which may occur during and post treatment, why and how to deal with them

❏ **10.** **Understand how to use stone therapy equipment**

❏ **10.1** explain the types of safe, purpose-built stone heating equipment and how to use and position them safely

❏ **10.2** explain the insurance implications of using non-professional stone heating equipment

❏ **10.3** explain methods of cooling stones

❏ **10.4** explain the types of stone, their properties and uses

❏ **10.5** explain how to select the correct size and shape of stone for the client's physical characteristics and the area being treated

❏ **10.6** explain how to dry and store different types of stone in a way that will effectively energise them

❏ **10.7** explain the types of suitable material used to protect the client's skin against extremes of temperature during stone therapy treatment

❏ **10.8** explain the recommended operating temperatures for hot and cold stones

❏ **10.9** explain the types of oil suitable for stone therapy treatment and its purpose

11. Understand the principles behind stone therapy techniques and how to use them

❏ **11.1** explain the historical and cultural background to stone therapy

❏ **11.2** explain the five elements of stone therapy

❏ **11.3** explain the basic principles and characteristics of the seven major chakras and their significance to the practice of stone therapy treatment

❏ **11.4** explain how to place stones on the seven major chakras to maximise client comfort and their benefits and purposes

❏ **11.5** explain how to place stones underneath the body to maximise their benefits, purposes and client comfort

❏ **11.6** explain how to place stones on the client's body during treatment and the importance of doing this in a careful, safe and considerate way

❏ **11.7** explain the importance of temperature and time management of the stones during treatment and how to carry this out

❏ **11.8** explain how to safely handle the stones to avoid excessive noise and disturbance during the treatment

❏ **11.9** explain how to recognise erythema and hyperaemia and their causes

❏ **11.10** explain why it is important to maintain correct posture during stone therapy treatment

❏ **11.11** explain the correct use and application of stone therapy techniques to meet a variety of treatment objectives

❏ **11.12** explain the importance of evaluating the effectiveness of stone therapy treatments

❏ **11.13** explain the correct use and application of stone therapy techniques to meet a variety of treatment objectives

❏ **11.14** summarise the benefits and effects of using hot and cold stones, either in isolation or combining the two temperatures during a treatment

❏ **11.15** explain how to adapt and combine stone therapy treatment techniques, depth and pressure to suit different client physical characteristics, areas of the body and preferences

❏ **11.16** explain how to adapt a stone therapy treatment for male and female clients

❏ **11.17** explain the areas of the body and body characteristics needing particular care when undertaking stone therapy treatments

❏ **11.18** evaluate the advantages of stone therapy treatments

❏ **11.19** explain how and why support and cushioning would be used during the treatment

❏ **11.20** explain how and when to safely reposition the client during treatment and the type of assistance which should be provided by the therapist

❏ **11.21** explain how stone therapy may be used to enhance other treatments e.g. manicure, pedicure, facial

❏ **11.22** explain the recommended recovery times for stone therapy treatments and why this is important

❏ **11.23** explain recommended timings for stone therapy treatments and how these should be adapted to meet the clients' individual needs and physical characteristics

12. Understand how to provide aftercare advice

❏ **12.1** evaluate the lifestyle factors and changes that may be required to improve the effectiveness of the treatment e.g. healthy eating, fluid intake and regular exercise etc

❏ **12.2** explain activities which should be avoided post-treatment

❏ **12.3** explain products for home use that will benefit and protect the client and those to avoid and why

❏ **12.4** recommend further treatments

Test yourself

1. What are the four different types of stone that can be used during stone massage treatment?

2. Where did stone therapy originate from?

3. When would you choose to use cold stones within a treatment?

4. What are the names of the seven different chakras?

5. What colour relates to the base chakra?

6. What is a chakra?

7. Give four contraindications that restrict treatment

8. Give four contraindications that prevent treatment

9. Give three contra-actions following treatment.

10. Explain the term 'tucking' of stones.

Index